Neuromuscular Disease Management and Rehabilitation, Part I: Diagnostic and Therapy Issues

Guest Editors

NANETTE C. JOYCE, DO
CRAIG M. MCDONALD, MD

PHYSICAL MEDICINE AND REHABILITATION CLINICS OF NORTH AMERICA

www.pmr.theclinics.com

Consulting Editor
GREGORY T. CARTER, MD, MS

August 2012 • Volume 23 • Number 3

SAUNDERS an imprint of ELSEVIER, Inc.

W.B. SAUNDERS COMPANY
A Division of Elsevier Inc.

1600 John F. Kennedy Boulevard • Suite 1800 • Philadelphia, Pennsylvania 19103

http://www.theclinics.com

PHYSICAL MEDICINE AND REHABILITATION CLINICS OF NORTH AMERICA Volume 23, Number 3
August 2012 ISSN 1047-9651, ISBN-13: 978-1-4557-4957-7

Editor: Jessica McCool

Reprints. For copies of 100 or more of articles in this publication, please contact the Commercial Reprints Department, Elsevier Inc., 360 Park Avenue South, New York, NY 10010-1710. Tel.: 212-633-3812; Fax: 212-462-1935; E-mail: reprints@elsevier.com.

Physical Medicine and Rehabilitation Clinics of North America (ISSN 1047-9651) is published quarterly by Elsevier Inc., 360 Park Avenue South, New York, NY 10010-1710. Months of issue are February, May, August, and November. Business and Editorial Offices: 1600 John F. Kennedy Blvd., Suite 1800, Philadelphia, PA 19103-2899. Customer Service Office: 3251 Riverport Lane, Maryland Heights, MO 63043. Periodicals postage paid at New York, NY and additional mailing offices. Subscription price per year is $248.00 (US individuals), $441.00 (US institutions), $132.00 (US students), $302.00 (Canadian individuals), $575.00 (Canadian institutions), $189.00 (Canadian students), $373.00 (foreign individuals), $575.00 (foreign institutions), and $189.00 (foreign students). Foreign air speed delivery is included in all *Clinics* subscription prices. All prices are subject to change without notice. **POSTMASTER:** Send address changes to *Physical Medicine and Rehabilitation Clinics of North America*, Customer Service Office: Elsevier Health Sciences Division, Subscription Customer Service, 3251 Riverport Lane, Maryland Heights, MO 63043. **Customer Service: 1-800-654-2452 (US). From outside of the United States, call 314-447-8871. Fax: 314-447-8029. E-mail: JournalsCustomer Service-usa@elsevier.com (for print support); JournalsOnlineSupport-usa@elsevier.com (for online support).**

Physical Medicine and Rehabilitation Clinics of North America is indexed in *Excerpta Medica, MEDLINE/PubMed (Index Medicus), Cinahl,* and *Cumulative Index to Nursing and Allied Health Literature.*

Printed and bound by CPI Group (UK) Ltd, Croydon, CR0 4YY

Transferred to Digital Print 2012 ,

Contributors

CONSULTING EDITOR

GREGORY T. CARTER, MD, MS
Medical Director, Muscular Dystrophy Association Regional Neuromuscular Center, Providence Medical Group, Clinical Neurosciences Division, Olympia, Washington; Department of Physical Medicine and Rehabilitation, University of California Davis, Sacramento, California

GUEST EDITORS

NANETTE C. JOYCE, DO
Assistant Professor, Department of Physical Medicine and Rehabilitation, Co-Director, ALS Clinic, Researcher, UC Davis Institute for Regenerative Cures, University of California Davis Health System, Sacramento, California

CRAIG M. MCDONALD, MD
Professor and Chair, Department of Physical Medicine and Rehabilitation; Professor of Pediatrics, University of California Davis School of Medicine; Director of Adult and Child Neuromuscular Disease Clinics, Director, NIDRR Rehabilitation Research and Training Center in Neuromuscular Diseases, University of California Davis Medical Center; Director, Neuromuscular Disease and Spina Bifida Programs, Department of Orthopaedic Surgery and Rehabilitation, Shriners Hospital for Children, Northern California, Sacramento, California

AUTHORS

R. TED ABRESCH, MS
Department of Physical Medicine and Rehabilitation, University of California at Davis, Sacramento, California

MICHAEL ALEXANDER, MD
Professor, Pediatrics and Physical Medicine and Rehabilitation, Thomas Jefferson University, Philadelphia, Pennsylvania; Chief of Pediatric Rehabilitation, Nemours/Alfred I duPont Hospital for Children, Wilmington, Delaware

W. DAVID ARNOLD, MD
Assistant Professor, Division of Neuromuscular Disorders, Department of Neurology, Wexner Medical Center at the Ohio State University, The Ohio State University, Columbus, Ohio

LAURA J. BALL, PhD, CCC/SP
Communication Sciences and Disorders, Massachusetts General Hospital Institute of Health Professions, Boston, Massachusetts

JOSEPH BASANTE, MA, MS, OTR/L, CHT
Occupational Therapist, Certified Hand Therapist, Nemours/Alfred I duPont Hospital for
Children, Wilmington, Delaware

GREGORY T. CARTER, MD, MS
Medical Director, Providence Regional Neuromuscular Center; Providence Hospice &
Palliative Medicine Program, Olympia, Washington; Department of Physical Medicine and
Rehabilitation, University of California Davis, Sacramento, California

RIMA EL-ABASSI, MD
Division of Neuromuscular Disorders, Department of Neurology, Louisiana State University Health Sciences Center, School of Medicine, New Orleans, Louisiana

SUSAN FAGER, PhD, CCC/SP
Assistant Director, Communication Center, Madonna Rehabilitation Hospital, Institute for
Rehabilitation Science and Engineering, Lincoln, Nebraska

KEVIN M. FLANIGAN, MD
The Center for Gene Therapy, Nationwide Children's Hospital; Professor of Pediatrics,
The Ohio State University, Columbus, Ohio

JULAINE M. FLORENCE, PT, DPT
Director, Clinical Studies, Neuromuscular Division; Research Professor of Neurology,
Research Professor of Physical Therapy, Department of Neurology, Washington
University School of Medicine, St Louis, Missouri

WILLIAM M. FOWLER, Jr, MD
Professor Emeritus and Founding Chair, Department of Physical Medicine and Rehabilitation, University of California Davis School of Medicine, Sacramento, California

MELANIE FRIED-OKEN, PhD, CCC/SP
Professor, Neurology, Pediatrics, ENT, BME; Oregon Health and Science University,
Portland, Oregon

JAY J. HAN, MD
Associate Professor, Director of the Neuromuscular Medicine Fellowship, Department of
Physical Medicine and Rehabilitation; Co-Director, Muscular Dystrophy Association
(MDA), Neuromuscular Disease Clinic, University of California Davis School of Medicine;
Lawrence J. Ellison Ambulatory Care Center, Sacramento, California

MARK P. JENSEN, PhD
Department of Rehabilitation Medicine, University of Washington School of Medicine,
Seattle, Washington

LEE-WAY JIN, MD, PhD
Professor and Director of Neuropathology, Department of Pathology and Laboratory
Medicine, University of California Davis School of Medicine, Sacramento, California

LINDA B. JOHNSON, BS, PT
Neuromuscular Medicine Clinical Evaluator, Department of Physical Medicine and
Rehabilitation, University of California Davis, Sacramento, California

NANETTE C. JOYCE, DO
Assistant Professor, Department of Physical Medicine and Rehabilitation, University of California Davis School of Medicine, Sacramento, California

BETHANY M. LIPA, MD
Neuromuscular Fellow, Department of Physical Medicine and Rehabilitation, University of California Davis School of Medicine; Lawrence J. Ellison Ambulatory Care Center, Sacramento, California

CRAIG M. MCDONALD, MD
Professor and Chair, Department of Physical Medicine and Rehabilitation; Professor of Pediatrics, University of California Davis School of Medicine; Director of Adult and Child Neuromuscular Disease Clinics, Director, NIDRR Rehabilitation Research and Training Center in Neuromuscular Diseases, University of California Davis Medical Center; Director, Neuromuscular Disease and Spina Bifida Programs, Department of Orthopaedic Surgery and Rehabilitation, Shriners Hospital for Children, Northern California, Sacramento, California

JORDI MIRÓ, PhD
Unit for the Study and Treatment of Pain - ALGOS, Centre de Recerca en Avaluació i Mesura del Comportament, Institut d'Investigació Sanitària Pere Virgili, Universitat Rovira i Virgili, Catalonia, Spain

BJÖRN OSKARSSON, MD
Assistant Professor, Department of Neurology, University of California Davis School of Medicine, Sacramento, California

TARIQ RAHMAN, PhD
Senior Research Engineer, Department of Biomedical Research, Nemours/Alfred I duPont Hospital for Children, Wilmington; Associate Research Professor, Department of Mechanical Engineering, University of Delaware, Newark, Delaware

ANDREW J. SKALSKY, MD
Assistant Professor of Pediatrics, Director, Pediatric Rehabilitation Program, Co-Director, MDA Neuromuscular Disease Clinic, Rady Children's Hospital, University of California San Diego School of Medicine, San Diego, California

Contents

The neuromuscular medicine and physiatry specialists are key health care
providers who work cooperatively with a multidisciplinary team to provide
coordinated care for individuals with neuromuscular diseases (NMDs). The
director or coordinator of the team must be aware of the potential issues
specific to NMDs and be able to access the interventions that are the foundations for proper care in NMD. Ultimate goals include maximizing health
and functional capacities, performing medical monitoring and surveillance
to inhibit and prevent complications, and promoting access and full integration into the community to optimize quality of life.

For diagnostic evaluation of a neuromuscular disease, the clinician must be
able to obtain a relevant patient and family history and perform focused
general, musculoskeletal, neurologic, and functional physical examinations
to direct further diagnostic evaluations. Laboratory studies for hereditary
neuromuscular diseases include the relevant molecular genetic studies.
The electromyogram and nerve-conduction studies remain an extension
of the physical examination, and help to guide further diagnostic studies
such as molecular genetics and muscle and nerve biopsies. All diagnostic
information needs to be interpreted within the context of relevant historical information, family history, physical examination, laboratory data, electrophysiology, pathology, and molecular genetics.

Electromyography (EMG) is an important diagnostic tool for the assessment of individuals with various neuromuscular diseases. It should be an

extension of a thorough history and physical examination. Some prototypical characteristics and findings of EMG and nerve conduction studies are discussed; however, a more thorough discussion can be found in the textbooks and resources sited in the article. With an increase in molecular genetic diagnostics, EMG continues to play an important role in the diagnosis and management of patients with neuromuscular diseases and also provides a cost-effective diagnostic workup before ordering a battery of costly genetic tests.

Molecular diagnosis is an important aspect in the care of patients with neuromuscular disorders. Because of the rapidly evolving nature of the field, the approach to obtaining a molecular diagnosis may be challenging. This article provides a general approach to molecular diagnostic testing while reviewing the principles of genetics and genetic disorders and the indications and limitations of testing methods in common hereditary neuromuscular disorders.

This article reviews the indications for a muscle biopsy, and then gives a step-by-step description of the processes of muscle selection through to interpreting the biopsy report. The article aims to aid the clinician in preparing for a muscle biopsy procedure to avoid common pitfalls and obtain optimal results from this minimally invasive procedure. The basic anatomic structure of normal muscle is reviewed to provide a foundation for understanding common patterns of pathologic change observed in muscle disease and common and disease-specific histopathologic findings are presented, focusing on a select group of neuromuscular diseases.

Neuromuscular disorders (NMDs) are a group of myopathic or neuropathic diseases that directly or indirectly affect the functioning of muscle. Physical therapists (PTs) have extensive specialized training in musculoskeletal evaluation and assessment that gives them the tools to meet the significant needs of this population. This article reviews the role of PTs in treating the NMD population with a discussion of available evaluation techniques and interventions and with an effort to differentiate between treatments known to apply to this population and conventional practice of PTs. The status of currently available outcome measures used for research and their applicability to clinics are presented.

This article reviews the current knowledge regarding the benefits and contraindications of exercise on individuals with neuromuscular diseases

(NMDs). Specific exercise prescriptions for individuals with NMDs do not exist because the evidence base is limited. Understanding the effect of exercise on individuals with NMDs requires the implementation of a series of multicenter, randomized controlled trials that are sufficiently powered and use reliable and valid outcome measures to assess the effect of exercise interventions—a major effort for each NMD. In addition to traditional measures of exercise efficacy, outcome variables should include measures of functional status and health-related quality of life.

Limb contractures are a common impairment in neuromuscular diseases. They contribute to increased disability from decreased motor performance, mobility limitations, reduced functional range of motion, loss of function for activities of daily living, and increased pain. The pathogenesis of contractures is multifactorial. Myopathic conditions are associated with more severe limb contractures compared with neuropathic disorders. Although the evidence supporting the efficacy of multiple interventions to improve range of motion in neuromuscular diseases in a sustained manner is lacking, there are generally accepted principles with regard to splinting, bracing, stretching, and surgery that help minimize the impact or disability from contractures.

Individuals with progressive neuromuscular disease often experience complex communication needs and consequently find that interaction using their natural speech may not sufficiently meet their daily needs. Increasingly, assistive technology advances provide accommodations for and/or access to communication. Assistive technology related to communication is referred to as augmentative and alternative communication (AAC). The nature of communication challenges in progressive neuromuscular diseases can be as varied as the AAC options currently available. AAC systems continue to be designed and implemented to provide targeted assistance based on an individual's changing needs.

This article presents an overview of occupational therapy assessments and treatment options for individuals with neuromuscular disabilities, with a particular focus on children with neuromuscular disorders. The discussion includes descriptions of standard treatments, commercial adaptive equipment, and homemade adaptive solutions. The state of the art in therapeutic and assistive robots and orthoses for the upper and lower extremity is also provided.

PHYSICAL MEDICINE & REHABILITATION CLINICS OF NORTH AMERICA

Foreword

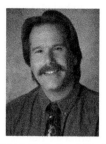

Gregory T. Carter, MD, MS
Consulting Editor

I am very pleased to introduce this outstanding issue of the *Physical Medicine and Rehabilitation Clinics of North America* on Neuromuscular Disease Management and Rehabilitation, Part I: Diagnostic and Therapy Issues. Our guest editors for this issue are Dr Craig M. McDonald, Professor and Chair of the Department of Physical Medicine and Rehabilitation at the University of California, Davis, and his protégé and junior faculty member, Dr Nanette C. Joyce. Dr McDonald is also the Director of the National Institute on Disability and Rehabilitation Research funded Neuromuscular Disease Research and Training Center at UC Davis. Craig has been doing cutting-edge research in neuromuscular disease (NMD) for over 20 years and I am honored to have been one of his collaborators on many projects. Craig is also one of my closest friends and we have literally "grown up together" in this field. Dr Joyce is truly a rising star in NMD and was a former NIDRR research fellow, actually doing the same fellowship I did 22 years ago!

They have picked a truly great bunch of authors to cover literally every aspect of NMD care. Indeed, this is such a comprehensive body of work it will be spread out over two issues.

Fittingly, this first issue starts out with an article on The Role of the Neuromuscular Specialist and Physiatry in the Management of Neuromuscular Disease, coauthored by Dr McDonald and Dr William M Fowler Jr. That is particularly fitting as Dr McDonald has chosen to dedicate this work to Dr Fowler, a decision I wholeheartedly support. It would be hard to overstate the influence Dr Fowler has had on Craig and I. Bill was really the first physiatrist to establish a large clinical and research program in NMD. He did this at UC Davis, shortly after he became the founding chair of the department there. Interestingly, one of the first faculty members Bill tried to recruit was Dr George Kraft! George chose to go to Seattle and carve a very similar path as Dr Fowler, although choosing multiple sclerosis as his disease to attack.

The next article is probably going to be the most useful text that any clinician who is caring for patients with NMD ever reads. Written by the guest editor himself, Dr McDonald's article really tells us "how to do it the right way." Craig puts nearly 25 years worth

Phys Med Rehabil Clin N Am 23 (2012) xiii–xv
http://dx.doi.org/10.1016/j.pmr.2012.06.014
1047-9651/12/$ – see front matter © 2012 Elsevier Inc. All rights reserved.

pmr.theclinics.com

of experience into this and his extensive experience and expertise shine through in all the clinical pearls he offers here. Following that is another rock-solid, core article on "Electrodiagnosis in Neuromuscular Disease," authored by my dear friend and former mentee, Dr Jay Han, along with Dr Bethany Lipa. Jay did a 3-year high-powered basic research fellowship in the lab of Dr Jeff Chamberlain. While there, Jay personally developed a novel and brilliant technique of doing motor unit analysis in mdx mice. Dr Han is now the director of the NMD Fellowship program at UC Davis and is an established, highly respected researcher himself.

Drs Kevin Flanigan and W. David Arnold provide a brilliant article on "A Practical Approach to Molecular Diagnostic Testing in Neuromuscular Diseases." Dr Flanigan has made huge breakthroughs in molecular assessment in NMD. He possesses an amazing intellect fueled by creative insight, as one might expect from a former music major and jazz horn player!

Dr Joyce and her colleagues, Björn Oskarsson, MD and Lee-Way Jin, MD, PhD, provide a very instructive and nicely illustrated article on "Muscle Biopsy Evaluation in Neuromuscular Disorders." Reading muscle biopsies is still a critical skill that any NMD specialist should possess and this article really provides helpful, immediately useful tips.

The next two articles on "Physical Therapy Evaluation and Management in Neuromuscular Diseases" and "Exercise in Neuromuscular Diseases" really address the core issues on how we can improve functional strength in our NMD patients. The authors include R. Ted Abresch. "Ted" recently retired after a magnificent 35-year career in NMD research. Ted and I have worked closely for my entire career and I credit Ted with teaching me so much about how to do research, from statistics to writing. Much of the success of the UC Davis NIDRR NMD RTC can be attributed to Ted Abresch. Dr Julaine Florence is also an author. Julaine is an internationally renowned expert and literally wrote the book on physical therapy protocol in pediatric NMD. Linda B. Johnson, BS, PT rounds out the picture nicely.

Another former UCD NMD fellow, Dr Andrew J. Skalsky, helps Craig author an excellent review on the "Prevention and Management of Limb Contractures in Neuromuscular Diseases."

My dear friend, Dr Melanie Fried-Oken, and her colleagues, Laura Ball and Susan Fager, do a great job providing an update on "Augmentative and Alternative Communication for People with Progressive Neuromuscular Disease." This is amazing material and helps our patients so much.

Speaking of amazing stuff, the next article, "Robotics, Assistive Technology, and Occupational Therapy Management to Improve Upper Limb Function in Pediatric Neuromuscular Diseases," written by Dr Tariq Rahman and colleagues, Joseph Basante MA, MS, OTR/L, CHT, and Michael Alexander, MD, really shows us a peek at the future of rehabilitation.

The final article on "Disease Burden in Neuromuscular Disease: The Role of Chronic Pain" deserves a nod to Dr Mark P. Jensen, and his former fellow, Dr Jordi Miró. Years ago I became very interested in looking at pain in the context of NMD. I knew I would need help with this and everyone I asked pointed me to Dr Jensen, and for good reasons. Mark has literally written the book on the biopsychosocial aspects of chronic pain across all forms of disease. Mark has his own Research Training Center on Chronic Pain and has produced the best, cutting-edge work in this area, bar none, and we are blessed to have him in our NMD group! Also authoring this article is Dr Rima El-Abassi, a very bright young protégé of Dr John England's.

Thanks to everyone who contributed to this great work, with special thanks to Drs McDonald and Joyce for all their hard work as guest editors. This is a wonderful addition to the literature, truly worthy of honoring Dr William M. "Bill" Fowler Jr, MD, the founding father of the "role of physiatry in the management of neuromuscular disease."

Gregory T. Carter, MD, MS
Regional Neuromuscular Center
Providence Medical Group
410 Providence Lane, Building 2
Olympia, WA 9806, USA

E-mail address:
gtcarter@uw.edu

Preface

Neuromuscular Disease Management and Rehabilitation, Part I: Diagnostic and Therapy Issues

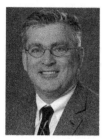 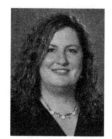

Craig M. McDonald, MD   Nanette C. Joyce, DO
Guest Editors

First let me say that Dr Nanette Joyce and I are quite honored to be the guest editors of this issue of the *Physical Medicine and Rehabilitation Clinics of North America* on Neuromuscular Disease Management and Rehabilitation, Part I: Diagnostic and Therapy Issues. This current issue in combination with the next issue of the *Clinics* (Part II), which focuses on multidisciplinary subspecialty management and therapeutics, are both intended to provide the reader with a comprehensive overview of the diagnostic approach, clinical characteristics, and care and management of patients with neuromuscular disease (NMD), with an emphasis on the most common hereditary and acquired neuromuscular disorders. Combining both hereditary and acquired NMDs, the prevalence exceeds 4 million, which is an impressive figure when compared, for example, to the prevalence of spinal cord injury, estimated to be between 239,000 and 306,000 in the United States. Virtually every physiatrist or neurologist who treats patients with significant impairments or who performs electrodiagnostic studies will encounter patients with either hereditary or acquired diseases of the peripheral neuromuscular system, including those that affect anterior horn cells, peripheral nerves, neuromuscular junctions, and muscle.

It is particularly rewarding for me to be collaborating on this important endeavor with Guest Editor, Dr Nanette Joyce, Assistant Professor of Physical Medicine and Rehabilitation at the University of California Davis and a rising star among physiatrists in the

Phys Med Rehabil Clin N Am 23 (2012) xvii–xx
http://dx.doi.org/10.1016/j.pmr.2012.06.013
1047-9651/12/$ – see front matter © 2012 Published by Elsevier Inc.

pmr.theclinics.com

United States in the new subspecialty of Neuromuscular Medicine. Nanette has followed one of the most impressive career training pathways ever embarked on by a PM&R specialist in the field of Neuromuscular Medicine. She completed a Fellowship in Neuromuscular Medicine in the ACGME-approved Fellowship at UC Davis (currently the only such approved Neuromuscular Medicine fellowship housed in a Department of PM&R) and she is Board certified in Neuromuscular Medicine, which is a relatively new subspecialty of the American Board of PM&R and the American Board of Psychiatry and Neurology. She then completed a 2-year Fellowship in Translational Medicine and Stem Cell Therapeutics in the UC Davis Institute for Regenerative Cures with her Fellowship being supported by the California Institute of Regenerative Medicine. In July of 2012, she was awarded a K12, early career development award, from the Association of Academic Physiatrists and the National Institutes of Health (NIH). She is currently participating in their associated Rehabilitation Medicine Scientist Training Program and is continuing her work in engineering stem cells to secrete trophic factors in a controllable manner and developing assays to characterize the cellular product. In ALS, for example, neuromuscular junction failure with motor neuron apoptosis leads to muscle weakness, atrophy, and severe disability from paralysis along with respiratory failure and death. Dr Joyce is bringing this novel therapeutic approach to treating motor neuron disorders from bench to bedside by performing proof-of-concept and preclinical studies. I am incredibly proud to have been one of the many mentors involved in Nanette's career development.

Tremendous advances in molecular genetics over the past three decades have led to a greater understanding of disease pathogenesis in a variety of neuromuscular diseases, but for most NMD conditions there remains no current therapy for the underlying cause. Many promising therapeutic strategies have recently been developed in animal models. Human trials of some of these strategies have recently started, leading to the hope of effective treatments for many of these currently incurable diseases. But while it is recognized that these diseases may remain incurable, NMDs are not untreatable. The last two decades have seen tremendous improvement in patient outcomes as a result of coordinated multidisciplinary care directed by the neuromuscular specialist. Improvements in disease management in Duchenne muscular dystrophy (DMD), for example, include treatment with corticosteroids, surgical management of spine deformity, noninvasive ventilation (specifically refined and popularized by Dr John Bach, a physiatrist), and more effective treatment of cardiomyopathy. These interventions have led to improved function and survival and a changing disease natural history in DMD. Similarly, ALS survival has been impacted by noninvasive and invasive ventilation and aggressive nutritional management. The neuromuscular medicine and physiatry specialists are key health care providers who work cooperatively with a multidisciplinary team to maximize health and functional capacities in NMD.

Much of our research in neuromuscular diseases over the years at UC Davis has been funded by the National Institute on Disability and Rehabilitation Research (NIDRR), the largest federal funding source for medical rehabilitation research and training. We recently received a NIDRR Advanced Rehabilitation Research Training Grant focused on training rehabilitation scientists in neuromuscular and neurodevelopmental disorders. NIDRR is to be commended for their long commitment to medical rehabilitation research and research training for persons with neuromuscular diseases.

It has been encouraging to see an increase in the NIH, Centers for Disease Control and Prevention (CDC), and Department of Defense (DOD) portfolios devoted to neuromuscular diseases. The situation in muscular dystrophy is a case in point. In 2001, as a result of effective lobbying efforts by a number of consumer advocacy groups such as Muscular Dystrophy Association (MDA), Parent Project Muscular Dystrophy

(PPMD), FSH Society, Myotonic Dystrophy Foundation, and others, landmark muscular dystrophy legislation was introduced in Congress. At the time the bill—the Muscular Dystrophy Community Assistance, Research, and Education Amendments (MD-CARE Act)—was unveiled in 2001, few bright spots existed for patients and families battling muscular dystrophy. Federal research for varied forms of muscular dystrophy was minimal; surveillance and data collection were nonexistent, and the federal government lacked a comprehensive muscular dystrophy research and care agenda. The MD-CARE Act forever changed this landscape.

The law created what are now multiple research Centers of Excellence—named after the late Sen. Paul Wellstone—funded by the NIH. It launched a data collection and surveillance program at the CDC. The law also created the Muscular Dystrophy Coordinating Committee to unite all relevant government and patient voices to develop an aggressive, milestone-driven action plan for all the muscular dystrophies. None of this would have been possible without the passionate, persistent, and informed advocacy of the muscular dystrophy community and a dedicated group of congressional champions. The tangible benefits from the MD-CARE Act are profound and have brought about improvements for patients and families that seemed far away when the legislation was introduced a decade ago, such as the following:

- Government and private sector funding for muscular dystrophy research has grown sharply, with hundreds of millions in NIH and CDC funding helping leverage private resources and yielding significant milestones.
- Multiple drugs and biologics are in varying phases of the discovery pipeline, including the critical phase III clinical trial stage.
- Early and correct diagnoses and evidence-based care standards mean more patients are receiving timely and improved care and more families benefit from genetic counseling.
- Advances in adaptive and communication technologies permit patients to live more engaged and connected lives.
- Improved life expectancy for individuals with muscular dystrophies and many other NMDs means more are pursuing college education and entering the workforce.

Similar advocacy efforts by the MDA, the ALS Association, Families of SMA, CMT Association, and many other advocacy groups are producing great awareness, improved care standards, and increased nonprofit and federal funding for a variety of other NMDs.

The emphasis of this Part I issue is on the diagnostic evaluation of NMDs and therapy issues. Effective management and anticipatory guidance for NMDs require an accurate diagnosis. It is critical for physiatrists and other clinicians who treat NMDs to understand key points to the initial clinical evaluation, electrodiagnostic evaluation, molecular genetic testing, and the role of muscle biopsy in diagnosis. A focus on therapy issues is an appropriate additional focus for this first issue, since physiatrists are experts in the rehabilitation and multidisciplinary management of disabling conditions, collaborating with allied health professionals such as physical therapists, occupational therapists, speech pathologists, orthotists, augmentative communication and assistive technology specialists, exercise scientists, recreational therapists, and rehabilitation engineers. In addition, physiatrists often participate with the multidisciplinary team in the management of chronic pain syndromes in NMDs, so the last article on "Disease Burden in Neuromuscular Disease: The Role of Chronic Pain" is particularly relevant to the PM&R specialist.

The number of MDA-sponsored neuromuscular disease clinics that have active participation by a PM&R specialist remains a substantial minority. While over 20 ACGME-approved Neuromuscular Medicine Fellowships have been developed in US Neurology Departments, there remains just one such training program housed in a Department of Physical Medicine and Rehabilitation (at UC Davis). Our hope is these two issues will demonstrate the value of physiatry to current practicing Neuromuscular Medicine specialists, increase participation of PM&R specialists in NMD clinics, spur physiatry residents to consider subspecialty training in Neuromuscular Medicine, motivate the young faculty in PM&R who have graduated from our program and other neurology-based fellowship programs to develop their own fellowship training programs in Neuromuscular Medicine, and ultimately expand the rehabilitation expertise among all Neuromuscular Medicine specialists. The ultimate goal of these two issues focusing on clinical management and rehabilitation is to improve the quality of life for people with neuromuscular diseases and their families.

This issue is dedicated to William M. Fowler Jr, MD, a pioneer in the rehabilitation management of persons with neuromuscular diseases (see Dedication). No physiatrist in history has been as instrumental as Dr Bill Fowler, my mentor and colleague for decades, in advancing the scientific basis of the rehabilitation management of neuromuscular diseases.

Finally, Dr Nanette Joyce and I wish to personally thank all of the contributing authors for all their time and hard work invested in the articles in Parts I and II, which will provide you with a tremendous wealth of clinical expertise that can be directly applied to your practice.

Craig M. McDonald, MD
Professor and Chair
Department of Physical Medicine and Rehabilitation
University of California Davis School of Medicine
Director
NIDRR Rehabilitation Research and
Training Center in Neuromuscular Diseases
Director
Neuromuscular Disease Clinics
University of California Davis Health System
Sacramento, CA 95817, USA

E-mail address:
craig.mcdonald@ucdmc.ucdavis.edu

Dedication

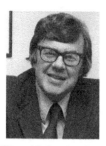

William M. Fowler, Jr, MD

This issue is dedicated to Dr William M. Fowler, Jr, a pioneer in the rehabilitation management of persons with neuromuscular diseases. Dr Fowler was on the medical faculty of the University of California (at UCLA and UC Davis) from 1964 to 1991. He was the Founding Chair of the Department of PM&R at UC Davis in 1968 and served as Chair there from 1968 to 1984. He was President of the American Academy of PM&R in 1980 and 1981. He was Founding Director of the NIDRR funded Rehabilitation Research and Training Center (RRTC) in Neuromuscular Diseases. The UC Davis RRTC in Neuromuscular Diseases remains the longest continuously funded RRTC in NIDRR history. Subsequent to his retirement, Dr Fowler served as an active Professor Emeritus at the UC Davis School of Medicine for decades, where he helped recruit Drs Greg Carter and David Kilmer to join the faculty in 1991, and helped recruit me to join the faculty in 1992. Dr Fowler is a past recipient of the Krusen Award, the American Academy of PM&R's highest honor. He previously authored a number of seminal articles on the natural history of NMDs, the role of creatine kinase for diagnosis and screening in muscular dystrophy, contraction-induced injury and overwork weakness in muscular dystrophy, physical activity and exercise training in neuromuscular diseases, manual muscle testing and quantitative strength testing, progressive resistive exercises, aerobic exercise, quantification of muscle contractility, management of contractures, natural history of scoliosis, cognitive assessment, employment, and quality of life in neuromuscular diseases.

It should be noted that Bill Fowler remains "sharp as a tack today," a coauthor at age 86 on the first article of this issue, and a valued source of wisdom and counsel for me and other colleagues at UC Davis for decades. Dr Fowler most importantly has left a lasting legacy by helping to train generations of PM&R and neuromuscular medicine specialists, who have developed a focus on the clinical management and rehabilitation of neuromuscular diseases. In addition, Dr Fowler deeply impacted the field of PM&R by counseling the Chairs of Departments of PM&R throughout the country to develop improved research capacity of their junior faculty and inspiring PM&R academicians in a variety of rehabilitation subspecialty areas to develop

Phys Med Rehabil Clin N Am 23 (2012) xxi–xxii
http://dx.doi.org/10.1016/j.pmr.2012.06.012
1047-9651/12/$ – see front matter © 2012 Elsevier Inc. All rights reserved.

pmr.theclinics.com

a more scientific and evidence-based approach to their practice. To quote from his American Academy of PM&R Presidential Address on November 3, 1981:

"Research is the single most important factor that will directly determine the acceptance of academic PM&R, and the viability of physiatry."

With sincere gratitude,

Craig M. McDonald, MD
Professor and Chair, Department of Physical Medicine and Rehabilitation
Director, NIDRR Rehabilitation Research and Training Center
in Neuromuscular Diseases
Director, Neuromuscular Disease Clinics
University of California Davis Health System
Sacramento, CA 95817, USA

E-mail address:
cmmcdonald@ucdavis.edu

The Role of the Neuromuscular Medicine and Physiatry Specialists in the Multidisciplinary Management of Neuromuscular Disease

Craig M. McDonald, MD*, William M. Fowler, Jr, MD

KEYWORDS

- Neuromuscular medicine specialist • Physiatry • Neuromuscular disease
- Management

KEY POINTS

- Both neuromuscular medicine specialists and physiatrists are key health care providers who work cooperatively with a multidisciplinary team to provide coordinated care for individuals with neuromuscular diseases (NMDs).
- Ongoing input from different specialties is important because the specific assessments and interventions that are necessary will change as the NMD progresses.
- Addressing the many complications of NMDs in a comprehensive and consistent way is also crucial for planning and determining eligibility for clinical trials and for improving care worldwide.
- The development and implementation of standardized care recommendations for NMDs will lead to improved health, function, participation, and quality of life.

This issue of the *Physical Medicine and Rehabilitation Clinics of North America* is intended to provide the reader with a comprehensive overview of the diagnostic approach, clinical characteristics, and care and management of patients with neuromuscular disease (NMD), with an emphasis on the most common hereditary and acquired neuromuscular disorders. NMDs, a classification category that describes hereditary and acquired

The authors have nothing to disclose.
This work was supported by grant H133B0900001 from the National Institute of Disability and Rehabilitation Research.
The authors take full responsibility for the contents of this article, which does not represent the views of the National Institute of Disability and Rehabilitation Research or the United States Government.
Department of Physical Medicine and Rehabilitation, University of California Davis School of Medicine, 4860 Y Street, Suite 3850, Sacramento, CA 95817, USA
* Corresponding author.
E-mail address: cmmcdonald@ucdavis.edu

Phys Med Rehabil Clin N Am 23 (2012) 475–493
http://dx.doi.org/10.1016/j.pmr.2012.06.010
1047-9651/12/$ – see front matter © 2012 Elsevier Inc. All rights reserved.

diseases of the peripheral neuromuscular system, includes those that affect anterior horn cells, peripheral nerves, neuromuscular junctions, and muscle.

The estimated total prevalence of the most common NMDs in the United States is 500,000.[1-7] Combined with all forms of acquired NMDs, the prevalence exceeds 4 million, which is an impressive figure when compared, for example, with the prevalence of spinal cord injury, which is estimated to be between 239,000 and 306,000.[8-11] There is tremendous diversity of the causes for both acquired and hereditary NMDs. Some NMDs are acquired with diverse causes distinct from genetic causes, such as autoimmune, infectious, metabolic, toxic, or paraneoplastic (eg, amyotrophic lateral sclerosis [ALS], myasthenia gravis, Lambert-Eaton syndrome, botulism, Guillain-Barré syndrome, or diabetic peripheral neuropathy). There are more than 500 distinct NMDs identified to date that have specific genes that have been linked causally to these conditions.[12-14] Limb girdle muscular dystrophy, for example, has more than 20 genetically distinct subtypes that have been identified to date. The genetic heterogeneity of hereditary NMDs has created challenges for clinicians and researchers.

Although currently incurable, NMDs are not untreatable. The neuromuscular medicine and physiatry specialists are key health care providers who work cooperatively with a multidisciplinary team to maximize health; maximize functional capacities, including mobility, transfer skills, upper limb function, and self-care skills; inhibit or prevent complications, such as disuses weakness, skeletal deformities, disuses weakness, airway clearance problems, respiratory failure, cardiac insufficiency and dysrhythmias, bone health problems, excessive weight gain or weight loss, metabolic syndrome; and promote access to full integration into the community with optimal quality of life.

The molecular basis of hereditary NMDs has been emerging and coming into sharper focus over the past 3 decades. Many promising therapeutic strategies have since been developed in animal models. Human trials of these strategies have started, leading to the hope of definitive treatments for many of these currently incurable diseases. Although specific treatments for NMDs have not yet reached the clinic, the natural history of these diseases can be changed by targeting interventions to known manifestations and complications. The diagnosis can be swiftly reached, families and patients can be well supported, and individuals who have NMDs can reach their full potential in education and employment. In Duchenne muscular dystrophy (DMD), for example, corticosteroid, respiratory, cardiac, orthopedic, and rehabilitative interventions have led to improvements in function, quality of life, health, and longevity, with children who are diagnosed today having the possibility of a life expectancy into their fourth decade.[15-28]

Advocacy organizations report variable and inconsistent health care for individuals with NMD. Although anticipatory and preventive clinical management of NMDs is essential, recommendations exist in only a few areas. Addressing the many complications of NMDs in a comprehensive and consistent way is also crucial for planning multicenter trials and for improving care worldwide. The development and implementation of standardized care recommendations have been emphasized by stakeholders in heterogeneous NMD communities, including government agencies, clinicians, scientists, academicians, volunteer health agencies, and advocacy organizations. The purpose of this issue is to provide a framework for recognizing the primary manifestations and possible complications and for planning the optimum treatment across different specialties with a coordinated multidisciplinary team.

REPORTED NEEDS OF INDIVIDUALS WITH NMDS

The greatest needs of the population of individuals with NMDs were recently evaluated by the National Institute on Disability and Rehabilitation Research–funded

Rehabilitation Research and Training Center in NMDs at the University of California (UC) Davis Medical Center. The authors performed a comprehensive quality-of-life survey of more than 1000 individuals with NMDs.[29,30] The most frequent problems impacting quality of life in NMDs are shown in **Table 1**. Consumers with NMDs reported that the most significant problems impacting their health, function, and quality of life were secondary conditions, including weakness, fatigue and poor endurance, weight management, sleep disturbances, muscle contractures, and breathing problems. These problems translate into functional issues that consumers with NMDs note to be significant, such as difficulty walking, exercising, controlling weight, and doing activities of daily living (ADLs).

THE MULTIDISCIPLINARY NMD TEAM

The comprehensive management of all of the varied clinical problems associated with NMDs is a complex task. For this reason, the multidisciplinary or interdisciplinary approach is critical. The two terms are often used interchangeably with inter-discipline communication being the key. It takes advantage of the expertise of many clinicians rather than placing the burden on one. This interdisciplinary approach to caring for patients with NMD, and participation by committed providers that have NMD-specific expertise are key ingredients to the provision of optimal care (**Fig. 1**).[31,32] Patients and families/care providers should actively engage with the medical professional who coordinates clinical care. Depending on the patient's circumstances, such as area/country of residence or insurance status, this role might be served by, but is not limited to, a neurologist or pediatric neurologist, physiatrist/rehabilitation specialist, neurogeneticist, pediatric orthopedist, pediatrician, or primary care physician. In the United States, the neuromuscular medicine specialist often does the coordination of care (fellowships in neuromuscular medicine approved by the Accreditation Council for Graduate Medical Education now exist for subspecialty certification within the American Board of Psychiatry and Neurology and the American Board of Physical Medicine and Rehabilitation). The director or coordinator of the team must be aware of the potential issues specific to NMDs and be able to access the interventions that are the foundations for proper care in NMD. These foundations

Table 1
Selected problems impacting health-related quality of life in NMD (n = 1169)

How Much Difficulty Do You Have Performing the Following Functions?	Moderate or Severe (%)	Slight (%)	Not a Problem (%)
Difficulty with muscle weakness	72.4	11.6	6.0
Difficulty getting exercise	66.1	17.5	16.3
Difficulty with fatigue	70.8	21.7	7.6
Difficulty controlling weight	36.0	27.9	36.2
Difficulty with sleeping	36.2	28.6	35.1
Difficulty with muscle contractures	33.6	29.9	36.6
How Much Does Your Health Limit You in the Following Activities?	**A Lot (%)**	**A Little (%)**	**Not at All (%)**
Vigorous activities, such as running	93	3	4
Walking more than a mile	84	9	7
Walking several blocks	73	17	10
Walking one block	54	27	18

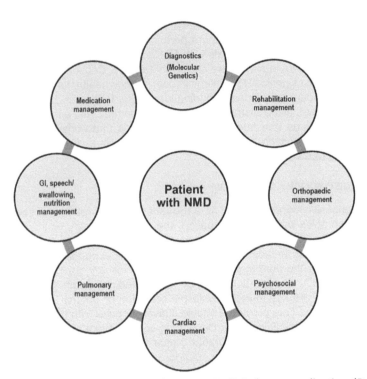

Fig. 1. "Multidisciplinary" or "interdisciplinary" NMD clinical care coordination. (*Data from* Bushby K, Finkel R, Birnkrant DJ, et al. Diagnosis and management of Duchenne muscular dystrophy, part 1: diagnosis, and pharmacologic and psychosocial management. Lancet Neurol 2010;9(1):77–93.)

include health maintenance and proper monitoring of disease progression and complications to provide anticipatory, preventive care, and optimum management.

NMD management is best performed by a team consisting of physicians; physical, occupational, and speech therapists; social workers; vocational counselors; and psychologists, among others. Ideally, owing to the significant mobility problems associated with most NMDs, the neuromuscular medicine specialist, physiatrist, and all the key clinical personnel should be available at each visit. Tertiary care medical centers in larger urban areas usually can provide this type of service. This may be an independent clinic or may be sponsored by one or more of the consumer-driven organizations that sponsor research and clinical care for people with NMDs, including the Muscular Dystrophy Association, the Amyotrophic Lateral Sclerosis Association, the Charcot-Marie-Tooth International and Association groups, and the Facioscapulohumeral Society, among others. Although the *physiatrist* (Greek for *physis* for "nature" and *iatrikos* for "healing") is well suited to direct the rehabilitation team and to oversee a comprehensive, goal-oriented treatment plan, physiatrists are the codirectors of less than 20% of the MDA clinics in the United States and a recent MDA Clinic Directors survey showed that fewer than one-half of MDA Clinics have a physiatrist as a member of the multidisciplinary team.[33,34] Bach[34] has previously described the many major advances physiatrists have contributed to the care of patients with NMD and has pointed out the rather significant need for more physiatric involvement in the care of these patients.

Toolkits of Assessments and Interventions for the Interdisciplinary NMD Team

There are varied toolkits of assessments and interventions applicable to NMD management (**Table 2**).[31] Input from different specialties and the specific assessments and interventions will change as the NMD progresses. Some measures, such as strength assessment, functional grading, timed function measures, and pulmonary function measures, are core measures performed at least annually for most NMDs. Others are performed regularly depending on the expected impairments for specific NMDs.

THE WORLD HEALTH ORGANIZATION INTERNATIONAL CLASSIFICATION OF FUNCTIONING FRAMEWORK

Although their degrees and severity can vary, the characteristics or complications of most NMDs include progressive weakness, limb contractures, spine deformity, and decreased pulmonary function; some patients suffer cardiac and intellectual impairment. In determining the severity of impairment and disability, a comprehensive evaluation of patients with NMDs should be done at routine intervals or as clinically indicated. The World Health Organization's International Classification of Functioning, Disability and Health (ICF)[35] provides a useful framework for evaluating the manifestations and complications of NMDs. The bioecological ICF framework[35] incorporates domains covering body structure and function, individual activities and participation, and environmental factors that impact the overall physical and mental health of the individual in a societal context. In this framework, *body structures* are anatomic parts of the body, such as organs, limbs, and their counterparts, and *body functions* are the physiologic functions of body systems, including physiologic functions. Impairments are problems in body structure or body function as a significant deviation from normal or loss. *Activity* is the execution of a task or action by an individual, and activity limitations are difficulties an individual may have in executing activities. *Participation* is the involvement in a life situation, and participation restrictions are problems an individual may have in the involvement in life situations. Although the ICF framework covers environmental domains, such as external barriers to participation, the authors typically do not include assessments of environmental domains of the ICF framework because of the limited ability of therapeutic agents, surgeries, or rehabilitation interventions evaluated in clinical trials to impact these domains.

Patient-reported outcomes (PROs) encompass self-perceived or caregiver-proxy–perceived concepts of health and well-being defined broadly including such concepts as health-related quality of life, satisfaction, physical functioning, basic mobility and transfers, sports and physical functioning, mobility and ambulation, upper extremity functioning and ADLs, pain, fatigue, quality of sleep, emotional health, social health, depression, anxiety, stigma, and so forth.

SELECTED ASSESSMENTS FOR NMD

There are diverse assessments that are performed in NMDs for clinical studies, natural history studies, and clinical trials. For example, **Table 3** summarizes the diverse nature of clinical endpoints and assessments that have been used clinically and in natural history studies involving individuals with DMD organized according to a modified ICF framework. Some core measures, such as manual muscle testing for strength, range of motion (ROM), timed function, pulmonary function, and selected cardiac measures, are routinely performed annually or more frequently if clinically indicated.

Important clinical data that should be obtained initially on each patient include the following: gender, birth date, family history, date of disease (symptom) onset, disease

Table 2
Multidisciplinary domains, assessments, and interventions for the NMD team

Multidisciplinary Domains	Tools/Assessments	Interventions
Diagnostics (neuromuscular medicine specialist, geneticist, pathologist)	Biomarkers (eg, creatine kinase) Electrodiagnostics Molecular genetics Muscle biopsy	Genetic counseling Family support
Medication management (neuromuscular medicine specialist, neurodevelopmental pediatrician, physiatrist)	Clinical evaluation Strength Function Range of motion	Considerations Age of patient Stage of disease Risk factors for side effects Available medications Choice of regimen Side-effect monitoring and prophylaxis Dose alteration
Rehabilitation management	Range of motion Strength Posture Function Alignment Gait	Stretching Positioning Splinting Orthoses Submaximum exercise/activity Seating Standing devices Adaptive equipment Assistive technology Strollers/scooters Manual/power wheelchairs
Orthopedic management	Assessment of range of motion Spinal assessment Spinal radiograph Bone age (left wrist and hand radiograph) Bone densitometry	Tendon surgery Osteotomies/arthrodesis Posterior spinal fusion
GI, speech/ swallowing, nutrition management	Upper and lower GI investigations Anthropometry	Diet control and supplementation Gastrostomy Pharmacologic management of gastric reflux and constipation
Pulmonary management	Spirometry Static airway pressures (MIP/MEP) Peak cough flow Pulse oximetry Capnography/end tidal carbon dioxide ABG Sleep studies/ polysomnography	Volume recruitment Noninvasive ventilation (via mask and nasal interfaces) Invasive ventilation (via tracheostomy) Airway clearance (Cough Assist Mechanical Insufflator-Exsufflator [Phillips Respironics, Andover, MA, USA], The Vest Airway Clearance System (Hill-Rom, St. Paul, MN, USA) Immunizations

(continued on next page)

Table 2 (continued)		
Multidisciplinary Domains	**Tools/Assessments**	**Interventions**
Cardiac management	ECG Echo Holter Cardiac MRI	ACE inhibitors Angiotensin receptor blockers β blockers Diuretics Inotropes Other heart failure medication Antiarrhythmics
Psychosocial management	Coping Neurocognitive Speech and language Autism Social work	Psychotherapy Pharmacologic interventions Social support Educational support Palliative/Supportive care

Abbreviations: ABG, Arterial Blood gas; ACE, angiotensin-converting enzyme; ECG, electrocardiogram; GI, gastrointestinal; MEP, maximal expiratory pressure; MIP, maximal inspiratory pressure; MRI, magnetic resonance imaging.

duration, dominant limb, weight and height, cardiovascular and pulmonary symptoms and findings, presence of contractures and spine deformity, muscle strength, ambulatory status (including age at cessation of ambulation and years of wheelchair use), and any treatment interventions. When relevant, these data should be updated at each patient visit. In large clinics, data can be recorded on a standardized form and entered into a computer database or electronic health record. Records of respiratory and cardiovascular symptoms and findings should be maintained at each clinic visit. The history should include questions relating to shortness of breath with ambulation, at rest, and during sleep; palpitations; dyspnea; and chest pain. A thorough systems review should be made of cardiopulmonary complications, including pneumonia, prolonged upper respiratory tract infections, respiratory compromise requiring assisted ventilation, and heart failure.

Strength Assessments

Precise measures of strength are important for evaluating clinical progression in NMD and assessing the efficacy of any interventions. Strength traditionally has been assessed with manual muscle testing (MMT) using the Medical Research Council (MRC) scale for muscle grading (**Table 4**), although this is not reliable in muscles that are only mildly affected.[36–42] Care must be exercised for consistent interexaminer measures of the antigravity muscles.

Quantitative strength measurements are somewhat more labor intensive but provide more sensitive and reproducible information.[38,40–42] These measurements include static (isometric) and dynamic (isokinetic) measurements, most often done in selected muscle groups (usually bilateral knee, elbow, shoulder, and neck flexors and extensors) with a force transducer that displays force output through a digital force monitor. Static pinch strength and grip strength also may be measured using a force transducer and these measurements should be followed serially at clinic visits. The highest score from 3 maximal trials is usually recorded. The handheld dynamometer (HHD) is perhaps the most practical yet reliable way to obtain quantitative strength testing in the clinic. The HHD is a small device equipped with an internal load cell that operates as a force transducer. The HHD is capable of measuring the force generated by a patient against the examiner who holds the device firmly against the patient and

Table 3
Clinical endpoints used in DMD prospective natural history studies and clinical trails (ICF framework)

Body Structure/Function[35]

Molecular diagnostics	Strength: quantitative grip strength
Dystrophin analysis by muscle biopsy (immunohistochemistry)	Strength: quantitative tip pinch and key pinch strength
Health status/review of systems	Strength: isometric strength with handheld devices
Medications, clinical complications	Strength: isometric strength with fixed devices
Anthropometric measures (standing height, weight, ulnar length, tibial length, skinfolds)	Strength: isokinetic strength with fixed devices
Vital signs	Strength: manual muscle testing (or MRC%)
Body composition (DEXA)	Pulmonary function tests: FVC, FEV1, PEFR, peak cough flow, MIP, MEP
Body composition (bioelectrical impedance)	Cardiac: ECG
Magnetic resonance imaging	Cardiac: echocardiography
Magnetic resonance spectroscopy (muscle)	Cardiac: Holter monitoring
Ultrasound imaging (muscle)	Cardiac: magnetic resonance imaging
Bone health (DEXA)	Cognitive and neuropsychological testing
Passive range of motion (goniometry)	
Spine deformity evaluation	

Activities (Clinical Evaluator-Determined Scales)[35]

Vignos lower extremity functional grade	Hammersmith Functional Motor Scale
Brooke upper extremity functional grade	Modified-Hammersmith Functional Motor Scale (extended)
North Star Ambulatory Assessment	Gross motor function measure
French Motor Function Measure	Egen Klassifikation Scale (version 2)
Bayley Scales of Infant Development	

Activities (Functional Tests with Timed Dimension)[35]

Time to rise from the floor (supine to stand)	6-min walk test
Time to climb 4 steps (beginning and ending standing with arms at sides)	2-min walk test
Time to walk/run 10 m or 30 ft (as fast as compatible with safety)	10-min walk test with energy expenditure using COSMED K4B2 (COSMED srl, Rome, Italy)
Time to stand from a chair (chair height should allow feet to touch floor)	Gait kinematics, kinetics with time-distance parameters
Time to propel a manual wheelchair 10 m or 30 ft	StepWatch step activity monitoring (Orthocare Innovations, LLC, Oklahoma, OK, USA)
Time to put on a T-shirt	ActiCal physical activity monitoring (Phillips Home Health Solutions, Bend, OR, USA)
Time to cut out a premarked square (3 in × 3 in) from a piece of paper with safety scissors (lines do not need to be followed precisely)	9-hole peg test
	Jebsen Taylor Hand Function Test

Participation measures[35]

Pediatric evaluation of disability inventory	Preferences for activities of children
Children's assessment of participation and enjoyment	Assessment of preschool children's participation

Patient-reported outcome measures

Pediatric quality of life questionnaire generic core scale	Individualized neuromuscular QoL
POSNA pediatric musculoskeletal functional health questionnaire/pediatric outcomes data collection instrument	Child Behavioral Checklist
	Canadian Occupational Performance Measure (COPM)
PedsQL Neuromuscular Module	Caregiver Burden Scale
PedsQL Multidimensional Fatigue Scale	WHO quality of life: Bref
NeuroQoL patient-reported quality of life	SF-36
Life satisfaction scale (life satisfaction scale for adolescents)	Pittsburgh Sleep Quality Index

Abbreviations: DEXA, Dual-Energy X-Ray Absorptiometry; ECG, electrocardiogram; FEV1, forced expiratory volume in the first second of expiration; FVC, forced vital capacity; MEP, maximal expiratory pressure; MIP, maximal inspiratory pressure; NeuroQoL, Neurological Diseases Quality of Life Instrument; PedsQL, Pediatric Quality of Life Inventory; PEFR, peak expiratory flow rate; POSNA, Pediatric Orthopaedic Society of North America; SF-36, 36-Item Short Form Health Survey; WHO, World Health Organization.

Table 4	
MRC grade degree of strength	
5	There is normal strength.
5-	There is barely detectable weakness.
4S	This grade is the same as 4 but stronger than the reference muscle.
4	The muscle is weak but moves the joint against a combination of gravity and some resistance.
4W	This grade is the same as 4 but weaker than the reference muscle.
3+	The muscle is capable of transient resistance but collapses abruptly. This degree of weakness is difficult to put into words but it is a muscle that is able to move the joint against gravity and an additional small amount of resistance. It is not to be used for muscles capable of sustained resistance throughout their whole range of movement.
3	The muscle cannot move against resistance but moves the joint fully against gravity. With the exception of knee extensors, the joint must be moved through its full mechanical range against gravity. If patients have contractures that limit movement of the joint, the mechanical range obviously will be to the point at which the contractures cause a significant resistance to the movement.
3-	The muscle moves the joint against gravity but not through the full extent of the mechanical range of the joint.
2	The muscle moves the joint when gravity is eliminated.
1	A flicker of movement is seen or felt in the muscle.
0	There is no movement.

provides stabilization (counter-resistance). The maximum force is recorded. Although it does not replace formal quantitative strength testing, the HHD has reasonably good reliability in NMD for weaker muscle groups and is a good alternative to MMT.

Dynamic strength may be assessed using an isokinetic dynamometer at a fixed speed (eg, 30°/s) for both concentric (shortening) and eccentric (lengthening) contractions.[40] Flexors and extensors should be evaluated through a full range of motion. Parameters that can be measured include peak torque, total work, work per repetition, peak-torque-to-body-weight ratio, joint angle at peak torque, ROM, and fatigue index (decrement in work performance over the exercise bout).

ROM Assessments

Passive joint ROM (PROM) measurements should be done with a standard goniometer following the protocol used by Brooke and colleagues[4] and Fowler and colleagues.[40] The joints to be evaluated for contractures include elbow and wrist extension, hip adduction for iliotibial band tightness, hip and knee extension, and ankle dorsiflexion. The definition of clinically significant contractures varies according to the joint. In some joints, even as little as a 7° flexion contracture can result in the center of gravity falling to an unstable plane (eg, anterior to the hip joint and posterior to the knee center of rotation). Care must be taken to measure the ROM of 2-joint muscles in the position of function (eg, ankle ROM measured with the knee fully extended).

Active ROM (AROM) assesses the participant's ability to recruit muscle strength to perform a muscle contraction through an available ROM. PROM is first performed by a clinical evaluator to assess the extensibility of muscle, tendons, and ligaments passively through a ROM. This assessment is followed by the evaluation of AROM. The assessment of ROM must be performed taking into account what PROM is available because of contracture. AROM and PROM are necessary for appropriate biomechanics in activities, such as walking and using the upper extremities for functional activities.

Timed Function Tests

Time to rise from the floor (supine to stand)

The time to rise from the floor from a supine position (in seconds) follows the protocol reported previously by The Clinical Investigation of Duchenne Dystrophy (CIDD),[36] University of California (UC), Davis,[40] and the Cooperative International Neuromuscular Research Group (CINRG).[42] The assessment is performed in all ambulatory study participants who can perform the test. For standing from supine, the velocity is calculated as 1 divided by the time to complete the task. Patients are given 30 to 60 seconds to complete the task. Patients who are unable to complete the task are given a score of 99 and a velocity that approaches zero.

Time to climb 4 stairs

The time to climb 4 standard stairs follows the protocol as described previously by CIDD,[36] UC Davis,[40] and CINRG.[42] The assessment is performed in children aged 2 years and older. For the total task of climbing 4 standard stairs, the velocity was calculated as 1 divided by the time to complete the task. Patients are given 30 to 60 seconds to complete the task. Patients who are unable to complete the task are given a score of 99 and a velocity that approaches zero.

Time to walk/run 10 m

The time to walk/run 10 m follows the protocol reported by CIDD,[36] and UC Davis for 30 ft,[40,43] and CINRG for 10 m.[42] The assessment is performed in children aged 2 years and older. The timed function test velocities were calculated as distance divided by completion time. The velocity for the 10-m walk/run test is determined by dividing distance (10 m) by the time to complete the task (in seconds). Patients are given 30 to 60 seconds to complete the task. Patients who are unable to complete the task are given a score of 99 and a velocity that approaches zero.

Other timed function tests

These tests may include the time to stand from a chair, time to propel a manual wheelchair 10 m or 30 ft, time to put on a T-shirt, and time to cut out a premarked square (3 in $\times$ 3 in) from a piece of paper with safety scissors.

Six-minute walk test

The authors have recently modified the American Thoracic Society (ATS) version of the 6-minute walk test (6MWT) and validated the test as a clinical endpoint for DMD.[44–46] Subsequently, there has been widespread use of this measure and success of the measure as a primary endpoint in multicenter clinical trials. The modified 6MWT uses standard video instructions, a safety chaser to assist patients up in the event of a fall, and constant rather than intermittent encouragement. Patients walk around 2 cones placed 25 m apart. For the CINRG DMD natural history study, the 6MWT is performed in all participants who can be expected to walk at least 75 m. Patients who are unable to ambulate 10 m on a 10-m walk/run test are given a zero value for the 6MWT. Using this protocol,[44] the authors determined the 6MWT to be reliable and valid in DMD at a single center. The primary variable derived from the 6MWT is the 6-minute walk distance (6MWD) in meters. For clinical trials whereby patients are tested serially, lower values of 6MWD can be obtained in more marginal ambulators. To account for maturational influences we have described the use of age- and height- based percent predicted values for 6MWT.[46] For patients with DMD, the authors also measure the number of steps taken during the 6MWT with a tally counter or with a stepwatch (Orthocare Innovations, LLC, Oklahoma, OK, USA) activity monitor placed on the right ankle. This practice allows the calculation of average stride length and cadence. The 6MWT takes approximately 15 minutes to complete.

Nine-hole peg test

The 9-hole peg test (9-HPT) is a commercially available, easy and quick-to-administer portable test that is used to measure upper limb function and dexterity.[47–52] The 9-HPT records the time to pick up 9 pegs from a container, put them into the holes, and then return them to the container. The test has been validated in all age groups and has high interrater and test-retest validity. The 9-HPT shows concurrent and convergent validity and the measure seems sensitive to change in adults with neuromuscular and musculoskeletal disorders.[51,52] Both adult and pediatric norms are available.[49,50] It has been chosen by the National Institutes of Health Toolbox as a measure of dexterity because it is a viable tool for longitudinal epidemiologic studies and intervention trials (www.nihtoolbox.org). The primary variable derived from the 9-HPT is the completion time in seconds. The total time for the administration of the 9-HPT is 10 minutes or less.

Disease-Specific Functional Rating Scales

Disease-specific functional rating systems exist for many NMDs. For example, the ALS Functional Rating scale (ALSFRS) is commonly obtained in patients with ALS.[53] In DMD, functional classifications use the upper extremity scale reported by Brooke and colleagues[36] and the lower extremity scales used by Vignos and colleagues.[54,55]

ALSFRS-revised

The ALSFRS-revised (ALSFRS-R) assesses patients' levels of self-sufficiency in areas of feeding, grooming, ambulation, communication, and respiratory.[53] The assessment determines the degree of impairment in the abilities of patients with ALS to function independently in ADLs, locomotion, communication, and breathing. It consists of 12 items to evaluate bulbar function, motor function, and respiratory function; each item is scored from 0 (unable) to 4 (normal). The ALSFRS has been validated both cross-sectionally and longitudinally against muscle strength testing, the Schwab and England ADL rating scale, the Clinical Global Impression of Change scale, and independent assessments of patients' functional status. The ALSFRS-R is an attractive primary outcome measure in clinical trials of ALS because it is validated, easy to administer, minimizes dropout, reduces cost, and correlates with survival. Unlike the other standard outcome measures currently used, the ALSFRS-R is also a measure of global function.[53]

Vignos lower extremity functional grade

The following functional grade was originally described by Vignos[54,55]: (1) walks and climbs stairs without assistance; (2) walks and climbs stairs with the aid of a railing; (3) walks and climbs stairs slowly with the aid of a railing (more than 12 seconds for 4 standard stairs); (4) walks unassisted and rises from chair but cannot climb stairs; (5) walks unassisted but cannot rise from chair or climb stairs; (6) walks only with the assistance or walks independently with long leg braces; (7) walks in long leg braces but requires assistance for balance; (8) stands in long leg braces but is unable to walk even with assistance; (9) is in a wheelchair; (10) is confined to bed.

Brooke upper extremity functional grade

The following functional grade was originally described by Brooke and colleagues[36]: (1) starting with arms at the sides, the patient can abduct the arms in a full circle until they touch above the head; (2) can raise arms above the head only by flexing the elbow (ie, shortening the circumference of the movement or using accessory muscles); (3) cannot raise hands above head but can raise an 8-oz glass of water to mouth using both hands if necessary; (4) can raise hands to mouth but cannot raise an 8-oz glass of water to mouth; (5) cannot raise hands to mouth but can use hands to hold pen or pick up pennies from the table; (6) cannot raise hands to mouth and has no useful function of hands. As an optional measure, if the patients have a Brooke grade of 1 or 2 measured by the therapist, it is determined how many kilograms of weight can be placed on a shelf above eye level, using 1 hand.

North Star Ambulatory Assessment

The North Star Ambulatory Assessment (NSAA) is a clinician-rated 17-item functional scale designed for ambulant boys with DMD who are able to stand.[56–61] This evaluation tool assesses functional activities, including standing, getting up from the floor, negotiating steps, hopping, and running. The assessment is based on a 3-point rating scale: 2 (ability to perform the test normally), 1 (modified method or assistance to perform test), 0 (unable to perform the test). Thus, the total score can range from 0 (completely nonambulant) to 34 (no impairment on these assessments). The NSAA is also currently used in several other countries and international clinical trials.[62] NSAA has shown good reliability and validity in multicenter studies and good clinical validity through Rasch analysis.[57,59]

Motor function measure

The motor function measure (MFM) is a recently developed instrument to assess motor function in ambulant and nonambulant patients with NMDs aged 6 to 62 years.[63] The scale is comprised of 32 items in 3 dimensions: D1, standing position and transfers (13 items); D2, axial and proximal motor function (12 items); and D3, distal motor function (7 items). Each test is scored by the therapist on a 4-point Likert scale. The scores for subscales and the composite total score range from 0% (worse) to 100% (better). In patients with heterogeneous NMD, internal consistency, intrarater and interrater reliability for the global scale and the subscales was excellent, and face validity, convergent validity and discriminant validity were good.[63] Vuillerot and colleagues[64] showed that the MFM was able to measure changes in motor function over time in DMD and the total score predicted a loss of ambulation. The MFM takes 30 to 40 minutes to complete.

Egen Klassifikation scale

The Egen Klassifikation (EK) scale was developed by the Danish Muscular Dystrophy Association as a clinical tool to assess overall functional ability in nonambulatory patients with DMD.[65] This tool includes assessments comprised of functional ability measuring upper extremity grade, muscle strength measured with the manual muscle test, and forced vital capacity defined as a percentage of normal values (FVC%). The construct is based on the interaction of physical components, such as muscle strength, ROM, respiratory status, wheelchair dependence, and age. The EK scale assesses 10 functional categories (EK 1–10), each on a scale of 0 (normal) to 3 (very impaired), contributing to an overall function score of 0 to 30. The EK scale has shown high interrater and intrarater reliability (Intraclass Correlation Coefficient [ICC] = 0.98) and good construct validity.[65,66]

Spine Deformity Evaluations

For many patients with NMD, spine deformity should be evaluated at every clinic visit. Data obtained at the time of the first patient visit and thereafter should include the presence or absence of spine deformity, any interventions, and the patients' age at the time of the observation. Radiographs should be reviewed, and the results for kyphosis and scoliosis should be recorded along the guidelines recommended by Carman and colleagues,[67] Fon and colleagues,[68] and Gupta and colleagues.[69]

Pulmonary Evaluations

Depending on the specific NMD diagnosis, pulmonary evaluations by a pulmonologist may be indicated. Pulmonary function tests (PFTs) include forced vital capacity (FVC), forced expiratory volume in 1 second (FEV$_1$), FEV$_1$/FVC, maximal voluntary ventilation, residual volume (RV), peak expiratory flow rate, and peak cough flow. Measurements are made using a spirometer (eg, KoKo spirometer and digidoser, nSpire Health, Inc, Longmont, CO, USA) and the pulmonary function data may be interpreted using the Crapo and colleagues[70] and Polgar[71] normative reference set for 6- to 7-year-old participants or the Hankinson and colleagues[72] normative reference set for participants aged 8 years or older. Maximal inspiratory pressure (MIP) and maximal expiratory pressure (MEP) are helpful and are measured near RV and total lung capacity, respectively, following the technique described by Black and Hyatt[73] using a direct ready dial gauge force meter and ventilated T-tube assembly. Three technically satisfactory measurements should be obtained and the maximum reading recorded. The interpretation of MIP and MEP values can be based on Wilson and colleagues[74] and Domenech-Clar and colleagues[75] normative pediatric reference sets. Participants are evaluated in a seated position with support for the back and feet and they wear nose clips or have their noses held closed by hand during testing. If necessary, cardboard mouthpiece adapters can be used to enable participants to make a full lip seal. PFTs should be done at least yearly and more frequently if clinical indications exist. If clinically indicated, arterial blood gas studies, pulse oximetry, or capnography (carbon dioxide monitoring) should be obtained. Formal sleep studies may be indicated depending on the NMD diagnosis and results of regular screening studies, such as overnight pulse oximetry.

Cardiac Evaluations

Depending on the specific NMD diagnosis, cardiac evaluations by a cardiologists may be indicated. Regular assessments may include electrocardiograms (ECG), echocardiography, Holter monitoring, and cardiac magnetic resonance imaging. Standard 12-lead ECGs should be obtained at 1-year intervals. In some diseases, particularly the myopathies with associated cardiomyopathy, echocardiograms are indicated.

Neuropsychological Tests

Neuropsychologic measurements may be helpful in some of these diseases, particularly if there are educational and vocational problems. However, previous reports that used some of the standard measurement tools suggested that subtle physical impairments may have negatively affected the test results. Therefore, caution is advised in interpreting these tests. Tools, such as the Category Test, Seashore Rhythm Test, and Speech-Perception Test should be used, if possible, because performance on these instruments is not dependent on motor function.[76–78]

PROS

Consumers, clinical researchers, the Food and Drug Administration (FDA), and industry have increasingly recognized the importance of PRO measures in the determination of clinically meaningful outcomes and validation of clinical and surrogate endpoints for therapeutic trials.[79] There are regulatory requirements that registration studies must incorporate primary endpoints that objectively measure clinically meaningful life-changing events with significant impact on health and well-being. In addition, the FDA has strongly recommended the inclusion of PRO measures, such as health-related quality of life (HRQOL) assessments, as endpoints in all clinical trials.[80,81] Both global measures of HRQOL and disease-specific NMD measures have been used in NMD populations.

ONGOING MANAGEMENT/ANTICIPATORY GUIDANCE

Once the diagnosis is confirmed, patients and families should be thoroughly educated about the expected outcome and what problems may be encountered. The neuromuscular specialist or physiatrist should then assess the goals of the patients and families and develop a medical management and rehabilitative program that matches those goals. Palliative care focuses on living well with optimized quality of life despite life expectancy.

Major advances in the understanding of the molecular basis of many NMDs have greatly enhanced the diagnostic accuracy and provide the basis for novel therapeutic interventions. There have also been major pharmacologic advances in the treatment of some NMDs, particularly ALS and DMD. The physiatrist may become involved in the prescription of disease-altering medications for the various NMDs and, therefore, should familiarize him or herself with the appropriate pharmacologic agents available. In addition, if not directly involved in research, the physiatrist should nonetheless encourage enrollment in experimental protocols, which not only furthers science but also provides some hope for patients. Education and employment are important with respect to self-esteem, quality of life, and integration into the community and should be emphasized in people with slowly progressive NMD. Patients should be referred to a support group. Support groups are often a great resource, not only for psychologic support but also for problem solving and recycling of equipment.

Given the many advances that have occurred in the management of people with NMD, many patients will survive through their childbearing years, possibly having children, and can expect to enjoy a good quality of life. The physiatrist can play a critical role during important life transitions and provide care that can maximize function and quality of life.

SUMMARY

Although currently incurable, NMDs are not untreatable. The neuromuscular medicine and physiatry specialists are key health care providers who work cooperatively with a multidisciplinary team to maximize health and functional capacities, inhibit or prevent complications, and provide access to resources that promote full integration into the community to optimize quality of life. Addressing the many complications of NMDs in a comprehensive and consistent way is also crucial for improving care worldwide and keeping patients in optimal health. This will allow persons with NMDs the best opportunity to participate in clinical trials which may further ameliorate the disease process. The development and implementation of standardized care recommendations have been emphasized by government agencies, clinicians, scientists, academicians, volunteer health agencies, and advocacy organizations. The neuromuscular medicine and physiatry specialists are well suited to working cooperatively to provide this type of multidisciplinary care and they can play a significant role in improving care for patients.

REFERENCES

1. Emery AE. Population frequencies of inherited neuromuscular diseases: a world survey. Neuromuscul Disord 1991;1(1):19–29.

2. Fedele D, Comi G, Coscelli C, et al. A multicenter study on the prevalence of diabetic neuropathy in Italy. Italian Diabetic Neuropathy Committee. Diabetes Care 1997;20(5):836–43.
3. De Domenico P, Malara CE, Marabello L, et al. Amyotrophic lateral sclerosis: an epidemiological study in the Province of Messina, Italy, 1976-1985. Neuroepidemiology 1988;7:152–8.
4. Somnier FE. Myasthenia gravis. Dan Med Bull 1996;43(1):1–10.
5. Hughes MI, Hicks EM, Nevin NC, et al. The prevalence of inherited neuromuscular disease in Northern Ireland. Neuromuscul Disord 1996;6(1):69–73.
6. Ahlstrom G, Gunnarsson LG, Leissner P, et al. Epidemiology of neuromuscular disease, including the postpolio sequelae in a Swedish country. Neuroepidemiology 1993;12(5):262–9.
7. Shoenberg BS, Melton LJ. Epidemiologic approaches to peripheral neuropathy. In: Dyck PJ, Thomas PK, Griffin JW, Low PA, Poduslo JF, editors. Peripheral neuropathy. Philadelphia: Saunders; 1993. p. 775–83.
8. DeVivo MJ, Fine PR, Maetz HM, et al. Prevalence of spinal cord injury: a re-estimation employing life table techniques. Arch Neurol 1980;37:707–8.
9. Harvey C, Rothschild BB, Asmann AJ, et al. New estimates of traumatic SCI prevalence: a survey-based approach. Paraplegia 1990;28:537–44.
10. Lasfarques JE, Custis D, Morrone F, et al. A model for estimating spinal cord injury prevalence in the United States. Paraplegia 1995;33:62–8.
11. LaPlante M. Disability in the United States: prevalence and causes. Washington (DC): U.S. Dept. of Education and the National Institute on Disability and Rehabilitation Research; 1992.
12. Kaplan JC. The 2009 version of the gene table of neuromuscular disorders. Neuromuscul Disord 2009;19:77–98.
13. Mitochondrial encephalopathies: gene mutation. Neuromuscul Disord 2004;14:107–16.
14. Available at: http://www.worldmusclesociety.org/news/read/85. Accessed June 2, 2012.
15. Manzur AY, Kuntzer T, Pike M, et al. Glucocorticoid corticosteroids for Duchenne muscular dystrophy. Cochrane Database Syst Rev 2008;1:CD003725.
16. Moxley RT 3rd, Ashwal S, Pandya S, et al. Practice parameter: corticosteroid treatment of Duchenne dystrophy: report of the Quality Standards Subcommittee of the American Academy of Neurology and the Practice Committee of the Child Neurology Society. Neurology 2005;64:13–20.
17. Jeppesen J, Green A, Steffensen BF, et al. The Duchenne muscular dystrophy population in Denmark, 1977–2001: prevalence, incidence and survival in relation to the introduction of ventilator use. Neuromuscul Disord 2003;13:804–12.
18. Yasuma F, Konagaya M, Sakai M, et al. A new lease on life for patients with Duchenne muscular dystrophy in Japan. Am J Med 2004;117:363.
19. Eagle M, Bourke J, Bullock R, et al. Managing Duchenne muscular dystrophy—the additive effect of spinal surgery and home nocturnal ventilation in improving survival. Neuromuscul Disord 2007;17:470–5.
20. Eagle M. Report on the muscular dystrophy campaign workshop: exercise in neuromuscular diseases Newcastle, January 2002. Neuromuscul Disord 2002;12:975–83.
21. Markham LW, Kinnett K, Wong BL, et al. Corticosteroid treatment retards development of ventricular dysfunction in Duchenne muscular dystrophy. Neuromuscul Disord 2008;18:365–70.
22. American Academy of Pediatrics Section on Cardiology and Cardiac Surgery. Cardiovascular health supervision for individuals affected by Duchenne or Becker muscular dystrophy. Pediatrics 2005;116:1569–73.

23. Bushby K, Muntoni F, Bourke JP. 107th ENMC International Workshop: the management of cardiac involvement in muscular dystrophy and myotonic dystrophy. 7th–9th June 2002, Naarden, the Netherlands. Neuromuscul Disord 2003;13:166–72.

24. Duboc D, Meune C, Lerebours G, et al. Effect of perindopril on the onset and progression of left ventricular dysfunction in Duchenne muscular dystrophy. J Am Coll Cardiol 2005;45:855–7.

25. Brooke MH, Fenichel GM, Griggs RC, et al. Duchenne muscular dystrophy: patterns of clinical progression and effects of supportive therapy. Neurology 1989;39:475–81.

26. Vignos PJ, Wagner MB, Karlinchak B, et al. Evaluation of a program for long-term treatment of Duchenne muscular dystrophy. Experience at the University Hospitals of Cleveland. J Bone Joint Surg Am 1996;78:1844–52.

27. Rahbek J, Werge B, Madsen A, et al. Adult life with Duchenne muscular dystrophy: observations among an emerging and unforeseen patient population. Pediatr Rehabil 2005;8:17–28.

28. Tatara K, Shinno S. Management of mechanical ventilation and prognosis in Duchenne muscular dystrophy. IRYO Jap J Natl Med Serv 2008;62(10):566–71.

29. Abresch RT, Seyden NK, Wineinger MA. Quality of life. Issues for persons with neuromuscular diseases. Phys Med Rehabil Clin N Am 1998;9:233–48.

30. McDonald CM. Physical activity, health impairments, and disability in neuromuscular disease. Am J Phys Med Rehabil 2002;81:S108–20.

31. Bushby K, Finkel R, Birnkrant DJ, et al. Diagnosis and management of Duchenne muscular dystrophy, part 1: diagnosis, and pharmacological and psychosocial management. Lancet Neurol 2010;9(1):77–93.

32. Bushby K, Finkel R, Birnkrant DJ, et al. Diagnosis and management of Duchenne muscular dystrophy, part 2: implementation of multidisciplinary care. Lancet Neurol 2010;9(2):177–89.

33. Results of Muscular Dystrophy Association Clinic Directors Survey, presented at the 2012 MDA Clinical Conference. Las Vegas (NV), March 6, 2012.

34. Bach JR. The historical role of the physiatrist in the management of Duchenne muscular dystrophy. Am J Phys Med Rehabil 1996;75(3):239–41.

35. World Health Organization. International Classification of Functioning, Disability, and Health: ICF. Copyright World Health Organization, Geneva, Switzerland, 2001. (ISBN 92 4 154542 9). Available at: http://www.who.int/classifications/icf/en. Accessed June 2, 2012.

36. Brooke MH, Griggs RC, Mendell JR, et al. Clinical trial in Duchenne dystrophy. I. The design of the protocol. Muscle Nerve 1981;4(3):186–97.

37. Brooke MH, Fenichel GM, Griggs RC, et al. Clinical investigation in Duchenne dystrophy: 2. Determination of the "power" of therapeutic trials based on the natural history. Muscle Nerve 1983;6(2):91–103.

38. Aitkens SG, Lord J, Bernauer E, et al. Relationship of manual muscle testing to objective strength measurements. Muscle Nerve 1989;12:173–7.

39. Kilmer DD, Abresch RT, Fowler WM Jr. Serial manual muscle testing in Duchenne muscular dystrophy. Arch Phys Med Rehabil 1993;74:1168–71.

40. Fowler WM Jr, Abresch RT, Aitkens S, et al. Profiles of neuromuscular diseases. Design of the protocol. Am J Phys Med Rehabil 1995;74(Suppl 5):S62–9.

41. Escolar DM, Henricson EK, Mayhew J, et al. Clinical evaluator reliability for quantitative and manual muscle testing measures of strength in children. Muscle Nerve 2001;24(6):787–93.

42. Mayhew JE, Florence JM, Mayhew TP, et al. Reliable surrogate outcome measures in multicenter clinical trials of Duchenne muscular dystrophy. Muscle Nerve 2007;35(1):36–42.

43. McDonald CM, Abresch RT, Carter GT, et al. Profiles of neuromuscular diseases. Duchenne muscular dystrophy. Am J Phys Med Rehabil 1995;74(Suppl 5):S70–92.
44. McDonald CM, Henricson EK, Han JJ, et al. The 6-minute walk test as a new outcome measure in Duchenne muscular dystrophy. Muscle Nerve 2009;41(4): 500–10.
45. McDonald CM, Henricson EK, Han JJ, et al. The 6-minute walk test in Duchenne/ Becker muscular dystrophy: longitudinal observations. Muscle Nerve 2010;42(6): 966–74.
46. Henricson E, Abresch R, Han, JJ, et al. Percent-predicted 6-minute walk distance in Duchenne muscular dystrophy to account for maturational influences. Version 2. PLoS Curr. 2012 Jan 25 [revised 2012 Feb 2];4:RRN1297.
47. Backman C, Cork S, Gibson G, et al. Assessment of hand function: the relationship between pegboard dexterity and applied dexterity. Can J Occup Ther 1992; 59:208–13.
48. Smith YA, Hong E, Presson C. Normative and validation studies of the nine-hole peg test with children. Percept Mot Skills 2000;90(3 Pt 1):823–43.
49. Michimata A, Kondo T, Suzukamo Y, et al. The manual function test: norms for 20- to 90-year-olds and effects of age, gender, and hand dominance on dexterity. Tohoku J Exp Med 2008;214(3):257–67.
50. Poole JL, Burtner PA, Torres TA, et al. Measuring dexterity in children using the nine-hole peg test. J Hand Ther 2005;18(3):348–51.
51. Svensson E, Hager-Ross C. Hand function in Charcot Marie Tooth: test retest reliability of some measurements. Clin Rehabil 2006;20(10):896–908.
52. Eklund E, Svensson E, Hager-Ross C. Hand function and disability of the arm, shoulder and hand in Charcot-Marie-Tooth disease. Disabil Rehabil 2009; 31(23):1955–62.
53. Gordon PH, Miller RG, Moore DH. ALSFRS-R. Amyotroph Lateral Scler Other Motor Neuron Disord 2004;5(Suppl 1):90–3. Review.
54. Vignos PJ Jr, Spencer GE Jr, Archibald KC. Management of progressive muscular dystrophy of childhood. JAMA 1963;184:89–96.
55. Vignos PJ. Management of musculoskeletal complications in neuromuscular disease: limb contractures and the role of stretching, braces and surgery. In: Fowler WM, editor. Advances in the rehabilitation of neuromuscular diseases. Philadelphia: Hanley & Belfus; 1988. p. 509–36.
56. Scott E, Mawson SJ. Measurement in Duchenne muscular dystrophy: considerations in the development of a neuromuscular assessment tool. Dev Med Child Neurol 2006;48(6):540–4. Review.
57. Mazzone ES, Messina S, Vasco G, et al. Reliability of the North Star Ambulatory Assessment in a multicentric setting. Neuromuscul Disord 2009;19(7):458–61.
58. Mazzone E, Martinelli D, Berardinelli A, et al. North Star Ambulatory Assessment, 6-minute walk test and timed items in ambulant boys with Duchenne muscular dystrophy. Neuromuscul Disord 2010;20(11):712–6.
59. Mayhew A, Cano S, Scott E, et al. Moving towards meaningful measurement: Rasch analysis of the North Star Ambulatory Assessment in Duchenne muscular dystrophy. Dev Med Child Neurol 2011;53(6):535–42.
60. Mazzone E, Vasco G, Sormani MP, et al. Functional changes in Duchenne muscular dystrophy: a 12-month longitudinal cohort study. Neurology 2011; 77(3):250–6.
61. Scott E, Eagle M, Mayhew A, et al. Development of a functional assessment scale for ambulatory boys with Duchenne muscular dystrophy. Physiother Res Int 2011. http://dx.doi.org/10.1002/pri.520.

62. Cirak S, Arechavala-Gomeza V, Guglieri M, et al. Exon skipping and dystrophin restoration in patients with Duchenne muscular dystrophy after systemic phosphorodiamidate morpholino oligomer treatment: an open-label, phase 2, dose-escalation study. Lancet 2011;378(9791):595–605.

63. Berard C, Payan C, Hodgkinson I, et al. A motor function measure for neuromuscular diseases. Construction and validation study. Neuromuscul Disord 2005; 15(7):463–70.

64. Vuillerot C, Girardot F, Payan C, et al. Monitoring changes and predicting loss of ambulation in Duchenne muscular dystrophy with the motor function measure. Dev Med Child Neurol 2010;52(1):60–5.

65. Steffensen B, Hyde S, Lyager S, et al. Validity of the EK scale: a functional assessment of non-ambulatory individuals with Duchenne muscular dystrophy or spinal muscular atrophy. Physiother Res Int 2001;6(3):119–34.

66. Steffensen B, Hyde SA, Attermann J, et al. Reliability of the EK scale, a functional test for non-ambulatory persons with Duchenne dystrophy. Adv Physiother 2002; 4(1):37–47.

67. Carman DL, Browne RH, Birch JG. Measurement of scoliosis and kyphosis radiographs. J Bone Joint Surg Am 1990;72:328–33.

68. Fon GT, Pitt MJ, Thies AC Jr. Thoracic kyphosis: range in normal subjects. AJR Am J Roentgenol 1980;134(5):979–83.

69. Gupta MC, Wijesekera S, Sossan A, et al. Reliability of radiographic parameters in neuromuscular scoliosis. Spine 2007;32(6):691–5.

70. Crapo RO, Morris AH, Gardner RM. Reference spirometric values using techniques and equipment that meet ATS recommendations. Am Rev Respir Dis 1981;123(6):659–64.

71. Polgar G. Pulmonary function tests in children. J Pediatr 1979;95(1):168–70.

72. Hankinson JL, Odencrantz JR, Fedan KB. Spirometric reference values from a sample of the general U.S. population. Am J Respir Crit Care Med 1999; 159(1):179–87.

73. Black LF, Hyatt RE. Maximal respiratory pressures: normal values and relationship to age and sex. Am Rev Respir Dis 1969;99:696–702.

74. Wilson SH, Cooke NT, Edwards RH, et al. Predicted normal values for maximal respiratory pressures in Caucasian adults and children. Thorax 1984;39(7): 535–8.

75. Domenech-Clar R, Lopez-Andreu JA, Compte-Torrero L, et al. Maximal static respiratory pressures in children and adolescents. Pediatr Pulmonol 2003; 35(2):126–32.

76. Fowler WM, Abresch RT, Aitkens SA, et al. Impairment and disability profiles of neuromuscular diseases: design of the protocol. Am J Phys Med Rehabil 1995; 74(2):S62–9.

77. Fowler WM. Rehabilitation management of muscular dystrophy and related disorders. II. Comprehensive care. Arch Phys Med Rehabil 1982;63(7):322–8.

78. Fowler WM, Goodgold J. Rehabilitation management of neuromuscular diseases. In: Goodgold J, editor. Rehabilitation medicine. St Louis (MO): CV Mosby; 1988. p. 298–316.

79. Mendell JR, Csimma C, McDonald CM, et al. Challenges in drug development for muscle disease: a stakeholders' meeting. Muscle Nerve 2007;35(1):8–16.

80. Food and Drug Administration: Center for Drug Evaluation and Research (CDER) in cooperation with the Center for Biologics Evaluation and Research (CBER) and the Center for Devices and Radiological Health (CDRH). Guidance for Industry on Patient-Reported Outcome Measures: Use in Medical Product Development to

Support Labeling Claims. Federal Register 2009;74(235):65132–3. Available at: http://www.fda.gov/Drugs/GuidanceComplianceRegulatoryInformation/Guidances/default.htm. Accessed June 3, 2012.

81. Acquadro C, Berzon R, Dubois D, et al. Incorporating the patient's perspective into drug development and communication: an ad hoc task force report of the Patient-Reported Outcomes (PRO) Harmonization Group meeting at the Food and Drug Administration. Value Health 2003;6:522–31.

Clinical Approach to the Diagnostic Evaluation of Hereditary and Acquired Neuromuscular Diseases

Craig M. McDonald, MD[a,b],*

KEYWORDS

- Neuromuscular disease • Diagnostic evaluation • History • Physical examination
- Motor neuron disease • Neuropathy • Neuromuscular junction • Myopathy

KEY POINTS

- Progressive acquired or hereditary neuromuscular diseases (NMDs) are disorders caused by an abnormality of any component of the lower motor neuron: anterior horn cell, peripheral nerve, neuromuscular junction (presynaptic or postsynaptic region), or muscle.
- Many NMDs are multisystem disorders affecting multiple organ systems.
- In the context of diagnostic evaluation of NMD, the clinician still must be able to obtain a relevant patient and family history and perform focused general, musculoskeletal, neurologic, and functional physical examinations to direct further diagnostic evaluations.
- Laboratory studies often include relevant molecular genetic studies in certain instances; however, specific genetic entities need to be strong diagnostic considerations, as these studies may be expensive and with limited sensitivity.
- Early diagnosis is facilitated by knowledge of the common initial clinical presentations of specific NMDs, and in many cases the early diagnosis has potential implications for treatment and prevention of secondary conditions.

The author has nothing to disclose.

This work was supported by grant H133B0900001 from the National Institute of Disability and Rehabilitation Research.

The author takes full responsibility for the contents of this article, which does not represent the views of the National Institute of Disability and Rehabilitation Research or the United States Government.

[a] Department of Physical Medicine and Rehabilitation, University of California Davis Medical Center, 4860 Y Street, Suite 3850, Sacramento, CA 95817, USA; [b] Department of Pediatrics, University of California Davis Medical Center, 2516 Stockton Blvd, Sacramento, CA 95817, USA
* Department of Orthopaedic Surgery and Rehabilitation, Shriners Hospital for Children Northern California, 2425 Stockton Blvd, Sacramento, CA 95817.
E-mail address: cmmcdonald@ucdavis.edu

INTRODUCTION

Progressive acquired or hereditary neuromuscular diseases (NMDs) are disorders caused by an abnormality of any component of the lower motor neuron: anterior horn cell, peripheral nerve, neuromuscular junction (NMJ; presynaptic or postsynaptic region), or muscle. The notion that a pathologic abnormality in an NMD may be purely isolated to one anatomic region of the lower motor neuron with primary or secondary changes isolated to muscle is only true for selected conditions. Many NMDs are multisystem disorders affecting multiple organ systems. For example, RNA toxicity generated from expansion of trinucleotide repeat sequences in myotonic muscular dystrophy (MMD) gives rise to skeletal muscle, smooth muscle, myocardial, endocrine, brain, and ocular abnormalities; Duchenne muscular dystrophy (DMD) gives rise to abnormalities of skeletal and cardiac muscle, the cardiac conduction system, smooth muscle, and the brain; Fukuyama congenital muscular dystrophy affects skeletal muscle and brain; mitochondrial encephalomyelopathies may affect the mitochondria of multiple tissues.

The most common NMDs are acquired peripheral neuropathies. Other acquired NMDs include amyotrophic lateral sclerosis (ALS), poliomyelitis, Guillain-Barré syndrome, myasthenia gravis, and polymyositis. Hereditary NMDs are also quite common and include such disorders as spinal muscular atrophy (SMA), Charcot-Marie-Tooth disease (CMT), congenital myasthenia, and DMD. Clinical NMD syndromes described over the decades in the literature have recently been redefined based molecular genetic advances and documentation of genetic heterogeneity within specific syndromes. For example, at least 70 genetically distinct subtypes of CMT have been described, some with undetermined gene loci; more than 14 genetically distinct subtypes of autosomal recessive limb-girdle muscular dystrophy (LGMD) have been identified; and 3 genetically distinct subtypes of Emery-Dreifuss muscular dystrophy exist.[1] In fact, the gene loci for more than 500 distinct neuromuscular and mitochondrial disorders have been identified at the time of writing. The basis for the use of molecular genetic studies for diagnosis is well described by Arnold and Flanigan in their article elsewhere in this issue.

In the context of diagnostic evaluation of NMD, the clinician still must be able to obtain a relevant patient and family history and perform focused general, musculoskeletal, neurologic, and functional physical examinations to direct further diagnostic evaluations. Laboratory studies often include relevant molecular genetic studies in certain instances; however, specific genetic entities need to be strong diagnostic considerations, as these studies may be expensive and with limited sensitivity.

Electrodiagnostic studies including electromyography (EMG) and nerve conduction studies remain an extension of the physical examination and help to guide further diagnostic evaluation such as molecular genetic studies (as in the case of CMT), muscle and nerve biopsies, or even motor point biopsies applied to the evaluation of congenital myasthenic syndromes. All diagnostic information needs to be interpreted not in isolation, but within the context of relevant historical information, family history, physical examination findings, laboratory data, electrophysiologic findings, and pathologic information if obtained.

A skilled synthesis of all available information may provide the patient and family with: (1) a precise diagnosis or as accurate a diagnosis as is medically possible; (2) prognostic information (if available for a specific entity); (3) information as to eligibility for molecular based therapeutic agents such as antisense oligonucleotides or morpholinos for exon skipping, or stop-codon read-through agents; and (4) anticipatory guidance for the near future. Knowledge of the natural history of specific NMD conditions helps in the ongoing rehabilitative management of progressive impairments, activity limitations, and disabilities.

This article briefly reviews the clinical approach to the diagnostic evaluation of progressive NMDs, including relevant history, family history, clinical examination findings, laboratory studies, and situations whereby pathologic studies play a role diagnostically.

NEUROMUSCULAR DISEASE HISTORY

Important elements of NMD history taking are shown in **Box 1**.

The common presenting chief complaints from parents of children with suspected neuromuscular disorders may include infantile floppiness or hypotonia, delay in motor milestones, feeding and respiratory difficulties, abnormal gait characteristics, frequent falls, difficulty ascending stairs or arising from the floor, muscle cramps, or stiffness. Adults often present with chief complaints of strength loss, fatigue or decreasing endurance, falls, difficulty ascending stairs, exercise intolerance, episodic weakness, muscle cramps, focal wasting of muscle groups, breathing difficulties, or bulbar symptoms relating to speech and swallowing.

Respiratory failure due to NMD has been reported in myasthenia gravis, myosin-loss myopathy, acid maltase deficiency, amyloidosis, desmin polymyositis (Jo-1), congenital myopathy (eg, rod; centronuclear), hydroxychloroquine toxicity, neural injury (specifically phrenic lesions), ALS, DMD, and SMA. NMDs with associated cardiac disorders include DMD, BMD, LGMD 1B, LGMD 1C, sarcoglycanopathies, MMD; McLeod, Emery-Dreifuss, Barth syndromes; desmin deficiency; Polymyositis; nemaline rod myopathy; Acid maltase deficiency; debrancher enzyme deficiency; carnitine deficiency; some mitochondrial myopathies; amyloid deficiency; drug-related disorders (metronidazole, emetine, and chloroquine, clofibrate, colchicine); cardiomyopathies; and some periodic paralyses.

Information should be obtained regarding the recent course of the chief complaint, specifically whether the process is getting worse, staying the same, or getting better. If strength is deteriorating, it is important to ascertain the rate of progression (ie, is weakness increasing over days, weeks, months, or years?). It is critical to determine whether the distribution of weakness is predominantly proximal, distal, or generalized. It is also useful to identify factors that may worsen or help the primary symptoms. A history of twitching of muscles may reflect fasciculations. Tremor or balance problems may be due to distal weakness or superimposed cerebellar involvement.

Bulbar involvement may be identified if the individual has difficulty chewing, swallowing, or articulating speech. Visual complaints (blurriness or diplopia) may indicate presence of cataracts or possibly involvement of extraocular musculature. Distal stocking glove or focal sensory complaints may be consistent with a peripheral neuropathy or focal nerve entrapment.

A comprehensive medical history and surgical history should be obtained. A history of recent illnesses should be carefully elucidated, including respiratory difficulties, aspiration pneumonias, or recurrent pulmonary infections. In addition, cardiac symptoms, such as dizziness, syncope, chest pain, orthopnea, or exertional cardiac complaints may indicate superimposed involvement of the myocardium. A pulmonary review of symptoms should be obtained. A history of weight loss may be due to recurrent illnesses, nutritional compromise, swallowing difficulty, or progressive lean tissue atrophy.

For the pediatric patient, a detailed history regarding pregnancy (eg, quality of fetal movement or pregnancy complications) and perinatal problems (evidence of fetal distress, respiratory difficulties in the delivery room, need for resuscitation or ventilation

Box 1
Clinical history in NMDs

- Distribution of Weakness
  - Anatomic distribution/pattern of weakness and focal wasting or hypertrophy of muscle groups (arms versus legs, proximal versus distal, symmetric versus asymmetric)
  - Myopathies have weakness that is usually proximal greater than distal with rare exceptions
- Course of weakness
  - Acute onset (days to weeks)
  - Chronic (months to years)
  - Episodic
  - Is the weakness getting worse, staying the same, or getting better?
  - Ascertain the rate of progression (days, weeks, months, or years)
- Fatigue or lack of endurance
- Muscle cramps or stiffness
- Lack of sensory loss
- Gait characteristics
  - Toe walking, excessive lordosis, Trendelenburg or gluteus maximus lurch, and so forth
- Functional difficulties
  - Ambulatory distances
  - Frequency of falls
  - Transitions from the floor to standing
  - Problems climbing stairs
  - Problems dressing
  - Problems reaching overhead
  - Difficulty lifting
  - Running ability, problems in physical education, and recreational or athletic performance
- Onset age (neonatal, childhood, teen, adult [20–60 years], or geriatric)
- Identify factors that worsen or help primary symptoms
- History of recent illnesses (eg, recent viral illnesses, respiratory difficulties, pneumonia, pulmonary infections)
- Pain
- Feeding difficulties, dysphagia, nutritional status, and body composition
- Cardiac symptoms (dizziness, syncope, chest pain, orthopnea, cardiac complaints with exertion)
- Pulmonary symptoms (breathing difficulties, sleep disturbance, morning headaches)
- Anesthetic history (eg, malignant hyperthermia)
- History regarding the child's acquisition of developmental milestones
  - Ascertain when the child was able to control his or her head, sit independently, crawl, stand with and without support, walk with and without support, gain fine motor prehension, and acquire bimanual skills (bringing objects to midline, transfer of objects)
  - History regarding language acquisition, mental development and school performance
- History regarding pregnancy and neonatal period
- Quality of fetal movement, pregnancy complications, perinatal complications, evidence of fetal distress, respiratory difficulties in the recovery room, need for resuscitation or ventilation problems in early infancy, infantile hypotonia, weak cry, poor feeding

problems in early infancy, ongoing respiratory difficulties, swallowing/feeding difficulties, and persistent hypotonia) should be obtained. Perinatal respiratory distress in the delivery room may be seen in acute infantile type I SMA, myotubular myopathy, congenital hypomyelinating neuropathy, congenital infantile myasthenia, transitory neonatal myasthenia, and severe neurogenic arthrogryposis.

In children, history regarding the acquisition of developmental milestones should be ascertained relating to head control, independent sitting, crawling, standing with and without support, walking with and without support, fine prehension, bimanual skill acquisition (bringing objects to midline, transfer of objects), and language acquisition. Information regarding gait characteristics (toe walking, excessive lordosis, and so forth), running ability, transitions from floor to standing, stair climbing, falls, recreational/athletic performance, pain or muscle cramps, and easy fatigue or lack of endurance may be important clues to the presence of a neuromuscular disorder. History regarding mental development, type of school, and school performance may be important indicators of superimposed central nervous system (CNS) involvement.

For the adult, detailed history regarding the age of onset of symptoms, age when bracing was provided to maintain ambulation, age to use of wheelchair (if applicable), pattern of progression, distribution of weakness, presence of muscle cramps, fatigue, or episodic weakness, presence of atrophy or fasciculations, performance in physical education, military or vocational performance and pursuits, current and past ambulatory distances, ability to transition from floor to standing, problems climbing stairs, and problems reaching overhead or dressing may all be important functional information.

Potential causes of muscle cramps are shown in **Box 2**. Muscle cramps in the setting of an elevated creatine kinase (CK) value and no skeletal muscle weakness has been reported, and a pedigree with mild Becker muscular dystrophy.[2] The etiology of myalgias can be quite varied, and a definitive cause is found in only one-fourth of those patients presenting with muscle pain as a chief complaint.[3] Patterns of weakness in myopathies, NMJ disorders, anterior horn cell disorders, and diagnostic considerations are outlined in **Box 3**, and selective anatomic distribution of peripheral neuropathies and neuronopathies are listed in **Box 4**.

A history should be obtained regarding dark-colored urine or hematuria as a clue regarding rhabdomyolysis. Myoglobinuria may be associated with: glycogenolysis; CPT II; LPIN1; malignant hyperthermia; central core disease; King-Denborough; DMD (some); hypokalemia; licorice; Li; thiazide; amphotericin; laxatives; infections; mitochondrial myopathy; muscle trauma; ischemia; overactivity; polymyositis, neuroleptic malignant syndrome; drugs (heroin, phencyclidine, ε-aminocaproic acid, clofibrate + renal failure, cyclosporine A+ lovastatin); toxins (eg, venoms; intravenous drugs; oral drugs [Haff]; mushrooms; ethanol).

A thorough anesthetic history should be obtained, as malignant hyperthermia is associated with one of the many subtypes of primary familial malignant hyperthermia (hypokalemic periodic paralysis, or one of the malignant hyperthermia susceptibility (MHS) loci, including MHS1: ryanodine receptor, 19q13 [allelic with central core congenital myopathy]; MHS2: Na^+ channel [SCNA4], 17q11; MHS3: Ca^{2+} channel [CACNL2A], 7q21; MHS4: 3q13; MHS5: Ca^{2+} channel [CACNA1S], 1q32; MHS6: 5p; CPT2: 1p32) and King-Denborough syndrome. Other NMD conditions occasionally reported to be associated with malignant hyperthermia include DMD, BMD, Fukuyama congenital muscular dystrophy, LGMD, facioscapulohumeral muscular dystrophy (FSHD), periodic paralysis, myotonia congenita, mitochondrial myopathy, minimal change myopathy, myoadenylate deaminase deficiency, and Schwartz-Jampel syndrome.

Box 2
Causes of muscle cramps

1. Cramps at rest (usually not a neuromuscular disorder)
   a. Benign nocturnal leg cramps
   b. Diurnal cramps related to exercise
2. Cramps occurring with exertion, relieved by rest (may be associated with myoglobinuria)
   a. Muscular dystrophy, Duchenne, Becker, limb-girdle muscular dystrophy (LGMD)
   b. Myopathy: rippling muscle syndromes (RMD)
      i. RMD1: chromosome 1q41; dominant
      ii. RMD2: caveolin-3; chromosome 3p25.3; dominant
   c. Metabolic disorders
      i. Glycogenoses
         1. Myophosphorylase deficiency (type V; McArdle disease)
         2. Phosphofructokinase deficiency (type VII)
         3. Phosphorylase b kinase deficiency (type VIII)
         4. Phosphoglycerate kinase deficiency (type IX)
         5. Phosphoglycerate mutase deficiency (type X)
         6. Lactate dehydrogenase deficiency (type XI)
         7. Myoadenylate deaminase deficiency
      ii. Lipid metabolism disorders
         1. Carnitine palmityl transferase deficiency
      iii. Uremia
      iv. Electrolyte abnormality: hyponatremia, hypocalcemia, hypomagnesemia, hypoglycemia
      v. Hypothyroidism
      vi. Hypoadrenalism
      vii. Paroxysmal myoglobinuria
      viii. Idiopathic rhabdomyolysis
   d. Toxic myoglobinuria
      i. Alcohol
      ii. Barbiturates
      iii. Heroin
      iv. Carbon monoxide
      v. Amphotericin B
      vi. Toxic venoms
   e. Inflammatory myositis
      i. Acute dermatomyositis, polymyositis
      ii. Viral myositis (Coxsackie and so forth)
      iii. Bacterial myositis (staphylococci, clostridia)

f. Acute extracellular volume depletion

    i. Perspiration

    ii. Diarrhea, vomiting

    iii. Diuretic therapy

    iv. Hemodialysis

g. Other lower motor neuron disorders

    i. Amyotrophic lateral sclerosis (ALS), old polio, other motor neuron disorders

    ii. Radiculopathy and neuropathy

FAMILY HISTORY

Whenever a neuromuscular disorder is suspected with a potential genetic origin, a detailed family history and pedigree chart is absolutely essential. Autosomal dominant conditions may have pedigrees with multiple generations affected with equal predilection to males and females. Typically one-half of offspring within a pedigree are affected. In autosomal recessive conditions, only one generation may be affected with equal proportions of males and females. Proportionally, one-fourth of offspring are clinically affected. Parents in earlier generations may be unaffected and the parents of affected children are presumptive heterozygote carriers of the condition. In many instances of autosomal recessive inheritance, no other family members within the nuclear family unit are affected, making the confirmation of inheritance pattern difficult without a molecular genetic marker being present or protein abnormality confirmed by immunohistochemistry techniques. In X-linked recessive conditions, males on the maternal side of the family are affected in approximately 50% of instances and females are carriers in 50% of instances.

Often it is valuable to examine affected relatives who may be either earlier or later in the course of their NMD relative to the patient. In addition, medical records and diagnostic evaluations of affected family members should be reviewed and the diagnosis confirmed if possible.

In some instances, the examination of a parent can help establish the diagnosis in an affected infant or child, as is frequently the case in MMD. In this disorder, genetic anticipation with abnormal CTG trinucleotide expansion of unstable DNA results in progressively earlier onset of the disease in successive generations with increasing severity, as described elsewhere in this issue.[1]

In the case of dystrophic myopathies, a definitive molecular genetic or pathologic diagnosis established in a sibling or close relative may allow the clinician to establish the diagnosis in a child or adult based on clinical examination and laboratory data such as CK or molecular genetic testing, thus allowing the avoidance of further invasive testing such as a muscle biopsy.

PHYSICAL EXAMINATION
Inspection at Rest

Simple inspection allows the observation of focal or diffuse muscle wasting, or focal enlargement of muscles as with the "pseudohypertrophy" seen in dystrophic myopathies such as DMD and BMD (**Fig. 1**), LGMD, and lipodystrophy. Cros and colleagues[4] have demonstrated that the increase in calf circumference in DMD is caused by an increase in fat and connective tissue, and is not secondary to true muscle fiber hypertrophy in the gastrocnemius. By contrast, the reduced bulk of the quadriceps in DMD

Box 3
Patterns of weakness in myopathies, neuromuscular junction (NMJ) pathology, and motor neuron disorders

Extraocular Muscles (EOM) Weak

- Myasthenia gravis (MG)
- Thyroid
- Botulism
- Mitochondrial: Kearns-Sayre; progressive external ophthalmoplegia (PEO); MNGIE
- Myopathy: centronuclear; multicore
- Oculopharyngeal muscular dystrophy
- Inclusion body myositis (IBM) + contracture
- Oculopharyngodistal myopathy
- Congenital ophthalmoplegias

Periocular Without EOM Weakness

- Dystrophies: myotonic; facioscapulohumeral muscular dystrophy (FSHD); oculopharyngeal
- NMJ: MG
- Congenital myasthenic syndromes
- Congenital myopathies
- Inflammatory myopathy: polymyositis
- Rule out: VII nerve lesion

Bulbar Dysfunction

- NMJ: MG; congenital myasthenic syndromes
- Thyroid
- Cranial nerve Δ
- Oculopharyngeal muscular dystrophy
- Distal myopathy (MPD2)
- Polymyositis: IBM; scleroderma
- Motor neuron Δ: ALS; bulbospinal muscular atrophy (BSMA)
- Pseudobulbar; Fazio-Londe
- Brown-Vialetto-van Laere

Posterior Neck Weak

- Common: MG; polymyositis; ALS
- Focal myopathy: neck; paraspinous
- Rare: FSHD; LMN (lower motor neuron) syndrome; IBM rod; proximal myotonic myopathy (PROMM); acid maltase deficiency; hypo K^+; carnitine deficiency; endocrine deficiency; desmin deficiency

Proximal Arms Weak

- Dystrophy: scapuloperoneal; FSHD
- Inflammatory: brachiocervical inflammatory myositis (BCIM)
- Absent muscles; Shoulder joint Δ
- NMJ: MG
- Neuropathic: ALS; pure LMN
- Brachial plexopathy

Distal and Proximal Weakness

- Dystrophy: myotonic; FSH, scapuloperoneal
- Myopathy: congenital; distal
- Glygogenoses: debrancher
- Phosphorylase b kinase
- Neuropathy + Myopathy: paraneoplastic; sarcoid; mitochondria; human immunodeficiency virus (HIV)
- Drugs (amiodarone; doxorubicin; colchicine; chloroquine)

Acute Weakness

- NMJ: MG
- Myoglobinuria
- Myosin-loss myopathy
- Carnitine deficiency
- Periodic paralysis: X-episodic Xp22
- Hypo K^+: CACNA1S; SCN4A; KCNE3
- Hyper K^+: SCN4A; KCNE3
- Andersen: KCNJ2
- Electrolyte disorders: Hyperkalemia, hypokalemia, hypermagnesemia or hypophosphatemia
- Barium
- Rule out: Neuropathy (acute inflammatory demyelinating polyradiculoneuropathy [AIDP]), chronic inflammatory demyelinating polyradiculoneuropathy [CIDP]); spinal cord

Wasting > Weakness

- Pathology: type II atrophy
- Cachexia: weight loss >15%, aging/sarcopenia
- Disuse
- Steroid myopathy
- Paraneoplastic

Weakness > Wasting

- Polymyositis
- Myoglobinuria
- Periodic paralysis
- NMJ: MG; Congenital myasthenia
- Neuropathy + conduction block

Quadriceps Weak

- LGMD: 1B; 2B; 2H; ring fiber
- Becker
- Myositis: IBM; mitochondria; focal
- Nerve: femoral; lumbosacral plexopathy
- Diabetic amyotrophy; L3-L4 root

Adapted from Pestronk A. Neuromuscular Disease Center Web site. St Louis (MO): Washington University; 2011. Available at: http://neuromuscular.wustl.edu.

Box 4
Selective anatomic distribution of peripheral neuropathies and neuronopathies (most peripheral neuropathies are symmetric and maximal distally in the lower extremities)

Extraocular Muscle
- Botulism
- Diabetes
- Miller-Fisher
- Diphtheria
- Rule out: MG; myopathy

Proximal Motor
- Immune demyelinating: Guillain-Barré syndrome; CIDP; SMA; porphyria
- Plexopathy: brachial; lumbar
- Rule out: joint pain; myopathy

Proximal Sensory
- Hereditary: porphyria; Tangier
- Neuronopathy: Hu; Sjögren; thoracic neuropathy
- Rule out: myelopathy

Skin Temperature–related
- Leprosy
- Upper extremity
- Immune: multifocal motor neuropathy (MMN); vasculitis; CIDP variant
- Amyloid: Carpal tunnel
- Entrapment: hereditary neuropathy with liability to pressure palsies (HNPP); other
- Toxic: lead; vincristine; ALS; LMN
- Rule out: spinal; CNS

Asymmetric
- Mononeuritis multiplex
- Neuronopathy: ALS; sensory
- Entrapments
- Plexopathies
- Toxic

Mononeuritis Multiplex
- Vasculopathy
- Amyloid
- Leprosy
- Diabetes
- Cytomegalovirus
- Waldenström
- Perineuritis
- Demyelinating: HNPP; multifocal CIDP; MMN

- Compression: multiple

- Lymphoma: intraneural

- Wartenberg

CNS

- Spinal: organophosphate; hexacarbon; Adrenomyeloneuropathy (AMN); metachromatic leukodystrophy (MLD); lymphoma; Cuban; Vernant

- Optic: disulfiram; CS2; Hg; drugs; Neuropathy, ataxia, and retinitis pigmentosa (NARP); Charcot Marie Tooth 6 (CMT6); Post col & Retinitis pigmentosa (RP); Cuban; Vernant

- Hearing loss: Hereditary Motor Sensory Neuropathy X (HMSN X), 1A, 1B, 4D, 6; mitochondrial; sarcoid

- Cerebellum: Friedreich ataxia (FA); Ataxia Telangectasia (AT); Metachromatic Leukodystrophy (MLD); refsum; A-β-lipoproteinemia; Spinocerebellar Ataxia (SCA) 2, 3, 4; Infantile Onset Spinocerebellar Ataxia (IOSCA); Hu & CV-2 autoantibodies

- Supratentorial: mitochondrial; thyroid; Hu; B12; vasculitis; neoplastic; sarcoid

- Infection: Lyme; HIV; rabies; syphilis; West Nile

- Hereditary: polyglucosan; Fabry; HexA; porphyria; prion; ALS; Cowchock; Nicotinamide adenine dinucleotide (NAD); Krabbe; MLD

Face

- Bell palsy; Melkersson; Tangier

- Polyradiculopathies: sarcoid; Lyme; Guillain-Barré syndrome

- Motor neuron disorders: ALS; Kennedy; Möbius

- Rule out: MG; myopathy

Adapted from Pestronk A. Neuromuscular Disease Center Web site. St Louis (MO): Washington University; 2011. Available at: http://neuromuscular.wustl.edu.

was caused by more severe fiber loss in a more active dystrophic process affecting the knee extensors. In DMD, pseudohypertrophy may be present in other muscle groups such as the deltoid (**Fig. 2**).

Other neuromuscular disorders may show calf pseudohypertrophy.[5] Calf hypertrophy is particularly prominent in childhood type of acid maltase deficiency. In SMA type III (Kugelberg-Welander syndrome), calf enlargement has been occasionally noted but wasting of affected musculature is typically more prominent. Other NMDs with enlarged muscles include myotonia conditions with overusage; hypothyroidism, acromegaly, infection with cysticercosis, trichinosis and schistosomiasis, anabolic drugs (eg, β2-adrenergic; androgen), glycogen storage diseases, amyloidosis, accumulation of gangliosides, and Schwartz-Jampel syndrome.

Children aged 6 to 11 years with DMD have been noted to exhibit an unusual clinical examination sign caused by selective hypertrophy and wasting in different muscles of the same region.[6] When viewing these patients posteriorly with their arms abducted to 90° and elbows flexed to 90°, the DMD patients demonstrated a linear or oval depression (due to wasting) of the posterior axillary fold with hypertrophied or preserved muscles on its 2 borders (ie, infraspinatus inferomedially and deltoid superolaterally), as if there was a valley between the 2 mounts, as seen in **Fig. 2**.

There are several characteristic facial features of MMD that may be noted on inspection (**Fig. 3**). The adult with long-standing MMD often has facial features so characteristic that it is often easy to make a tentative diagnosis from across the

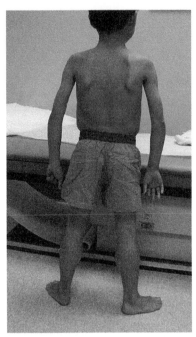

Fig. 1. A child with Duchenne muscular dystrophy. Note the calf hypertrophy, mild equinus posturing at the ankles, shoulder retraction, and mild scapular winging.

room. The long thin face with temporal and masseter wasting is drawn and described by some as lugubrious. Adult males often exhibit frontal balding. Infants and young children with a variety of myopathies may exhibit a tent-shaped mouth (see **Fig. 3**).

Focal atrophy of particular muscle groups may provide diagnostic clues to specific neuromuscular disorders. SMA shows diffuse muscle atrophy or focal atrophy in more slowly progressive subtypes. Emery-Dreifuss may present with striking wasting of the biceps, accentuated by sparing of the deltoids and forearm muscles. There may also be wasting of the calf muscles in this condition. Quadriceps-selective weakness and atrophy may be a presenting sign in a variety of myopathies such as BMD, LGMD 1B; 2B; 2H; 2L (11p13 LGMD 2L: recessive, anoctamin 5 [ANO5, MEM16E,

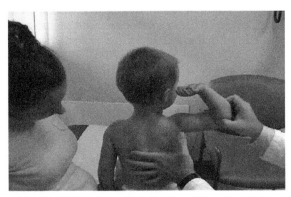

Fig. 2. Pseudohypertrophy of the posterior deltoid muscle and posterior axillary depression sign in Duchenne muscular dystrophy.

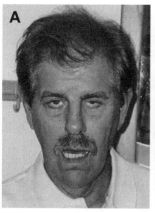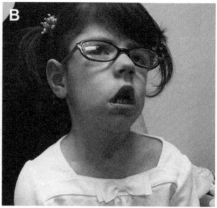

Fig. 3. (*A*) An adult with characteristic facial characteristics associated with myotonic muscular dystrophy (DM1). Note the long-drawn face, temporal wasting, and male pattern baldness. (*B*) A 4-year-old child with congenital DM1. Note the triangular or tent-shaped mouth and slight temporal wasting.

GDD1]; chromosome 11p14.3; recessive, Emery-Dreifuss: lamin A/C hereditary IBM3), inflammatory myopathies, sporadic inclusion body myositis (IBM), polymyositis with mitochondrial pathology, focal myositis, myopathy with ringed fibers, and SMA types III and IV, 5q types III and IV, femoral neuropathy, diabetic amyotrophy, and L3-L4 radiculopathy.

Patients with focal shoulder girdle weakness, as in FSHD and LGMD, may show characteristic patterns of muscle atrophy and scapular displacement. In FSHD, involvement of the latissimus dorsi, lower trapezius, rhomboids, and serratus anterior results in a characteristic appearance of the shoulders with the scapula positioned more laterally and superiorly, giving the shoulders a forward-sloped appearance. The upper border of the scapula rises into the trapezius, giving it a hypertrophied appearance falsely. From the posterior view, the medial border of the scapula may exhibit profound posterior and lateral winging (**Fig. 4**). The involvement of shoulder girdle musculature in FSHD may also be quite asymmetric.

Most weakness in neuromuscular disorders is associated with focal atrophy. Those with CMT, particularly those with the type II axonal forms, demonstrate distal atrophy or "stork-leg appearance" relatively early in the disease course. Those with primarily demyelinating type I forms of CMT may show distal wasting later in the disease course.

Muscle fasciculations may be seen as nonspecific findings of a variety of lower motor neuron disorders. Fasciculations are particularly common in motor neuron disorders, such as ALS and SMA. Distal essential tremor may be seen in a large proportion of CMT patients (30%–50%),[7] and other patients with weakness such as SMA. Polyminimyoclonus, another variant of muscle fasciculations, characterized by a fine tremor of the fingers and hands, may be evident in SMA I and II.

Palpable nerves in the cubital tunnel, posterior auricular region, or around the fibular head may indicate onion bulbs seen in CMT I subtypes, or Dejerine-Sottas disease (CMT III).

General Examination

Important aspects of the cardiac and pulmonary assessment pertaining to NMD conditions are described in the next issue of this journal. Hepatomegaly may be

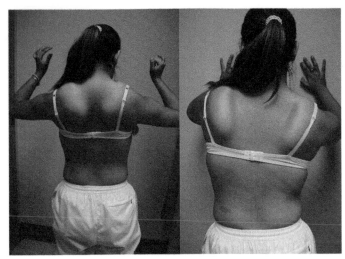

Fig. 4. A young adult with facioscapulohumeral muscular dystrophy (FSHD). Note the posterior and lateral scapular winging, the high-riding appearance of the scapula, and the asymmetry of winging in the photo on the right.

seen in metabolic myopathies such as acid maltase deficiency (type 2 glycogenosis) and types 3 and 4 glycogenosis. Characteristic rashes and nail-bed capillary changes may be present in dermatomyositis. Patients with Ullrich congenital muscular dystrophy who have a collagen VI abnormality often show hyperkeratosis pilaris in the extensor surfaces of the upper arms (**Fig. 5**). Craniofacial changes and dental malocclusion are commonly seen in congenital MMD, congenital myopathies, congenital muscular dystrophy, and type II SMA.

Cognitive Assessment

Some NMDs such as congenital and noncongenital MMD (DM1), PROMM (DM2), Fukuyama congenital muscular dystrophy, selected cases with mitochondrial encephalomyelopathies, and a small proportion of DMD cases may have significant intellectual impairment. In addition, other NMDs with significant cognitive involvement include hereditary IBM (9pp13), selected mitochondrial encephalomyopathies, congenital muscular dystrophy (Santavuori, POMGnT1 1p32; merosin 6q22; Fukuyama fukutin

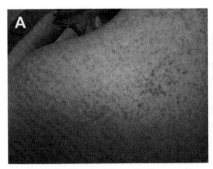
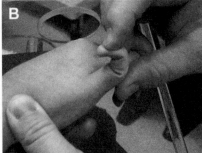

Fig. 5. Hyperkeratosis pilaris (a fine erythematous popular rash on the back and extensor surface of the upper arm) on the left (*A*) and distal joint hyperlaxity on the right (*B*) in a patient with Ullrich congenital muscular dystrophy.

9q31; and integrin-α7 12q13), and phosphoglycerate kinase deficiency. In these instances referral for neuropsychological testing, a neurodevelopmental evaluation, and/or a pyschoeducational evaluation may be helpful.[8]

Cranial Nerve Examination

Neuromuscular disorders tend not to have optic nerve involvement; however, an evaluation of vision and a fundoscopic examination can be exceedingly important. For example, MMD patients (DM1) may have cataracts giving significant visual impairment. These cataracts may have multicolored subcapsular opacities noted on a careful slit-lamp examination. In addition to the lens opacities, retinal degeneration characterized by peripheral pigmentary changes in the macula may be present in MMD. Other ocular abnormalities, including low intraocular pressure, enophthalmos, blepharitis, and corneal lesions have been described in this disorder. All MMD patients should have regular ophthalmologic evaluations.

Ptosis is a finding described in myasthenia gravis, congenital myasthenic syndromes, transient autoimmune neonatal myasthenia, oculopharyngeal muscular dystrophy, and occasionally MMD.

Ophthalmoparesis may be a finding seen in myasthenia gravis, congenital myasthenic syndromes, and oculopharyngeal muscular dystrophy. In addition, extraocular muscle involvement may occur in some of the congenital myopathies, particularly myotubular myopathy, and some of the mitochondrial myopathies. For example, progressive external ophthalmoplegia (PEO) is a mitochondrial disorder that may present with bilateral ophthalmoplegia with or without limb weakness. Congenital fibrosis of the extraocular muscles, or congenital familial external ophthalmoplegia, is an autosomal dominant, congenital, nonprogressive disorder of the ocular muscles with primary findings of bilateral ptosis and external ophthalmoplegia. Affected individuals with PEO often have associated facial weakness. Gaze is limited in all directions, eye movement speed is slow. the disorder is associated with ptosis and is slowly progressive.

Facial weakness is an important clinical feature of FSHD. The initial weakness affects the facial muscles, especially the orbicularis oculi, zygomaticus, and orbicularis oris. These patients often have difficulty with eye closure but not ptosis (**Fig. 6**). The individual may assume an expressionless appearance and exhibit difficulty whistling, pursing the lips or drinking through a straw, or smiling. Even in the very early stages, forced closure of the eyelids can be easily overcome by the examiner. Masseter, temporalis, extraocular, and pharyngeal muscles are characteristically spared in FSHD.

Facial weakness may also be observed in oculopharyngeal muscular dystrophy, myasthenia gravis, congenital myasthenic syndromes, Möbius syndrome, congenital myopathies, and myotubular myopathy. Rare cases with FSHD have been described, secondary to a hereditary neuropathy with weakness in predominantly a scapuloperoneal distribution, with involvement of the facial muscles and other limb muscles such as the shoulder girdle, ankle dorsiflexors, and ankle everters.

A sensorineural hearing deficit was originally observed in Coats syndrome (early-onset FSHD). These individuals have a myopathy presenting in infancy. The disease progression is fairly rapid, with most individuals becoming wheelchair reliant by the late second or third decade; they may also have a progressive exudative telangiectasia of the retina. Early recognition and photocoagulation of the abnormal retinal vessels may prevent visual loss. Several studies of later-onset FSHD using audiometry have demonstrated hearing deficits in many patients in addition to those with Coats syndrome, suggesting that impaired hearing function is more common than expected in FSHD.[9–11] Thus, all patients with FSHD should have screening audiometry and ophthalmologic evaluation.

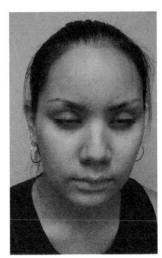

Fig. 6. Facial weakness of orbicularis oculi in FSHD. Eye closure is weak and weakness of orbicularis oris produces difficulty smiling, puffing out the cheeks, and pursing the lips.

Involvement of palatal, pharyngeal, and laryngeal muscles may produce dysarthria and dysphagia. Patients at particular risk include those with ALS, SMA, myasthenia gravis, congenital myasthenic syndromes, and congenital myopathies such as myotubular myopathy, oculopharyngeal muscular dystrophy, late-stage DMD, and late-stage LGMD with autosomal recessive inheritance. The function of the swallowing mechanism is best evaluated with a fluoroscopic video-dynamic evaluation of swallowing.

Vocal cord paralysis is a relatively uncommon finding in hereditary neuromuscular disorders; however, distal infantile spinal muscular atrophy with diaphragm paralysis (DSMA1; SMARD1; HMN 6) is linked to chromosome 11q13.3.[12,13] Vocal cord paralysis has also been described as a complication of dermatomyositis.

Examination of the tongue for muscle bulk and presence of fasciculations should be performed. Tongue fasciculations are a common finding in ALS and SMA types I, II, and III. However, tongue fasciculations are not an absolute finding in ALS or SMA. For example, 56% to 61% of SMA I patients, 30% to 70% of SMA II, patients and roughly half of SMA III patients late in the disease course show tongue fasciculations.[14–17] Thus, absence of tongue fasciculations does not necessarily exclude these motor neuron disorders. The bulk of the tongue may be increased in some metabolic diseases such as acid maltase deficiency, and often in later stages of DMD.

Tone

Hypotonia (**Fig. 7**) is an important clinical examination finding in children with neuromuscular disorders. The most common etiology for infantile hypotonia is central, accounting for approximately 80% of cases. Hypotonia remains the most common reason for referral to the pediatric electrodiagnostic laboratory. A differential diagnosis of infantile hypotonia is shown in **Box 5**.

Strength Assessment

The distribution of weakness is often a critical piece of information that allows the clinician to categorize a patient into a specific neuromuscular diagnostic syndrome. The distribution of weakness should be noted (predominantly proximal versus distal; lower

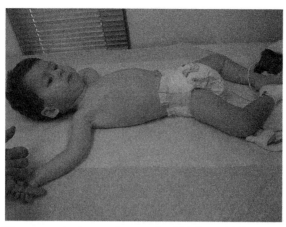

Fig. 7. A child with severe spinal muscular atrophy (SMA) II, with hypotonia and chest-wall wasting, creating a bell-shaped chest.

extremity versus upper extremity; focal versus generalized; isolated peripheral nerve distribution versus multiple peripheral nerves; or single versus multiple roots/ myotomes). It should be noted whether extraocular, facial, and bulbar muscles are involved or spared. In addition to appendicular (limb) strength, the strength of axial musculature should also be noted.

A common finding in myopathies, particularly dystrophic myopathies, is the early and selective weakness of the neck flexors as opposed to the neck extensors. For example, the neck flexors are the earliest muscle group to show weakness in DMD.[18,19] Clinical examination of a child or adult with a suspected dystrophic myopathy should always include an evaluation of neck-flexor strength (**Fig. 8**). Quantitative isometric strength measurements of neck strength in normal subjects with grade 5 neck flexors and extensors on manual muscle testing show the neck extensors to be stronger than the neck flexors. Absolute muscle strength is directly proportional to the physiologic cross-sectional area of muscle fiber.[20,21] The cross-sectional area of the neck extensors is much greater than the cross-sectional area of the neck flexors. Seventeen muscle groups act bilaterally as neck extensors, whereas only 6 muscle groups act bilaterally as neck flexors. Thus, with dystrophic myopathies the progressive loss of muscle fiber over time results in significant clinically detectable weakness of the neck flexors earlier than the neck extensors. This weakness is often accentuated in children by the large proportional size of the head relative to the rest of their body.

Predominantly distal lower extremity weakness is highly suggestive of an acquired or inherited peripheral neuropathy, the differential for which is quite broad. There are several other inherited neuromuscular disorders that can present with distal lower extremity weakness. Anterior horn cell disorders include distal chronic SMA. Myopathies include inflammatory myopathies, such as inclusion body myositis, scapuloperoneal syndromes including scapuloperoneal muscular dystrophy, late adult-onset autosomal dominant distal myopathy, Finnish tibial muscular dystrophy, early adult-onset autosomal recessive distal myopathy (types I and II) and, occasionally, metabolic myopathies. Distal upper extremity weakness may be seen initially in Asian-variant distal SMA, and Welander-type late adult-onset autosomal dominant distal myopathy.

Box 5
Differential diagnosis of infantile hypotonia

1. Cerebral hypotonia
   a. Chromosome disorders
      i. Trisomy
      ii. Prader-Willi syndrome
   b. Static encephalopathy
      i. Cerebral malformation
      ii. Perinatal CNS insult
      iii. Postnatal CNS insult
   c. Peroxisomal disorders
      i. Cerebrohepatorenal syndrome (Zellweger)
      ii. Neonatal adrenoleukodystrophy
   d. Inborn errors of metabolism
      i. Glycogen storage disease type II (Pompe disease)
      ii. Infantile GM1, gangliosidosis
      iii. Tay-Sachs infantile GM2 gangliosidosis)
      iv. Vitamin dependency disorders (many) and so forth
   e. Amino acid and organic acid disorders
      i. Maple syrup disease
      ii. Hyperlysinemia
      iii. Nonketotic hyperglycinemia
      iv. Propionyl-CoA carboxylase deficiency and so forth
   f. Other genetic disorders
      i. Familial dysautonomia
      ii. Cohen syndrome
      iii. Oculocerebrorenal syndrome (Lowe)
   g. Benign congenital hypotonia
2. Spinal cord
   a. Trauma (obstetric; postnatal)
      i. Hypotonia early with acute paraplegia
      ii. Hypertonia
   b. Tumor or arteriovenous malformation
      i. Hypertonia may occur later or with slow growing tumor
   c. Anterior horn cell
      i. SMA type I (Werdnig-Hoffman)
      ii. SMA type II
      iii. Poliomyelitis
      iv. Neurogenic arthrogryposis

3. Polyneuropathies
   a. Congenital hypomyelinating neuropathy
   b. Chronic inflammatory demyelinating polyneuropathy
   c. AIDP (Guillain-Barré)
   d. Hereditary motor-sensory neuropathies (eg, I, III)
   e. Toxic polyneuropathy
   f. Leukodystrophies (Krabbe; Nieman-Pick)
   g. Leigh syndrome
   h. Giant axonal neuropathy
   i. Dysmaturation neuropathy
4. Neuromuscular junction
   a. Presynaptic
      i. Infantile botulism
      ii. Hypermagnesemia: eclampsia
      iii. Aminoglycoside antibiotics
      iv. Congenital myasthenia
      v. Acetylcholine vesicle paucity
      vi. Decreased quantal release
   b. Postsynaptic
      i. Neonatal (autoimmune)
      ii. Congenital myasthenia
      iii. Acetylcholinesterase deficiency
      iv. Slow changes
      v. Acetylcholine receptor deficiency
5. Myopathies
   a. Congenital myopathies
      i. Nemaline rod
      ii. Central core
      iii. Myotubular (centronuclear)
      iv. Congenital fiber type disproportion
   b. Congenital myotonic dystrophy
   c. Congenital muscular dystrophy
      i. Fukuyama type (CNS involvement)
      ii. Merosin deficiency (with or without CNS involvement)
      iii. Atonic-sclerotic type (Ulrich disease)
      iv. Undifferentiated
   d. Inflammatory myopathies
      i. Infantile polymyositis
   e. Metabolic myopathies
      i. Acid maltase deficiency (type II)

ii. Muscle phosphorylase deficiency (type V)

iii. Phosphofructokinase deficiency (type VII)

iv. Cytochrome c oxidase

v. Carnitine deficiency

f. Endocrine myopathies

i. Hypothyroidism

ii. Hypoparathyroidism

The differential diagnosis of the limb-girdle syndromes presenting in childhood and adulthood, and characterized by predominantly proximal weakness of shoulder and pelvic girdle muscles, remains large and may include LGMD subtypes, polymyositis, dermatomyositis, congenital myasthenic syndromes, IBM, type III SMA, manifesting carrier of DMD, BMD, FSHD, scapuloperoneal myopathy, Emery-Dreifuss muscular dystrophy, congenital myopathies occasionally presenting later in childhood or adulthood (ie, adult-onset nemaline rod disease, central core disease, centronuclear myopathy, fiber type disproportion, multicore disease, sarcotubular myopathy, fingerprint myopathy, reducing body myopathy), mitochondrial myopathies with limb-girdle weakness, other metabolic myopathies that may present in adulthood (ie, adult-onset acid maltase deficiency, debrancher enzyme deficiency, McArdle disease, carnitine deficiency), myopathy with tubular aggregates, and myopathy with cytoplasmic bodies.

Quantitative strength testing

Strength is difficult to objectively evaluate in children with motor impairments. Kilmer and colleagues[22] have demonstrated strength measurement to be more stable and reproducible in children older than 5 years. Quantitative strength measurements have been demonstrated to be far more sensitive than clinical strength testing for detecting weakness in children and adults with motor impairments.[23,24] The author and his colleagues at the University of California Davis Research and Training Center in Neuromuscular Disease have published several studies using isometric and isokinetic quantitative strength testing as a measure of impaired strength in patients with neuromuscular disorders,[22–33] and have shown quantitative strength testing to be a more sensitive measure of weakness than clinical examination, particularly when strength is grade 4 to 5 on manual muscle testing. At age 6, the reduction in tension

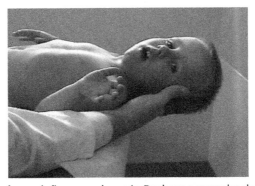

Fig. 8. Examination for neck flexor weakness in Duchenne muscular dystrophy.

developed by the knee extensors of DMD subjects was approximately 50% of control values for knee extension while knee extension was between grade 4 and 5 on same-day clinical manual muscle testing. Thus, by the time patients have progressed to grade 4 strength by manual muscle testing, substantial weakness is present.

Repetitive strength testing

When suspecting episodic weakness with a fatigue component, the examiner may have the patient repetitively contract a muscle against resistance for 10 to 15 contractions through a functional range of motion. This exercise often brings about obvious fatigue and progressive weakness after several contractions in myasthenic syndromes, such as myasthenia gravis or congenital myasthenia; this can also be accomplished more quantitatively with isokinetic dynamometry, comparing peak torque with initial contractions versus later contractions (eg, the fifth contraction or tenth contraction).

Sensory Examination

A stocking-glove loss of sensation or vague distal dysesthesias may be present in a peripheral neuropathy. Focal sensory changes in one or more peripheral nerve distributions can indicate focal entrapments, which are commonly seen in hereditary neuropathy with predisposition to pressure palsy (HNPP), one of the CMT subtypes.

Cerebellar Examination

The presence of tremor, dysdiadachokinesia (problems with rapid alternating movements), or axial and appendicular ataxia/balance problems can be important findings in syndromes such as ataxia telangiectasia, autosomal dominant spinocerebellar degeneration syndromes, and Friedreich ataxia.

Deep Tendon Reflexes

Whereas deep tendon reflexes (DTRs) are generally depressed or absent in many NMDs, they may be brisk in syndromes with superimposed upper motor neuron involvement such as ALS or some spinocerebellar degeneration syndromes. It is important to remember that the presence of DTRs does not necessarily exclude the presence of an NMD. For example, in one series,[14] DTRs were absent in all 4 extremities in 74% of SMA I cases, but present and depressed in 26% of cases. In SMA II and III, DTRs are invariably depressed and usually become absent over time.

Myotonia

The clinical finding common to all myotonic disorders is myotonia, which is a state of delayed relaxation or sustained contraction of skeletal muscle. Grip myotonia may be demonstrated by delayed opening of the hand with difficult extension of the fingers following tight grip. Paradoxic myotonia is the situation whereby myotonia becomes worse with successive movements instead of improving with activity. Percussion myotonia may be elicited by percussion of the thenar eminence with a reflex hammer, giving an adduction and flexion of the thumb with slow return (**Fig. 9**). Other sites that may give a local contraction with percussion include the deltoid, brachioradialis, and gluteal muscles. Occasionally, myotonia of the tongue draped over a tongue blade may be elicited with a midline tap of the finger, giving a bilateral contraction notch along the lateral portion of the tongue bilaterally with slow relaxation. Myotonic syndromes include MMD (Steinert disease), myotonia congenita (Thomsen disease), Becker-type myotonia congenita, paramyotonia

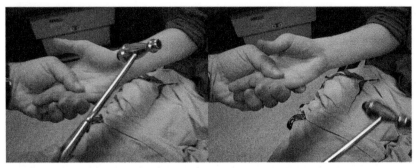

Fig. 9. Percussion myotonia in DM1.

congenita (Eulenburg disease), and Schwartz-Jampel syndrome (chondrodystrophic myotonia).

Schwartz-Jampel syndrome is usually distinguished by typical facial characteristics, blepharospasm, dwarfism, and other skeletal abnormalities, and the presence of hypertrophic and clinically stiff muscles. Muscle hypertrophy may also be seen in myotonia congenita and paramyotonia congenita.

Myotonia may be aggravated by cold in myotonia congenita, the dominant form of Becker-type myotonia congenita, and paramyotonia congenita. The myotonia seen in MMD is not typically exacerbated by cold.

Limb Contractures

A comprehensive description of the specific contractures most often present among the more common NMD conditions is presented by Skalsky and McDonald elsewhere in this issue. The presence of specific contractures can be helpful diagnostically, as in the clinical distinction between congenital muscular dystrophy, which often presents with contractures, versus other congenital structural myopathies, which frequently present with hypotonia but no contractures. The presence of isolated elbow flexion contractures can be a diagnostic clue to Emery-Dreifuss muscular dystrophy. In general, dystrophic myopathies have a greater predilection than other myopathies and neurogenic conditions toward the development of contractures.

Spinal Deformity

A discussion of the prevalence, natural history, and management of spinal deformity is discussed in the next issue of this journal. NMD populations at risk for scoliosis include DMD, severe childhood autosomal recessive muscular dystrophy (SCARMD), congenital muscular dystrophy, FSHD, congenital MMD, SMA, and Friedreich ataxia.

Functional Examination

A thorough functional examination is essential in the diagnostic evaluation of a patient suspected of an NMD. This examination includes an evaluation of head control, bed/mat mobility, transitions from supine-to-sit and sit-to-stand, sitting ability without hand support, standing balance, gait, stair climbing, and overhead reach.

An evaluation of overhead reach examining the patient from the front and from behind is helpful in evaluation of shoulder girdle weakness. Careful assessment of scapular winging, scapular stabilization, and scapular rotation is very helpful in the assessment of patients with FSHD and LGMD. The scapula is stabilized for overhead abduction by the trapezius, rhomboids, and serratus anterior. Abduction to 180° requires strong supraspinatus and deltoid in addition to strong scapular stabilizers.

Patients with proximal weakness involving the pelvic girdle muscles may rise off the floor using the classic Gower sign whereby the patient usually assumes a 4-point stance on knees and hands, brings the knees into extension while leaning forward on the upper extremities, substitutes for hip extension weakness by pushing off the knees with the upper extremities, and sequentially moves the upper extremities up the thigh until they have achieved an upright stance with full hip extension (**Fig. 10**). A Gower sign is not specific to any neuromuscular condition but may be seen in a variety of NMDs including DMD, BMD, LGMD 1, LGMD 2, SMA type III, congenital muscular dystrophy, congenital myopathy, myasthenic syndromes, severe forms of CMT (eg, CMT III and CMT IV), and other NMD conditions producing proximal weakness.

Patients with proximal lower extremity weakness often exhibit a classic myopathic gait pattern (**Fig. 11**A). Initially, weakness of the hip extensors produces anterior pelvic tilt and a tendency for the trunk to be positioned anterior to the hip joint. Patients compensate for this by maintaining lumbar lordosis, which positions their center of gravity/weight line posterior to the hip joints, thus stabilizing the hip in extension on the anterior capsule of the hip joint. Subsequently, weakness of the knee extensors produces a tendency for patients to experience knee instability and knee buckling with falls. Patients compensate for this by decreasing stance phase knee flexion and posturing the ankle increasingly over time into plantar flexion. This movement produces a knee extension moment at foot contact, and the plantar flexion of the ankle during mid to late stance phase of gait helps position the weight line/center of gravity anterior to the knee joint (thus producing a stabilizing knee-extension moment). Patients with DMD will progressively demonstrate initial foot contact with the floor increasingly forward onto the mid foot and finally the forefoot as they reach the transitional phase of ambulation before wheelchair reliance. Finally, weakness of the hip abductors produces a tendency toward lateral pelvic tilt and pelvic drop of the swing-phase side. Patients with proximal weakness compensate for this by bending or lurching their trunk laterally over the stance-phase hip joint (**Fig. 11**B). This action produces the so-called gluteus medius lurch or Trendelenburg gait pattern.

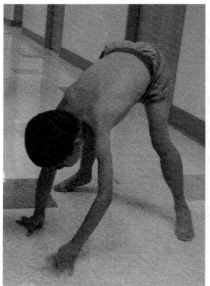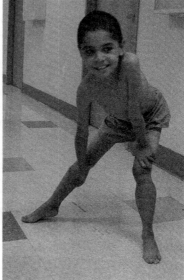

Fig. 10. Gower sign in a 7-year-old boy with Duchenne muscular dystrophy.

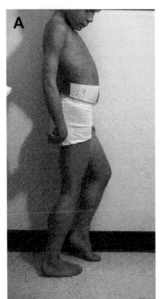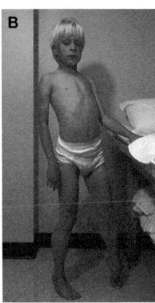

Fig. 11. Myopathic gait pattern in Duchenne muscular dystrophy, caused by weakness in pelvic girdle and knee extension. (*A*) Lumbar lordosis to keep center of mass posterior to hip joint; anterior pelvic tilt due to hip extensor weakness; weight line/center of mass maintained anterior to an extended knee; and forefoot ground contact with stance-phase plantar flexion (toe walking) to maintain a knee-extension moment and knee stability. (*B*) Trendelenburg or "gluteus medius gait" with lateral lean over the stance side due to hip abductor weakness; ankle dorsiflexion weakness necessitates swing-phase circumduction for clearance.

Patients with this classic gait pattern, secondary to proximal pelvic girdle weakness, often exhibit toe walking. The clinician may mistakenly provide an ankle-foot orthosis (AFO) with the ankle positioned at 90°, with the thought that the patient needs orthotic management of foot drop. However, this can produce a precipitous increase in falls because the orthotic blocks the ankle at 90°, thus compromising the patient's ability to stabilize the knee into extension with equinus posturing of the gastrocnemius-soleus complex.

Patients with distal weakness affecting the ankle dorsiflexors and ankle everters, and less severe proximal weakness (eg, CMT, Emery-Dreifuss muscular dystrophy, MMD, FSHD, and other conditions) often exhibit a foot slap at floor contact and a steppage gait pattern to facilitate swing-phase clearance of the plantar-flexed ankle. Alternatively, these patients may clear the plantar-flexed ankle using some degree of circumduction at the hip or vaulting on the stance-phase side. These patients often benefit from the provision of an AFO with either a solid ankle or articulated ankle with a plantar flexion stop at neutral. More mild distal lower extremity weakness may become clinically evident by testing heel walking and toe walking.

LABORATORY EVALUATIONS
Serum Laboratory Studies

A variety of NMDs, particularly those characterized by sarcolemmal muscle membrane injury, show significant elevations in transaminases, aldolase, and CK. The CK enzyme catalyzes the release of high-energy phosphates from creatine phosphate. It occurs mainly in muscle and leaks into the serum in large amounts in any disorder involving muscle fiber injury. The muscle membrane fraction is specific to skeletal muscle. The CK value may be significantly elevated in the early stages of DMD and BMD, with values up to 50 to 100 times normal. A normal CK value may help exclude DMD and BMD. Overlap in CK values occurs between DMD and BMD. Other forms of muscular dystrophy such as Emery-Dreifuss muscular dystrophy, LGMD, FSHD, and congenital muscular dystrophy may show moderate elevations in CK. However, in congenital muscular dystrophy the CK value may be extremely variable, ranging from normal values to a fairly marked elevation. There is no close association between disease severity and CK values. In all dystrophic myopathies, the CK values tend to decrease over time with increasing severity of the disease caused by progressive loss of muscle fiber and irreversible cell death. Thus, a 3-year-old with DMD may have a CK value of 25,000 whereas a 10-year-old with DMD may show a CK value of 2000. Other dystrophic myopathies with elevated CK values (>1000) values include: LGMD 2A to 2I; LGMD 1C; distal myopathy of the Miyoshi type; immune polymyopathy with signal recognition particle and HMG-CoA reductase antibody; paraneoplastic syndromes; acid maltase deficiency; acute damage from injection; rhabdomyolysis; and muscle trauma. In addition, myopathy from hypothyroidism may be associated with high CK values. Other conditions with significant elevations in CK may include polymyositis, dermatomyositis, acute rhabdomyolysis, and malignant hyperthermia. In many of the congenital structural myopathies, such as central core disease, nemaline rod myopathy, and fiber-type disproportion syndrome, a serum CK is likely to be normal or only mildly elevated.

CK levels have been found to be normal to elevated 2 to 4 times in SMA I and II.[34] SMA III patients have also been found to have normal to slightly elevated CK values with elevations generally in the range of 2 to 5 times normal. A serum CK level greater than 10 times the upper limit of normal generally is an exclusionary criteria for SMA[15,35,36] and, in this setting, workup for other disorders such as inflammatory or dystrophic myopathies should be pursued. Functional status and disease progression did not correlate with initial CK determination in one series of SMA III cases.[37]

Thus, in a child with muscle weakness, a normal CK does not exclude a myopathy or other NMD condition, a severely elevated CK is suggestive of but not diagnostic of a dystrophic myopathy, and a very high CK is no reflection of disease severity in both inflammatory and dystrophic myopathies. Normal CK values may be seen in the acute active phase of childhood dermatomyositis, even in the presence of severe weakness.

Serial CK measurement in the morning after several days of sedentary activity is still useful in the evaluation of potential female DMD carriers who do not have a detectable gene deletion on molecular genetic studies. Three normal CK values in a female is approximately 90% specific for ruling out carrier status. Even one abnormally elevated CK makes carrier status a possibility.

Lactate and pyruvate levels are useful in the setting of a possible metabolic myopathy. Presence of a lactic acidosis may be seen in mitochondrial encephalomyelopathies such as Kearns-Sayre syndrome, MERRF (myoclonus epilepsy and ragged-red fibers), and MELAS (mitochondrial encephalomyelopathy with lactic acidosis and strokelike episodes). Whenever clinical evidence suggests a disorder of oxidative metabolism, blood lactate and pyruvate values should be obtained. Arterial lactate values are more reliable. Lactate elevations under ischemic or exercise stress suggest mitochondrial dysfunction. In a setting of lactic acidemia, the lactate/pyruvate ratio may aid in the differential diagnosis. Children with suspected encephalomyelopathy should be evaluated with cerebrospinal fluid (CSF) lactate levels, as these values are less subject to flux than either venous or arterial values.

The ischemic forearm test, initially used by McArdle, is the most widely used means of assessing muscle anaerobic metabolism,[35,38,39] The hallmark of defects in muscle glycogenolysis is failure of the normal increase in lactate in venous blood flowing from ischemically exercised muscles. The increase in blood pyruvate is also attenuated or absent, as is the lactate/pyruvate (L/P) ratio, which normally rises roughly 5-fold. A virtually unchanged L/P ratio with exercise typifies myophosphorylase and muscle phosphofructokinase deficiency. In muscle lactate dehydrogenase deficiency, ischemic exercise causes a disproportionate increase in pyruvate relative to lactate, which is secondary to increasing levels of pyruvate behind the metabolic block. An exaggerated increase in ammonia and purine metabolites with heavy exercise typifies glycolytic defects. A normal lactate response but impaired ammonia production is characteristic of myoadenylate deaminase deficiency.

Laboratory Evaluation of Neuromuscular Junction Disorders

Patients suspected of Lambert-Eaton syndrome, infantile or late acquired botulism, myasthenia gravis, or presynaptic and postsynaptic congenital myasthenic syndromes may be evaluated electrodiagnostically with repetitive stimulation studies, as described by Lipa and Han elsewhere in this issue. Increasingly, molecular genetic studies are being employed to diagnose congenital myasthenic syndromes.

Those suspected of infantile botulism should have stool or a rectal irrigation sample sent for botulinum toxin. The stool studies are often helpful in establishing an early diagnosis, as the electrodiagnostic studies may have less sensitivity within the first few days of presentation.

Infants suspected of transient neonatal myasthenia or congenital myasthenic syndromes may show a clinical response to intravenous edrophonium (Tensilon) testing or neostigmine testing. The author prefers comparing the degree of decrement on repetitive stimulation studies before and serially (every 2 minutes) after neostigmine administration in infants with suspected myasthenic syndromes, as clinical response to neostigmine or edrophonium may be exceedingly difficult to judge in the intubated neonate. Decremental responses at slow rates of stimulation (2–3 Hz) are not specific to postsynaptic defects in infants with congenital myasthenic syndromes, and may be seen in presynaptic or postsynaptic subtypes. Motor point biopsy of the anconeus or intercostal muscle dissected with their motor branches allows for in-vitro electrophysiologic studies to measure miniature end-plate potentials, gated ion channels, and other parameters to characterize pre-synaptic, intrasynaptic, or post-synaptic pathology.

Children and adults with suspected myasthenia gravis should have acetylcholine receptor antibodies sent (binding or blocking, modulating, and striated muscle acetylcholine antibodies). Negative antibody studies do not rule out autoimmune myasthenia gravis, as some patients have antibodies of a different nature that cannot be measured with current laboratory techniques. Patients with myasthenia gravis should have a chest radiograph and/or chest computed tomography scan to rule out thymoma.

Muscle Imaging

Ultrasound imaging has been used as a screening tool to discern pathologic change in muscle.[40–44] More recently, magnetic resonance imaging (MRI) has been used to evaluate the extent and distribution of involvement in neuromuscular disorders as well as disease progression.[45–50] MRI has also been used to help differentiate between dystrophic myopathy and neurogenic atrophy caused by disorders such as SMA. A recent review describes the use of skeletal muscle MRI in diagnosis and monitoring of disease progression.[45]

Although muscle imaging is generally not used to delineate a specific diagnosis, these techniques are useful for the identification of appropriate sites for muscle biopsy, for determination of distribution and extent of involvement, and for monitoring disease progression.[40,45]

Body Composition by Dual-Energy X-Ray Absorptiometry

Both lean and fat tissue mass can be accurately and reliably estimated over wide age ranges using Dual-energy x-ray absorptiometry (DEXA). Subjects with myogenic atrophy have a significantly elevated fat/muscle ratio. Both functional activity scales and strength correlates with percentage of lean body mass measured by DEXA. Diffuse neurogenic atrophy is associated with decrease in the mass of all 3 compartments (lean mass, fat mass, and bone mineral content) but relatively normal fat/muscle ratios standardize to body mass index. Regional body composition by DEXA has been proposed as a monitor of disease progression in such entities as muscular dystrophy or in progressive denervating diseases such as SMA and peripheral neuropathies. Skalsky and colleagues[51] have recently extensively reviewed the use of regional and whole-body DEXA to guide treatment and monitor disease progression in NMD.

Electrodiagnostic Studies

Nerve conduction and electromyography are an extension of the clinician's physical examination and a powerful tool for the localization of abnormalities within the lower motor neuron. In addition, EMG and nerve conduction studies help to guide further evaluation such as molecular genetic studies (eg, to improve cost-effectiveness of molecular genetic panels in CMT by determining the nature of a peripheral neuropathy as demyelinating or axonal), and to help guide muscle biopsies by providing information regarding the most appropriate muscle site for biopsy. Lipa and Han[39] provide a comprehensive review of the role of electrodiagnostic studies regarding the diagnostic evaluation of NMDs elsewhere in this issue.

Molecular Genetic Studies

The application of molecular genetic techniques has resulted in enormous gains in our understanding of the molecular and pathophysiologic basis of hereditary NMDs. In addition, molecular genetic studies now aid in the diagnostic evaluation of many NMD conditions, as described in this issue by Arnold and Flanigan.[1] In MMD, the CTG repeat size of the DMPK gene inversely correlates with age of onset of DM1 (**Fig. 12**). In addition, complete sequencing of genes is critical for the determination of the potential value of genetics-based therapeutic agents for particular patients.

Evaluation of Muscle and Nerve Biopsy

Although molecular genetic testing has reduced the need for muscle biopsy, the appropriate acquisition of muscle biopsies is still valuable in the diagnostic evaluation of hereditary and acquired NMDs, and this topic is reviewed by Joyce and colleagues elsewhere in this issue. Nerve biopsies are somewhat useful in the characterization of more severe hereditary motor and sensory neuropathies, congenital hypomyelinating neuropathy, and neuroaxonal dystrophy. In addition, perineural immune complex deposition seen in some autoimmune neuropathies, or changes consistent with vasculitis, may also be useful diagnostically. Otherwise, nerve biopsies rarely add useful specific information to the diagnostic evaluation of the NMD patient beyond the information obtained from nerve conduction studies and EMG.

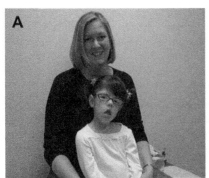 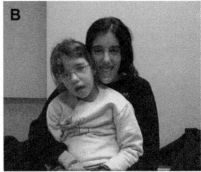

Fig. 12. Four individuals with MMD. The mother on the left (*A*) has 75 CTG repeats in the DM protein kinase (DMPK) gene loci on chromosome 19q13.3, and her daughter has 2538 CTG repeats. The mother on the right (*B*) is more symptomatic and has 450 CTG repeats, and her daughter has 1650 repeats. This status is an example of genetic anticipation with greater severity occurring in successive generations.

CLINICAL CLUES TO HELP WITH THE EARLY DIAGNOSIS OF COMMON NMD CONDITIONS: IMPLICATIONS FOR TREATMENT

Most NMD syndromes give very specific patterns of presentation and strength loss. For the most common NMD conditions, the patterns of strength impairment and natural history profiles for change in strength over time have been described in detail by the author and colleagues at the University of California, Davis Research and Training Center in Neuromuscular Disease.[26,27,29–32,52,53] Early diagnosis is facilitated by knowledge of the common initial clinical presentations of specific NMDs. This knowledge allows for streamlined and cost-effective laboratory evaluations, electrodiagnostic studies, molecular genetic diagnostic evaluations, imaging, and determination of whether muscle biopsies are necessary. Early diagnosis is facilitated by knowledge of the common initial clinical presentations of specific NMDs, and in many cases the early diagnosis has potential implications for treatment and prevention of secondary conditions.

MOTOR NEURON DISEASES
Amyotrophic Lateral Sclerosis

Sporadic amyotrophic lateral sclerosis
ALS can be defined as a rapidly progressive neurodegenerative disease characterized by weakness, spasticity, and muscular atrophy, with subsequent respiratory compromise leading to premature death. It is caused by the destruction of motor neurons in the primary motor cortex, brainstem, and spinal cord. Onset of ALS is insidious and most commonly presents with painless asymmetric limb weakness. ALS most often afflicts people between 40 and 60 years of age with a mean age of onset of 58 years.[54–56] Five percent of cases have onset before age 30. Men are affected more commonly than women at a ratio of 1.5:1.0. Patients with lower motor nerve (LMN) abnormality usually present complaining of muscle weakness. In addition, they may note muscle atrophy, fasciculations, and muscle cramping. Cramping may occur anywhere in the body, including the thighs, arms, and abdomen. Cramping of abdominal or other trunk muscles raises a red flag urging the clinician to consider a diagnosis of ALS. Patients with upper motor nerve (UMN) abnormality often complain of loss of dexterity or a feeling of stiffness in the limbs. Such patients may

note weakness, which is caused by spasticity resulting from disinhibition of brainstem control of the vestibulospinal and reticulospinal tracts. Signs and symptoms suggesting bulbar muscle weakness include dysarthria, dysphagia, drooling, and aspiration. These signs and symptoms may be caused by UMN and/or LMN dysfunction involving the bulbar muscles. Signs of spastic dysarthria, indicating UMN abnormality, include a strained and strangled quality of speech, reduced rate, low pitch, imprecise consonant pronunciation, vowel distortion, and breaks in pitch. LMN dysfunction creates flaccid dysarthria in which speech has a nasal and/or wet quality, pitch and intensity are monotone, phrases abnormally short, and inspiration audible. Patients may complain of intermittent gagging sensations attributable to muscle weakness with drooping of the soft palate. Complaints of difficulty chewing and swallowing, nasal regurgitation, or coughing when drinking liquids may all indicate dysphagia.

Other signs and symptoms frequently associated with ALS are cachexia, fatigue, and musculoskeletal complaints. The term ALS cachexia refers to a phenomenon experienced by some patients whereby weight loss occurs in excess of that caused by muscle atrophy and reduced caloric intake. Both subcutaneous fat and peritoneal fat are lost, presumably because of acceleration of the basal metabolic rate.[57] In patients with ALS cachexia, greater than 20% of body weight is typically lost over a 6-month period.

Familial ALS

The vast majority of ALS cases are presumably acquired and occur sporadically. However, approximately 5% to 10% of all ALS cases are familial (FALS) and most commonly have an autosomal dominant inheritance pattern, although autosomal recessive, X-linked, and mitochondrial inheritance patterns have been reported.[58–62] The age of onset of FALS occurs a decade earlier than for sporadic cases, and progression of the disease is more rapid. Males and females are equally affected. About 20% of FALS cases result from a copper-zinc superoxide dismutase (SOD1) gene defect.[63–65] Other disease-causing genetic mutations have more recently been identified. These mutations have been found in genes encoding for angiogenin, chromatin-modifying protein, dynactin, vesicle-associated membrane protein, and TAR-DNA binding protein.[65]

Predominantly Proximal Spinal Muscular Atrophy

In type I SMA, onset is generally up to 6 months, the patients never sit without support, and survival is usually less than 2 years. In SMA type II, onset is generally up to 18 months, patients sit independently but never stand or walk without aids, and survival is usually longer than 2 years and often into young adulthood. In SMA type III, onset is after 18 months, patients achieve standing or walking without support but may lose this milestone at a later age, and survival is essentially normal. In all SMA types, proximal muscles are weaker than distal muscles. Patients have symmetric weakness involving the lower extremities earlier and to a greater extent than the upper extremities.[52] The diaphragm is usually relatively preserved, relative to intercostal and abdominal musculature. In SMA I, this results in a diaphragmatic breathing pattern during respiration with abdominal protrusion, paradoxic thoracic depression, and intercostal retraction (see **Fig. 6**). Patients with SMA may have both neck flexor and neck extensor weakness. Clinical features of SMA I, II, and III are shown in **Table 1**.

Spinal muscle atrophy I (Werdnig-Hoffman disease)

The majority of cases of SMA I present within the first 2 months with generalized hypotonia and symmetric weakness. The age of onset of symptoms is less than 4 months

Table 1
Childhood-onset proximal spinal muscular atrophy (SMA)

	SMA I (Werdnig-Hoffman)	SMA II (Intermediate SMA)	SMA III (Kugelberg-Welander)
Onset	<6 mo	6–18 mo	>18 mo IIIa <3 y IIIb >3 y
Genetics	SMN1: AR homozygous SMN2: ≤2 copies	SMN1: AR homozygous SMN2: 3 copies	SMN1: AR homozygous SMN2: 4–8 copies
Phenotype	Severe hypotonia, weak suck, weak cry, proximal weakness, absent reflexes, respiratory failure common	Hypotonia, proximal weakness, muscle wasting, contractures, scoliosis, absent reflexes, tongue fasciculations	Proximal symmetric weakness, lordotic gait, Gower sign, decreased reflexes, tremor, tongue fasciculations
Milestones	Poor head control Never sit independently	Sit with head control Never stand unassisted May require ventilatory support	Stand & walk unassisted; may lose standing or continue to walk IIIa: onset 18 mo to <3 y (80% not walking at age 40) IIIb: onset >3 y (40% not walking at age 40)
Life expectancy	1–2 y 10% living at age 20	Most live to third decade; many live to fourth to fifth decade	Normal life expectancy

in the vast majority of cases. Weak sucking, dysphagia, labored breathing during feeding, frequent aspiration of food or secretions, and weak cry are frequently noted by history.

Examination shows generalized hypotonia and symmetric weakness involving the lower extremities earlier, and to a greater extent in the upper extremities. Proximal muscles are weaker than distal extremities. In the supine position, the lower extremities may be abducted and externally rotated in a "frog-leg" position (see **Fig. 6**). The upper extremities tend to be adducted and externally rotated at the shoulders with a semiflexed elbow. Volitional movements of fingers and hands persist well past the time when the shoulders and elbows cannot be flexed against gravity. The thorax is flattened anteroposteriorly and is bell-shaped as a result of intercostal weakness. Pectus excavatum may be variably present. The diaphragm is usually preserved, relative to the intercostal and abdominal musculature, resulting in a diaphragmatic breathing pattern during respiration with abdominal protrusion, paradoxic thoracic depression, and intercostal retraction. Neck flexor weakness may result in persistent posterior head lag when the trunk is lifted forward from the supine position. Neck extensor weakness may result in forward head lag when the infant is positioned in the horizontal prone position. With advanced disease, the mouth may remain open as a result of masticatory muscle weakness. Facial weakness may be noted in up to half of patients. The diagnostic criteria for SMA outlined by the International SMA Consortium[15] lists marked facial weakness as an exclusionary criterion for SMA, but this is not absolute. Tongue fasciculations have been reported in 56% to 61% of patients,[34] so the absence of this finding does not necessarily exclude the disease. In one series,[34]

DTRs were absent in all 4 extremities in 74% of cases. Thus, the preservation of DTRs does not exclude the diagnosis of SMA. Appendicular muscle fasciculations and distal tremor are also associated examination findings. Extraocular muscles are spared, as is the myocardium. Mild to moderate contractures of hip flexion, knee flexion, and elbow flexion may be observed in some patients along with wrist contractures and ulnar drift of the fingers. Severe arthrogryposis is not typically observed.

Spinal muscular atrophy II

Disease onset is usually more insidious than that of SMA I. The findings of generalized hypotonia, symmetric weakness, and delayed motor milestones are hallmarks of SMA II. Weakness also involves proximal muscles more than distal muscles, and lower extremity more than upper extremity. A fine tremor of the fingers and hands occurs in a minority of patients. This polyminimyoclonus may be attributed to spontaneous, repetitive rhythmic discharges by the motor neurons that innervate a large territory of muscle. Wasting tends to be more conspicuous in SMA II than in SMA I. DTRs are depressed and usually absent in the lower extremities. Appendicular or thoracic muscle wall fasciculations may be observed. Tongue fasciculations have been observed in 30% to 70% of SMA II patients.[15,17,34] Progressive kyphoscoliosis and neuromuscular restrictive lung disease is almost invariably seen in the late first decade. Contractures of the hip flexors, tensor fasciae latae, hamstrings, triceps surae, and elbow and finger flexors are quite common. Hypotonic hip dislocations have been noted commonly in SMA II patients. Sensory examination is completely normal, and extraocular muscles and the myocardium are spared. In a large series from Germany[44] of 104 cases classified as SMA II (sits alone, never walks), 98% survived to the age of 10 and 77% to the age of 20 years. Thus, a longer life span is possible with adequate supportive care.

Spinal muscular atrophy III (Kugelberg-Weilander syndrome)

In more chronic SMA III, also referred to as Kugelberg-Welander syndrome, weakness usually initially occurs between the ages of 18 months and the late teens. Motor milestones may be delayed in infancy. Proximal weakness is observed, with the pelvic girdle being more affected than the shoulder girdle.[52] There is an exaggerated lumbar lordosis and anterior pelvic tilt owing to hip extensor weakness. There is also a waddling gait pattern with pelvic drop and lateral trunk lean over the stance-phase side, secondary to hip abductor weakness. If ankle plantar flexion strength is sufficient, the patients may show primarily forefoot or toe contact and no heel strike, similar to patients with DMD. This measure is compensatory for knee extensor weakness to maintain a stabilizing knee extension moment at the knee. The patient may exhibit a Gower sign when arising from the floor; stair climbing is difficult because of hip flexor weakness. Facial weakness is sometimes noted. Fasciculations are noted in about half of the patients[15] and are more common later in the disease course. Fasciculations in the limb muscles and thoracic wall muscles are common. Calf pseudohypertrophy has been occasionally noted, but wasting of affected musculature is more prominent. DTRs are diminished and often become absent over time. Contractures are generally mild as long as patients remain ambulatory. Scoliosis may be observed in SMA III, but occurs less frequently and is less severe than scoliosis in SMA II. Although no survival data exist for patients with SMA III, cases have been followed into the eighth decade without mechanical ventilation.[52,66] Ventilatory failure due to neuromuscular restrictive lung disease is a rare event in SMA III, occurring only in adulthood.[18,52] Zerres and Rudnik-Schoneborn[66] have proposed further subtypes, including SMA IIIa (walks without support; age of onset before 3 years) and SMA IIIb (walks without support; age of onset 3–30 years). In their series, only 44% of SMA IIIa patients remained ambulatory 20 years after onset of weakness, whereas 89% of IIIb patients remained ambulatory after a similar 20-year duration.

Diagnosis of SMA is confirmed by a consideration of clinical findings, molecular genetic studies and, occasionally, electrodiagnostic studies. Muscle biopsy is generally not required to confirm the diagnosis. Genetic studies have now established that SMA is caused by mutations in the telomeric SMN1 gene, with all patients having at least one copy of the centromeric SMN2 gene. At least one copy of the SMN2 must be present in the setting of homozygous SMN1 mutations; otherwise, embryonic lethality occurs. The copy number of SMN2 varies in the population, and this variation appears to have some important modifying effects on SMA disease severity.[67–70] All SMA patients have more than 2 SMN2 genes. It appears that a higher number of SMN2 copies in the setting of SMN1 mutations is associated with a less severe clinical SMA phenotype: SMA I (severe): 2 or 3 gene copies of SMN2; SMA II: 3 copies of SMN2; SMA III: 4 to 8 copies of SMN2. However, substantial variations in SMA phenotype and disease severity can exist with a given SMN2 copy number, so it is not recommended that disease severity be predicted based solely on SMN2 copy numbers. Therapeutic interventions for SMA are reviewed by Skalsky and colleagues elsewhere in this issue.

HEREDITARY ATAXIAS
Friedreich Ataxia

Friedreich ataxia is a spinocerebellar degeneration syndrome with the onset of symptoms before age 20 years. This autosomal recessive condition has been linked in one subtype to chromosome 9q13-21.1 (FRDA), with the protein implicated being termed frataxin. A second subtype referred to as FRDA2 is linked to chromosome 9p23-p11.

The incidence of Friedreich ataxia is 1 in 25,000 to 50,000. Carrier frequency is 1 in 60 to 110. Age of onset is usually younger than 20 years, typically around puberty, with a range from 2 to 25 years. Obligate signs and symptoms include progressive ataxic gait, cerebellar dysfunction with tremor and dysmetria, dysarthria, decreased proprioception or vibratory sense (or both), muscle weakness, and absent DTRs. Other common signs include cavus foot deformity, cardiomyopathy, scoliosis, and upper motor neuron signs, such as a Babinski sign and spasticity. Weakness is progressive, and affects lower extremities and small muscles in the hands and feet. Sensory loss is typical and especially affects vibration and joint position sensation. Tendon reflexes are often absent. An occasional patient may have chorea without ataxia. With electrodiagnostic studies, sensory nerve potentials may be absent or reduced. Progression is slow, with mean time to wheelchair dependence 15 years of age; time of death from cardiomyopathy ranges from the third to seventh decade. The prevalence of scoliosis approaches 100%, but some cases have more severe progressive spinal deformity than others. Those cases of Friedreich ataxia with onset of disease before the age of 10 years generally have more severe progressive scoliosis. Those with the onset of disease during or after puberty have later-onset spinal deformity, which may not require surgical intervention.

Frataxin is a mitochondrial protein located on the inner mitochondrial membrane. It is likely required for maintenance of the mitochondrial genome, and is involved in iron homeostasis and iron transport into mitochondria. Idebenone is a power antioxidant and a synthetic analogue of coenzyme Q. It may improve iron homeostasis and mitochondrial function in Friedreich ataxia. In randomized clinical trials, longer-term idebenone treatment has been shown to prevent progression of cardiomyopathy and cardiac hypertrophy in both pediatric and adult patients with Friedreich ataxia.

Its stabilizing effect on neurologic dysfunction has been shown to be present only in the pediatric population, mainly before puberty. This finding suggests that the age at which idebenone treatment is initiated may be an important factor in the effectiveness of the therapy.[71]

Spinocerebellar Ataxias

The hereditary ataxias are a group of genetic disorders characterized by slowly progressive incoordination of gait, often associated with poor coordination of hands, speech, and eye movements. Atrophy of the cerebellum frequently occurs. A peripheral neuropathy can occur in many of the subtypes. The hereditary ataxias are categorized by mode of inheritance and causative gene or chromosomal locus. The genetic forms of ataxia are diagnosed by family history, physical examination, and neuroimaging. Molecular genetic tests are available for the diagnosis of many but not all spinocerebellar ataxias. More than 60 genetically distinct autosomal dominant and autosomal recessive subtypes of hereditary ataxia and spinocerebellar ataxia have been identified.

PERIPHERAL NERVE DISORDERS
Acute Inflammatory Demyelinating Polyradiculoneuropathy (Guillain-Barré Syndrome)

Acute inflammatory demyelinating polyradiculoneuropathy (AIDP) is a primarily demyelinating neuropathy with autoimmune etiology. Motor axons are affected more than sensory axons. Incidence in children is similar to that seen in adults. Children often have a prodromal respiratory or gastrointestinal infection occurring within 1 month of onset. Common precipitating infections include *Mycoplasma*, cytomegalovirus, Epstein-Barr virus, *Campylobacter jejuni*, and various vaccinations. Weakness generally begins distally in the lower extremity with a progressive ascending paralysis ultimately involving the upper limbs. Pain and sensory symptoms are not uncommon. The most common cranial nerve abnormality is an ipsilateral or bilateral lower motor neuron facial paralysis. Objective sensory loss has been documented in the minority of children.[72] In one series, only 15% required mechanical ventilation.[73] The maximal degree of weakness generally reaches a peak within 2 weeks of onset, and time to maximum recovery was 7 ± 5 months in one series.[74,75] Complete recovery occurs in most children. Classic criteria for poor recovery in adults (low median compound motor action potentials [CMAPs] and fibrillation potentials) may not apply to children.[74] Disturbances of the autonomic nervous system are common in children, including transient disturbances of bowel and bladder, excessive sweating or vasoconstriction, mild hypertension or hypotension, and occasionally cardiac arrhythmias.

The acute motor axonal neuropathy (AMAN) involves predominantly motor nerve fibers with a physiologic pattern suggesting axonal damage, whereas the AIDP involves both motor and sensory nerve fibers with a physiologic pattern suggesting demyelination. Another clinical variant is the Miller-Fisher syndrome, characterized by acute-onset ataxia, ophthalmoparesis, and areflexia.

Diagnosis is generally confirmed by electrodiagnostic studies,[39] and the CSF protein is characteristically elevated in a majority of children. Serum autoantibodies that may be elevated include immunoglobulin (Ig)M and IgG versus β-tubulin and heparan sulfate. AMAN patients may show increased IgG antibodies to GM1 ganglioside. The Miller-Fisher syndrome is associated with a high frequency of the IgG GQ1b antibodies. The major considerations in differential diagnosis of AIDP or AMAN include transverse myelitis, toxic neuropathies, tick paralysis, infantile botulism, myasthenia gravis, and dermatomyositis.

Treatment has typically included corticosteroids, plasma exchange, or more recently, intravenous immune globulin.[76-79] AIDP patients respond to both plasma exchange and intravenous immunoglobulin (IVIG). Patients with AMAN respond preferentially to IVIG over plasma exchange. Recovery is often reasonable in children without treatment. After standard IVIG therapy, children with axonal forms of Guillain-Barré syndrome recover more slowly than those with the demyelinating form, but outcome at 12 months appears to be equally favorable in both groups.[80]

Chronic Inflammatory Demyelinating Polyradiculoneuropathy

Children or adults with chronic inflammatory demyelinating polyradiculoneuropathy (CIDP) often have a presentation similar to AIDP; however, the disorder continues with a chronic or relapsing course. The disorder may begin as early as infancy, but is seen in children and adults. Electrophysiologic studies show focal conduction block, temporal dispersion of CMAPs, prolongation of distal motor latencies, markedly slow conduction velocities, and absent or prolonged H-wave and F-wave latencies. CIDP cases often demonstrate axonal loss on EMG. The CSF protein is elevated in most cases. The differential diagnosis usually includes CMT types I and III. The presence of acute relapsing episodes point toward CIDP. Because of the more severe involvement of proximal nerves and nerve roots, a distal sural nerve biopsy may not always show inflammatory changes and demyelination. Treatment may include corticosteroids (prednisone) and IVIG as first-line approaches, and subsequent plasma exchange.

Charcot-Marie-Tooth

CMT neuropathy (also called hereditary motor-sensory neuropathy [HMSN]) is a heterogeneous group of inherited disease of peripheral nerve that affects both children and adults and causes significant progressive neuromuscular impairment.[81,82] It has been estimated that 1 per 2500 to 3000 persons has a form of CMT. CMT 1 denotes individuals with a hypertrophic demyelinating neuropathy (onion bulbs) and reduced nerve conduction velocities, whereas CMT 2 refers to individuals with an axonal neuropathy and normal or slightly reduced nerve conduction velocities. Individuals with CMT 3 (Dejerine-Sotttas disease) have a primarily demyelinating peripheral neuropathy with a more severe phenotype presenting in infancy. Historically types 1, 2, and 3 were believed to be autosomal dominant conditions, with type 3 CMT patients exhibiting point mutations with frame shift and either dominant or recessive inheritance. CMT 4 refers to autosomal recessive CMT. However, recently axonal forms of CMT have been identified with autosomal recessive inheritance (deemed AR-CMT 2A, 2B, and so forth).

In general, in most CMT subtypes onset is usually during the first or second decade of life. Both motor and sensory nerve function are affected. The clinical features include distal muscle weakness, impaired sensation, and absent or diminished DTRs. Weakness usually is greatest initially present in the foot and hand intrinsics and distal lower extremities, and subsequently in the distal upper extremities. Slow progressive weakness, more proximally in the knees, elbows, and pelvic and shoulder girdles, may occur over decades.[26] There is variable penetrance in most subtypes. Weakness is usually initially greatest in the distal lower extremities and subsequently in the distal upper extremities. Slow progressive weakness more proximally in the knees, elbows, and pelvic and shoulder girdles may occur over decades.[52] The various gene locations and known protein abnormalities associated with various forms of CMT (HMSN) and the clinical subtypes are described in **Table 2**.

Table 2
Charcot-Marie-Tooth disease subtypes: comparison of clinical features

Disorder	Gene	Location	Usual Onset	Early or Distinct Symptoms	Tendon Reflexes	Average NCVs
CMT1: Dominant; Demyelinating						
CMT 1A	PMP-22	17p11-12	First decade	Distal weakness	Absent	15–20 m/s
CMT 1B	P0	1q22	First decade	Distal weakness	Absent	<20 m/s
CMT 1C	LITAF	16p13	Second decade	Distal weakness	Reduced	16–25 m/s
CMT 1D	EGR2	10q21	Second decade	Distal weakness	Absent	26–42 m/s
CMT 1E (Deafness)	—	17p11-12 (small mutations)	Late onset: fifth decade	Sensory loss: distal Weakness: Distal Vocal cord dysfunction in some patients	Reduced	NCV: axon loss
CMT 1F	Neurofilament light chain (NEFL)	8p21.2	<13 y	Weakness Legs & arms Distal > proximal May be severe Early: delayed motor milestones or gait disorder Dominant	Absent	Motor NCV: 15–38 m/s SNAPs: often absent F-waves: normal or slow
CMT X (S-D*)	Connexin-32	Xq13	Second decade	Distal weakness	Absent distal	25–40 m/s
HNPP	PMP-22	17p11	Third decade	Focal episodic weakness	Normal	Entrapments
Dejerine-Sottas (HMSN 3) Dominant or recessive	PMP-22 P0 EGR2	17p11-12 1q22 10q21	First 1-2 years	Severe weakness	Absent	<10 m/s
CMT Intermediate NCV	DNM2 10q24 1p34	19p12 10q24 1p34	First or second decade	Distal weakness	—	25–50 m/s

(continued on next page)

Table 2
(continued)

Disorder	Gene	Location	Usual Onset	Early or Distinct Symptoms	Tendon Reflexes	Average NCVs
	PO	1q22				
	CMT-X	Xq13				
CMT2: Dominant; Axonal						
CMT 2A	KIF1Bβ Mitofusin 2	1p36 1	10 y	Distal weakness	Absent distal	>38 m/s
CMT 2B	RAB7	3q13	Second decade	Distal weakness Sensory loss Acromutilation	Absent distal	Axon loss
CMT 2C	TRPV4	12q24	First decade	Vocal cord & distal weakness	Absent	>50 m/s
CMT 2D	GARS	7p15	16–30 y	Distal weakness Arms > legs	Reduced	Axon loss
CMT 2E	NF-68	8p21	1–40 y	Distal weakness	Reduced	Axon loss
CMT 2F/ Distal HMN	HSPB1 (HSP 27)	7q11	6–54 y	Difficulty walking	Reduced ankle	Axon loss
CMT 2G	—	12q12	15–25 y	Distal weakness	Reduced	CMAPs, SNAPs Small in legs 42–58 m/s
CMT 2I	PO	1q22	Late onset	Distal weakness Sensory loss (90%–100%) Severe Panmodal Distal > proximal Weakness (80%–100%) Legs (80%) > arms (35%) Distal Mild to severe	Reduced	Velocity: usually >20 m/s to normal Often not clearly demyelinating CMAPs & SNAPs: reduced amplitude or absent

CMT	Gene	Locus	Age/Clinical features	Additional features	Tendon reflexes	Electrophysiology
CMT 2J	P₀	1q22	Age: adult; usually after 30 y; Legs; Paresthesias, hypoesthesia (85%)	CMT with hearing loss & pupillary abnormalities	—	Predominantly axonal neuropathy (adult onset)
CMT 2K	Ganglioside-induced differentiation-associated protein 1 GDAP1	8q21	Weakness (100%) Distal Severe Feet > hands: hand onset later in first decade Proximal: moderate; Legs > arms	Vocal cord paralysis Onset: second decade Hoarseness (80%) Not present in some families Gait disorder	—	NCV: axon loss; velocities preserved
CMT 2L	HSPB8	12q24	15–33 y	Distal weakness	Reduced	Axon loss
CMT 2M	DNM2	19p13	Onset age: congenital to fourth decade Cataracts: early Neuropathy: childhood	Legs > arms Sensory: panmodal loss; sensory ataxia; paresthesias Weakness: distal; legs > arms Progression: mild	Reduced	NCV: axon loss
CMT 2N	AARS;	16q22	Onset age: mean 28 y; range 6–54 y	Leg weakness Occasional asymptomatic patient	Tendon reflexes Knees: reduced Ankles: absent reduced	Axonal to intermediate NCV: 32–50 m/s; CMAP amplitudes reduced SNAP amplitudes: small

(continued on next page)

Table 2
(continued)

Disorder	Gene	Location	Usual Onset	Early or Distinct Symptoms	Tendon Reflexes	Average NCVs
CMT 2O	DYNC1H1;	14q32	Onset: early childhood Delayed motor milestones	Delayed Weakness: distal; legs > arms Sensory loss: distal; panmodal; normal in some patients Pes cavus: some patients have CNS learning difficulties	Tendon reflexes: normal or reduced	—
CMT 2P	LRSAM1	9q33	Onset age: 27–40 y	Clinical Weakness & wasting Distal Legs > arms	Tendon reflexes: reduced	NCV: SNAP & CMAP amplitudes reduced
HMSN-P	—	3q13	17–50 y	Proximal weakness Cramps	Absent	Axon loss
HSMN + Ataxia	—	7q22	13–27 y	Gait ataxia	Absent	Axon loss
CMT 2 P0	P0	1q22	37–61 y	Leg weakness Pupil or hearing	Reduced	<38 m/s to normal
AR-CMT2: Recessive; Axonal						
AR-CMT2A	Lamin A/C	1q21	Second decade	Distal weakness	Reduced	Axon loss
AR-CMT2B	MED25	19q13.3	Third & fourth decade	Distal weakness	Absent distal	Axon loss
AR-CMT2 Ouvrier	—	Autosomal	Onset: early childhood; first decade	Weakness: distal; symmetric; legs before arms Sensory loss: mild Progression: slow; severe distal weakness by 20 y	Reduced	Axon loss

HMSN 3: Infantile

Dejerine-Sottas (HMSN 3)	P0 PMP-22 Periaxin	Autosomal Dominant/ recessive	2 y	Severe weakness	Absent	<10 m/s
Congenital Hypomyelinating Neuropathy	P0 EGR2 PMP-22	Autosomal Recessive	Birth	Severe weakness	Absent	<10 m/s
CMT4: Recessive; Demyelinating						
CMT 4A	GDAP1	8q13	Childhood	Distal weakness	Reduced	Slow
CMT 4B	MTMR2	11q22	2–4 y	Distal & proximal weakness	Absent	Slow
CMT 4B2	SBF2	11p15	First 2 decades	Distal weakness Sensory loss	Absent	15–30 m/s
CMT 4C	KIAA1985	5q23	5–15 y	Delayed walking	Reduced	14–32 m/s
CMT 4D (Lom)	NDRG1	8q24	1–10 y	Gait disorder	Absent	10–20 m/s
CMT 4E	EGR2	10q21	Birth	Infant hypotonia	Absent	9–20 m/s
CMT 4F	Periaxin	19q13	1–3 y	Motor delay	Absent	Absent
CMT 4H	FGD4	12q12	10–24 mo	Walking delay	Absent	<15 m/s
CCFDN	CTDP1	18q23	First or second decade	Distal leg weakness	Reduced	20–34 m/s

Abbreviations: AR, autosomal recessive; CMAP, compound motor action potential; CMT, Charcot-Marie-Tooth disease; CNS, central nervous system; NCV, nerve conduction velocity; SNAP, sensory nerve action potential.

CMT 1

The majority of CMT 1 pedigrees (70%) demonstrate linkage to chromosome 17p11.2-12 and are designated CMT 1A.[72] CMT 1A duplication results in increased expression of peripheral myelin protein-22 (PMP-22). Conduction velocities are uniformly slow in all nerves, with a mean of 17 to 20 m/s and a range 5 to 34 m/s. Onset is typically in the first decade with leg arreflexia, gait disorder (toe walking or steppage gait), foot muscle atrophy or pes cavus, occasionally short Achilles tendons, and enlarged nerves owing to onion-bulb formation in half of patients. Distal weakness develops initially in intrinsic muscles of the feet and hands. Weakness of ankle dorsiflexion, ankle eversion, and extensor hallucis longus develops with more normal strength proximally. Progress cavus foot deformities with clawing of the toes often develops. Orthopedic procedures are limited to soft-tissue procedures and correcting wedge osteotomies, and joint fusion should be avoided if possible to avoid late pain. Late in the disease diaphragm or bulbar weakness may develop in rare cases. Progression is slow over many decades. Defects in the human myelin zero gene (P_0) on chromosome 1q22-q23 leads to CMT 1B. P_0 is the major protein structural component of peripheral nervous system myelin. The clinical presentation is similar to CMT 1A; however, onset may lag into the second to third decade in a minority of patients and there is more variability in severity. Nerve conduction velocities are usually less than 20 m/s. P_0 mutations may lead to other clinical variants referred to as CMT 1E (demyelinating CMT with deafness), and predominantly axonal neuropathy with late adult onset (eg, CMT 2I and CMT 2J with hearing loss and pupillary abnormalities).

CMT 2

CMT 2 is a less common disorder than CMT 1. In general, CMT 2 patients demonstrate later age of onset, less involvement of the small muscles of the hands, and no palpably enlarged nerves. Wasting in the calf and anterior compartment of the leg may give rise to an "inverted champagne bottle" or "stork-leg" appearance. Conduction velocities are mildly reduced, and CMAP and sensory nerve action potential (SNAP) amplitudes are usually reduced. CMT 2A2 with mitofusin abnormality accounts for approximately 20% of CMT 2 probands. CMT 2C linked to chromosome 12q23-q24 has interesting features of early onset in the first decade, and diaphragm and intercostal weakness producing shortness of breath. Vocal cord paralysis may alter the voice of these patients. The disease may progress to proximal and face muscles. Arthrogryposis is present in some patients. Phrenic nerve CMAPs are often reduced. CMT 2E with abnormality in neurofilament light chain linked to chromosome 8p21 may have associated hearing loss in 30% of cases. Although most axonal CMT is autosomal dominant, emerging pedigrees are being identified with recessive inheritance.

CMT 3

Dejerine-Sottas disease (CMT 3) is a severe, hypertrophic, demyelinating polyneuropathy with onset in infancy or early childhood. Most patients achieve ambulation, but some may subsequently progress to wheelchair reliance. Nerve conduction velocities are greatly slowed (often less than 10 m/s), and elevations in CSF protein may be present. Dejerine-Sottas disease may be associated with point mutations in either the PMP-22, P_0, or EGR2 genes.[72] Although this disorder was previously thought to be autosomal recessive, many cases are due to de novo point mutations and actually have dominant inheritance.

Congenital hypomyelinating neuropathy

This severe and often fatal newborn disorder often presents with respiratory distress in the delivery room. These infants often have severe generalized hypotonia and associated arthrogryposis. Diagnostically these infants have absent sensory nerve action potentials (SNAPS) or low-amplitude SNAPS with prolonged distal latencies. CMAPs are either absent or of low amplitude, with motor conduction velocities ranging from 3 to 10 m/s. The disorder has been linked to PMP-22, P_0, and EGR2 genes. Sural nerve biopsy may be useful. Inheritance is usually autosomal recessive, with some dominant inheritance linked to EGR2.

CMT 4

Autosomal recessive CMT 4 is relatively rare. Most cases are demyelinating with more severe phenotypes, and onset is often in childhood. CMT 4C linked to 5q23 is a relatively more common form of CMT 4.

Toxic Neuropathies

Toxic polyneuropathies are rare occurrences in children in North America. Toxic exposure to heavy metals and environmental toxins may be more common in other regions of the world. Expeditious diagnosis is critical in identifying and removing the source of the toxicity and in establishing treatment with agents such as penicillamine.

Arsenic polyneuropathy

Arsenic toxicity produces is a sensorimotor neuropathy that may be axonal or, at times, predominantly demyelinating, simulating Guillain-Barré syndrome or CIDP. Gastrointestinal symptoms are common, as are tachycardia and hypotension. Mee lines may be seen in nails along with other skin changes and alopecia. The diagnosis is established by obtaining levels of arsenic in blood, urine, hair, and nail samples.

Lead polyneuropathy

Lead toxicity is most commonly observed in children who have ingested old lead-based paint. Acute exposures cause lead encephalopathy more commonly. Clinical findings may include anorexia, nausea and vomiting, gastrointestinal disturbance, fatigue, clumsiness and ataxia, and occasionally cognitive impairment, seizures, mental status changes, papilledema, and coma. The weakness is predominantly in the lower limbs, but the upper limbs may be involved. Electrophysiologic studies show a primarily axonal degeneration affecting motor greater than sensory axons. A microcytic hypochromic anemia with basophilic stippling of red blood cells establishes the diagnosis. Lead lines may be evident in long bone films. Lead levels may or may not be elevated in urine and blood, but levels of δ-aminolevulinic acid are usually elevated in the urine.

Mercury poisoning

Mercury poisoning may occur from the ingestion of mercuric salts, exposure to mercury vapor, or use of topical ammonia mercury ointments. Patients present with a generalized encephalopathy, fatigue, and occasionally a rash. A predominantly distal motor axonal neuropathy occurs. DTRs may be absent and the gait is often ataxic. Sensory examination is often normal, although patients may complain of distal paresthesias. Electrophysiologic studies show motor axonal degeneration with normal sensory conduction studies.

Organophosphate poisoning

This entity is caused by exposure to insecticides or high-temperature lubricants or softeners used in the plastic industry. Patients present with an encephalopathy manifested by confusion and coma. After acute exposure cholinergic crisis, manifested by sweating, abdominal cramps, diarrhea, and constricted pupils, may be present. A predominantly motor polyneuropathy is a late effect. However, the disorder may present as a rapidly progressive polyneuropathy mimicking Guillain-Barré syndrome. Severe paralysis with respiratory failure requiring ventilatory support may occur, and in this situation there may be a superimposed postsynaptic defect in neuromuscular transmission.

Glue sniffing (n-hexane)

Glue-sniffing neuropathy may be seen in teenage recreational glue sniffers. Repeated use may cause symptoms and signs of a predominantly distal motor and sensory polyneuropathy, which is predominantly demyelinating. Motor and sensory nerve conduction studies demonstrate moderate slowing.

Chemotherapeutic agents

Vincristine, in particular, often produces a relatively pure motor axonal polyneuropathy. Severity is dose dependent. Clinical findings include distal weakness, absent deep tendon reflexes, and at times foot drop. The disorder is often readily apparent by clinical examination, and electrophysiologic studies or nerve biopsy is usually not necessary. The neuropathy usually improves with discontinuation of the medication, although significant electrophysiologic abnormalities (reduced CMAP amplitudes and neuropathic recruitment) may persist. Vincristine may be particularly troublesome for children with hereditary motor-sensory neuropathy.

Metabolic Neuropathies

Uremic neuropathy

Uremic polyneuropathy often occurs in children and adults with end-stage renal disease. If clinical manifestations are present, they consist of a predominantly distal motor and sensory polyneuropathy with glove-and-stocking loss of sensation, loss of vibratory sense, and distal weakness, particularly involving peroneal innervated musculature. With successful renal transplantation, clinical findings and electrophysiologic abnormalities normalize.

Diabetic polyneuropathy

Diabetes produces is a mixed motor and sensory polyneuropathy with both axonal changes and mild demyelination. The polyneuropathy is less common in children with diabetes mellitus, in comparison with adults. The severity of the neuropathy may be related to the degree of glucose control.[83]

Alcoholic polyneuropathy

Chronic ethanol ingestion produces a polyneuropathy. Studies show that 9% of alcoholics clinically manifest polyneuropathy, with females showing more severe neuropathy. Alcohol abuse is generally severe over years with intakes of greater than 100 g of alcohol per day. Nutritional deficiency and skipped meals exacerbates the neuropathy. Those with ethanol neuropathy show weight loss of 30 to 40 lb (13.5–18 kg) in 50% of cases. The majority show clinical signs of polyneuropathy, but approximately 40% are asymptomatic. Muscles are thin and tender, distal tendon reflexes reduced, and there is variable loss of distal pain and temperature sensation. Patients complain of pain consisting of a dull ache and burning in feet and legs, and occasionally complain of lancinating pains. The distribution of signs is distal and symmetric. hyperesthesia is common. Weakness involves the legs more so than the hands. Tendon reflexes are reduced at the ankle in 80% of cases. Regarding autonomic findings, patients frequently exhibit hyperhidrosis in the feet and hands. Electrodiagnostic studies show distal axonal loss in sensory and motor nerves, small sensory potentials, and mildly slowed conduction velocities. Findings are more severe in the lower extremities. Nerve biopsy shows distal axonal loss. The disease course of the neuropathy shows slow improvement with reduced alcohol intake.

NEUROMUSCULAR JUNCTION TRANSMISSION DISORDERS
Autoimmune Myasthenia Gravis

This disorder is similar to the autoimmune myasthenia gravis observed in adults. The onset is often insidious, but at times patients may present with acute respiratory difficulties. Patients usually present with variable degrees of ophthalmoparesis and ptosis. In addition, patients may exhibit facial weakness, swallowing difficulties, speech problems, and weakness of the neck, trunk, and limbs. Proximal muscles are more affected than distal muscles, and the upper limits are more affected than the lower limits. Fluctuation in the disease course with relapse and remission is common. Patients often complain of fatigue and diplopia, as well as progressive difficulty with chewing or swallowing. Patients are often worse with fatigue toward the end of the day. Thymoma, which occurs in about 10% of adult cases, is not a feature of the childhood-onset disease.

Serum acetylcholine receptor (AChR) antibodies are an important diagnostic screening tool. Anti-AChR antibodies can be detected in the serum in about 85% to 90% of patients with generalized myasthenia gravis and in more than 50% of those with ocular myasthenia. The most common antibodies detected are AChR binding, followed by AChR modulation and then striational AChR antibodies. MUSK antibodies are an additional marker present in some seronegative patients and many patients with ocular myasthenia.

Diagnosis may also be confirmed by clinical response to an anticholinesterase drug such as edrophonium (Tensilon). Alternatively, neostigmine, a longer-acting agent, can be used. Repetitive nerve stimulation studies show a characteristic decrement in the CMAP, with slow stimulation rates (2–5 Hz) over a train of 4 to 5 stimuli. A decrement greater than 12% to 15% is often noted.

Congenital Myasthenia Syndromes

Congenital myasthenia syndromes (CMS) is a term used for a heterogeneous group of disorders that are genetically determined rather than autoimmune mediated. Patients may present in the neonatal period, later in childhood, or even in adult life. Patients often exhibit ptosis, external ophthalmoparesis, facial weakness, general hypotonia, proximal greater than distal muscle weakness, and variable degrees of functional impairment. Patients show absence of anti-AChR antibodies. More than 20 subtypes have been described, and congenital myasthenia may be classified according to the following: (1) presynaptic defects (eg, choline acetyltransferase [ChAT] deficiency causing CMS with episodic apnea; paucity of synaptic vesicles and reduced quantal release; or congenital Lambert-Eaton–like syndrome); (2) synaptic basal lamina defects (eg, endplate acetylcholinesterase [AChE] deficiency at NMJs); and (3) postsynaptic defects (eg, AChR disorders involving α, β, δ, ϵ subunits; kinetic abnormalities in AChR function caused by AChR deficiency; slow AChR channel syndromes; fast-channel syndromes; endplate rapsyn deficiency).

Several congenital myasthenic syndromes have been associated with arthrogryposis syndromes. For example multiple pterygium syndrome (Escobar syndrome) has been associated with AChR γ, $\alpha 1$, and δ subunit mutations.

For diagnostic workup, standard EMG with repetitive nerve stimulation is used initially, and subsequently stimulated single-fiber EMG may be useful. Ultrastructural evaluation of the NMJ with electron microscopy usually is performed on a biopsy of the deltoid or biceps, including the muscle region containing the NMJ or the motor point. For in vitro electrophysiologic and immunocytochemical studies of the NMJ, a short muscle usually is removed from origin to insertion along with its motor branch and NMJ (motor point biopsy). Muscles obtained have included the anconeus muscle near the elbow, the external intercostal muscle in the fifth or sixth intercostal space near the anterior axillary line, or the peroneus tertius muscle in the lower extremity. Such in vitro electrophysiologic studies allow specific delineation of the congenital myasthenic syndrome into one of the numerous specific subtypes. More recently the diagnostic evaluation of CMS has increasingly relied on molecular genetic studies.

For treatment of a CMS subtype a definitive diagnosis is important, because some CMS syndromes deteriorate with empiric treatment with AChE inhibitors such as pyridostigmine (Mestinon). For example, slow-channel syndromes may deteriorate on pyridostigmine, and endplate AChE deficiency may deteriorate or show no response. Some presynaptic syndromes may show response to 3,4-diaminopyridine, which increases release of acetylcholine at the presynaptic terminal. This drug has been used in Lambert-Eaton syndrome and in presynaptic CMS on a compassionate-use basis.

Infantile Botulism

Infants with botulism usually present between 10 days and 6 months of age with an acute onset of hypotonia, dysphagia, constipation, weak cry, and respiratory insufficiency. The neurologic examination shows diffuse hypotonia and weakness, ptosis, ophthalmoplegia with pupillary dilation, reduced gag reflex, and relative preservation of deep tendon reflexes. The diagnosis may be made by electrodiagnostic studies[78] or by measurement *Clostridium botulinum* toxin in a rectal aspirate–containing stool.

Noninfantile Acquired Botulism

Older children and adults acquire botulism through poorly cooked, contaminated food with the toxin or through a cutaneous wound that becomes contaminated with soil-containing *Clostridium botulinum*. The toxin can often be identified in the serum and the food source. Clinical findings include acute onset of constipation, ptosis, diplopia, bulbar weakness, respiratory difficulties, ophthalmoparesis, pupillary dilation, and diminished DTRs. Recovery may take months. The diagnosis is generally made from electrodiagnostic studies.

MYOPATHIES
Dystrophinopathies

Duchenne muscular dystrophy

DMD is an X-linked disorder caused by a gene abnormality at the Xp21 gene loci. The gene codes for dystrophin, which is a protein localized to the intracellular side of the plasma membrane of all myogenic cells, certain types of neurons, and in small amounts of other cell types. Dystrophin deficiency at the plasma membrane of muscle fibers disrupts the membrane cytoskeleton and leads to the secondary loss of other components of the muscle cytoskeleton. The primary consequence of the cytoskeleton abnormalities is membrane instability, leading to membrane injury from mechanical stresses, transient breaches of the membrane, and membrane leakage. Chronic dystrophic myopathy is characterized by aggressive fibrotic replacement of the muscle and eventual failure of regeneration, with muscle fiber death and fiber loss. In general, loss of the reading frame causes complete absence of dystrophin (<5% by Western blot) and a Duchenne phenotype.

While the history of hypotonia and delayed motor milestones are often reported in retrospect, the parents are often unaware of any abnormality until the child starts walking. There has been variability reported in the age of onset.[31,32] In 74% to 80% of instances, the onset has been noted before the age of 4 years.[31,32] The most frequent presenting symptoms have been abnormal gait, frequent falls, and difficulty climbing steps. In DMD the earliest weakness is seen in the neck flexors during preschool years. Parents frequently note the toe walking, which is a compensatory adaptation to knee extensor weakness and a lordotic posture to the lumbar spine, which is a compensatory change attributable to hip extensor weakness (see **Fig. 10**). The vast majority of cases are identified by 5 to 6 years of age. Occasionally, DMD is identified presymptomatically in situations where a CK value is obtained with a markedly elevated value, malignant hyperthermia occurs during general anesthesia for an unrelated surgical indication, or a diagnosis is pursued in a male with an affected older sibling. Difficulty negotiating steps is an early feature, as is a tendency to fall owing to the child tripping or stumbling on a plantar-flexed ankle, or the knee buckling or giving way because of knee extensor weakness. There is progressive difficulty getting up from the floor, with presence of a Gower sign (see **Fig. 9**).

Pain in the muscles, especially the calves, is a common symptom. Enlargement of muscles, particularly the calves (see **Fig. 1**), is commonly noted. The deltoid may also be hypertrophied. The tongue is also frequently enlarged. There is also commonly an associated wide arch to the mandible and maxilla with separation of the teeth, presumably secondary to the macroglossia.

Weakness in DMD is generalized but predominantly proximal early in the disease course. Pelvic girdle weakness predates shoulder girdle weakness by several years. Ankle dorsiflexors are weaker than ankle plantar flexors, ankle everters are weaker than ankle inverters, knee extensors are weaker than knee flexors, hip extensors are weaker than hip flexors, and hip abductors are weaker than hip adductors.[31,32] Molecular genetic studies to confirm DMD are summarized by Arnold and Flanigan[1] elsewhere in this issue, and muscle biopsy immunohistochemistry is summarized by Joyce and collegues[51] in this issue.

Glucocorticoid therapy had become the standard of care in DMD throughout the life span. The past several years have seen a markedly increased interest by pharmaceutical companies in conducting ground-breaking research and development into effective treatment agents for DMD. Therapeutic approaches under development for clinical trials in DMD include antisense oligonucleotide (AON) exon-skipping therapies, gene-therapy strategies, stem-cell therapies, and a host of small-molecule therapies (eg, compounds that induce read-through of premature stop-codon mutations, promotion of muscle growth via myostatin inhibition, utrophin upregulation, and steroid analogues with improved side-effect profiles). Diagnostic and clinical features of DMD are shown in **Table 3**.

Becker muscular dystrophy

In BMD, patients have similar distribution of weakness to those with DMD; however, onset may be delayed to the late first decade, second decade, or in mild BMD the third or fourth decade in some instances. Some patients with BMD may present initially in the late second or third decade with signs of cardiomyopathy with clinically normal strength or mild strength loss. Diagnostic and clinical features of BMD are shown in **Table 3**. In severe BMD, there can be overlap in the age at diagnosis with DMD.[31,32] For cases with a deletion mutation, the "reading-frame" hypothesis predicts that BMD patients with in-frame deletions produce a semifunctional, internally deleted dystrophin protein. Thus DMD patients with frameshift point mutations or "out-of-frame deletions," on the other hand, produce a severely truncated protein that is unstable.

Table 3
Characteristics of dystrophinopathies (DMD and BMD)

	DMD	BMD
USA prevalence (estimated)	15,000	3700–8300
Incidence rate	1/3500 male births	Unknown
Inheritance	X-linked	X-linked
Gene location	Xp21 (reading frame shifted)	Xp21 (reading frame maintained)
Protein	Dystrophin	Dystrophin
Onset	2–6 y	4–12 y (severe BMD) Late teenage to adulthood (mild BMD)
Severity & course	Relentlessly progressive Reduced motor function by 2–3 y Steady decline in strength Life span <35 y	Slowly progressive Severity & onset correlate with muscle dystrophin levels
Ambulation status	Loss of ambulation: 7–13 y (no corticosteroids) Loss of ambulation: 9–15 y (corticosteroids)	Loss of ambulation: >16 y
Weakness	Proximal > Distal Symmetric Legs & arms	Proximal > Distal Symmetric Legs & arms
Cardiac	Dilated cardiomyopathy first to second decade Onset of signs second decade	Cardiomyopathy (may occur before weakness); third to fourth decade frequent
Respiratory	Profoundly reduced vital capacity in second decade Ventilatory dependency in second decade	Respiratory involvement in subset of patients Ventilatory dependency in severe patients
Muscle size	Calf hypertrophy	Calf hypertrophy
Musculoskeletal	Contractures: ankles, hip, knees Scoliosis: onset after loss of ambulation	Contractures: ankles & others in adulthood
CNS	Reduced cognitive ability Reduced verbal ability	Some patients have reduced cognitive ability
Muscle pathology	Endomysial fibrosis and fatty infiltration Variable fiber size & myopathic grouping Fiber degeneration/regeneration Dystrophin: absent Sarcoglycans: secondary reduction	Variable fiber size Endomysial connective tissue and fatty infiltration Fiber degeneration Fiber regeneration Dystrophin: reduced (usually 10%–60% of normal)
Blood chemistry & hematology	CK: Very high (10,000–50,000) High AST & ALT (normal GGT) High aldolase	CK: 5000–20,000 Lower levels with increasing age

Abbreviations: ALT, alanine aminotransferase; AST, aspartate aminotransferase; BMD, Becker muscular dystrophy; CK, creatine kinase; DMD, Duchenne muscular dystrophy; GGT, γ-glutamyltransferase.

Facioscapulohumeral Muscular Dystrophy

FSHD is a slowly progressive dystrophic myopathy with predominant involvement of facial and shoulder girdle musculature. The condition has autosomal dominant inheritance with linkage to the chromosome 4q35 locus. It is the second most common inherited muscular dystrophy in the adult population, with a prevalence estimate of 1 to 5 in 100,000.[84] Overall, FSHD is the third most common of the dystrophies, behind DMD and MMD. Presentation ranges from congenital to late in life, but typical age of presentation is generally before 20 years. Initially, 85% of patients show predominant involvement of facial and shoulder girdle musculature with facial weakness commonly being the initial manifestation. Facial weakness (see **Fig. 6**) typically involves the orbicularis oris, zygomaticus, and orbicularis oculi. Patients often have an expressionless face. Even in the very early stages, forced closure of the eyelids can be easily overcome by the examiner. The patient will typically have difficulty burying the lashes and pursing the lips, smiling, drinking through a straw, or whistling. The face is spared in 5% to 15% of patients who usually exhibit later onset of facial weakness (in the fourth or fifth decade), and often have a smaller deletion. By age 30 years, 95% show facial weakness. The facial weakness predominates in approximately 7% of patients. Masseter, temporalis, extraocular, and pharyngeal muscles are characteristically spared in FSHD. Scapular stabilizers, shoulder abductors, and shoulder external rotators may be significantly affected, but at times the deltoids are surprisingly sparred if tested with the scapulae stabilized. Posterior and lateral scapular winging is common and scapulae are high riding (see **Fig. 4**). The biceps and triceps may both be more affected than the deltoids.[30] Over time, ankle dorsiflexion weakness often becomes significant in addition to pelvic girdle weakness, and some patients (approximately 13%) exhibit ankle dorsiflexion weakness very early in the disease course. Bilateral proximal lower extremity weakness occurs with disease progression, with female gender and larger deletions being risk factors. Late in the disease course of early onset FSHD, patients may show marked wrist extension weakness. Some investigators have found asymmetric weakness in the dominant upper extremity.[30] Lower abdominal weakness leads to a positive Beevor sign in many. Muscles usually spared include bulbar, extraocular, deltoid, and respiratory. Severe respiratory weakness does occur, but fewer than 5% will require ventilatory assistance. Pectus excavatum and progressive thoracolumbar hyperlordosis may occur. Wheelchair reliance occurs in 20% of patients. Prognosis is worse with younger onset. There is linear decline in strength between 20 and 50 years of age, but some reports question that declining strength stabilizes in later life. Life expectancy in FSHD is often normal. Clinical features of FSHD are shown in **Table 4**. Functional consequences for facial weakness include sleeping with eyes open, bulbar dysfunction using straws, blowing up balloons, dysarthria (especially labial consonants), transverse smile, and misinterpretation of patients having a dour or flat affect.

In FSHD with locus at 4q35 (95% of all FSHD), there are 2 different abnormalities in the D4Z4 DNA fragment. In 90% of FSHD patients termed FSHD1, there is deletion in units of the D4Z4 DNA repeat sequence (a D4Z4 contraction) resulting in a reduced D4Z4 fragment size; this allows increased expression of the DUX4 gene in the distal repeat. The D4Z4 contraction produces permissive sequences in the 4qA region distal to the repeats, which allows polyadenylation and stabilization of the distal DUX4 transcript. In some 5% of patients with facioscapulohumeral muscular dystrophy (FSHD), no D4Z4 repeat contraction on chromosome 4q35 is observed. Such patients, termed FSHD2, show loss of DNA methylation and heterochromatin markers at the D4Z4 repeat, similar to patients with D4Z4 contractions (FSHD1).[37] Thus, the D4Z4 DNA

Table 4
Clinical characteristics of facioscapulohumeral muscular dystrophy

	FSHD
USA prevalence (estimated)	15,000
Prevalence rate	1/20,000
Inheritance	70%–90% AD; 10%–30% sporadic
Gene location	4q35
Protein	FSHD1: deletion in units of the D4Z4 DNA repeat sequence (a D4Z4 contraction) FSHD2: N/A
Onset	Mean ~16 y Range: congenital to late age 25%–30% have signs but no symptoms
Severity & course	Variable progression Normal life expectancy Most exhibit weakness by age 20 One-third have no symptoms
Ambulation status	10%–20% become wheelchair dependent by age 50
Weakness	Presents with shoulder girdle and facial muscle weakness; often asymmetric Involvement of abdominal, foot extensor, and pelvic muscles; deltoids spared
Cardiac	Some conduction defects
Respiratory	Small percentage need ventilatory assistance (1%–2%)
Muscle size	Focal atrophy of shoulder girdle and facial muscles
Quality of life	Pain in 70%
Musculoskeletal	Sloped shoulder Scapular winging Mild scoliosis in one-third of patients
CNS	Hearing loss 75% Coats disease 60%
Muscle pathology	Nonspecific chronic myopathy, dystrophic changes Occasional small group of atrophied fibers Occasional moth-eaten fibers Mononuclear inflammatory reaction in 40% of patients
Blood chemistry & hematology	CK: normal to 5 times upper limit of normal range

Abbreviations: AD, autosomal dominant; FSHD, facioscapulohumeral muscular dystrophy; N/A, no data available.

methylation in both FSHD1 and FSHD2 patients is reduced, resulting in an open chromatin structure that polyadenylates and upregulates DUX4 transcriptional activity in the distal repeat. This commonality suggests that a change in D4Z4 chromatin structure and polyadenylated and upregulated DUX4 expression in myoblasts unifies FSHD1 and FSHD2. DUX4 is localized to the nucleus and is toxic by being proapoptotic, is involved in transcriptional regulation, creates sensitivity to oxidative stress, represses MyoD and its target genes diminishing myogenic differentiation, and interferes with Pax7 in satellite cells to inappropriately regulate Pax targets during muscle regeneration.

FSHD2 is identical to FSHD1 in its clinical presentation and clinical features. Notable differences include a higher incidence (67%) of sporadic cases in FSHD2, the absence of gender differences in disease severity in FSHD2, and possibly later symptom onset in FSHD2. Overall, average disease severity in FSHD2 was similar to that reported in FSHD1 and was not influenced by D4Z4 repeat size.[37] However, in FSHD2, a small effect of the degree of hypomethylation on disease severity was observed.[37] In approximately 5% of FSHD-like families, there is no linkage to 4q35.

Limb-Girdle Muscular Dystrophy

Before the advent of genetic testing, a group of patients commonly sharing a progressive pattern of greater proximal than distal muscular weakness with either autosomal dominant (LGMD1) or autosomal recessive (LGMD2) inheritance were said to have LGMDs. Recent advances in molecular and genetic analyses have now identified several distinct genetic mutations in these patients. In the various subtypes of LGMD, those patients with autosomal recessive inheritance (LGMD2) generally have earlier age of onset and are weaker than those with autosomal dominant inheritance and LGMD1. The lower extremities tend to be more affected than upper extremities. In autosomal dominant late-onset LGMD, distal upper extremity muscles tend to show little progressive weakness over the years.[53] In LGMD2, the distribution and pattern of weakness tends to be similar to DMD; however, the rate of progression tends to be slower than that observed in DMD.[31,32,53] In one series,[53] several differences between DMD and LGMD2 (SCARMD) were noted. The limb extensors were not weaker than limb flexors. In particular, ankle dorsiflexors were similar in strength to ankle plantar flexors, knee extensors showed similar strength compared with knee flexors, and hip extensors and hip flexors showed similar strength values. Clinical features of the more common LGMDs are shown in **Tables 5** and **6**.

Emery-Dreifuss Muscular Dystrophy

Emery-Dreifuss muscular dystrophy (EMD) refers to a group of muscular dystrophies with weakness, contractures, and cardiac conduction abnormalities. The inheritance pattern is variable among subtypes.

Emery-Dreifuss muscular dystrophy 1

EMD1 is an X-linked recessive progressive dystrophic myopathy caused by an abnormality of the protein emerin with a gene locus identified at Xq28.[85,86] Patients usually present in the teenage years, but age of presentation can vary from the neonatal period with hypotonia to the third decade. Early elbow flexion contractures are a hallmark of the disease.[86]

Severe contractures, including elbow flexion, ankle equinus, rigid spine, and neck extension contractures, are often more limiting than weakness, which begins in a scapulohumeral peroneal distribution. The biceps and triceps show wasting and weakness, and the deltoids and forearms are more spared. The calf frequently shows wasting. Ankle dorsiflexors often are weaker than ankle plantar flexors, leading to the equinus contractures.[86] Scapular winging is frequent. Tightness of the cervical and lumbar spinal extensor muscles, resulting in limitation of neck and trunk flexion, with inability to flex the chin to the sternum and to touch the toes, also has been reported in EMD. The face is either spared or affected late. Functional difficulties are experienced walking or climbing stairs. Progression is slow, and loss of ambulation is rare. Some cases with EMD1 can have nocturnal hypoventilation as a result of restrictive expansion of the chest in association with the rigid spine, and partly because of involvement of the diaphragm.

Progressive cardiac disease is almost invariably present with onset in the early second decade to the 40s. Arrhythmia can lead to emboli or sudden death in early

Table 5
Characteristics of common autosomal dominant limb-girdle muscular dystrophies (AD-LGMD)

	LGMD 1A	LGMD 1B	LGMD 1C
USA prevalence	4200	2850	675
Inheritance	AD	AD	AD
Gene location	5q31	1q11-q21	3p25
Protein	Myotilin	Lamin A/C	Caveolin-3
Onset	Variable Third to seventh decade Anticipation: age of onset decreases in succeeding generations	<20 y	5 y to adulthood
Severity & course	Slow progression	Slow progression Upper limbs involved by third or fourth decade	Moderate severity and progression Adults with Gower maneuver
Weakness	Legs and arms Symmetric Proximal at onset Early foot drop Distal with disease progression Wrist and finger extensors + deltoid Dysarthria (30%) Facial (17%) Neck extensors in some patients	Lower limb Symmetric Proximal Variant: quadriceps weakness with Arg377His mutation	Proximal

Ambulation status	Late loss of ambulation (>10 y after onset)		Mild: adults continue to ambulate with Gower maneuver
Cardiac	Cardiomyopathy 50% Onset sixth or seventh decade	Cardiomyopathy 62% Atrioventricular conduction block	No cardiomyopathy
Respiratory	Mild restrictive lung disease	Mild restrictive lung disease	Mild restrictive lung disease
Muscle size	—	—	Hypertrophy of calf
Musculoskeletal	Contractures: ankles (30%)	No contractures	Cramps after exercise
CNS	No intellectual defect reported	No intellectual defect reported	No intellectual defect reported
Muscle pathology	Myopathic Variable fiber size Fiber degeneration and regeneration Rimmed vacuoles Normal levels of myotilin or increased immunostaining Reduced laminin-γ1 Type I predominance with increasing weakness Normal dystrophin & sarcoglycan	Laminin A subcellular localization: Normal: nucleus; colocalizes with emerin Mutated: may aggregate in nucleus & be present in cytoplasm	Myopathic Reduced caveolin-3 staining: no 21-kDa band on Western blot
Blood chemistry	CK: 1–15 times normal; commonly twice normal	CK: normal to mildly elevated	CK: 4–25 times normal

Table 6
Characteristics of common autosomal recessive limb-girdle muscular dystrophies (AR-LGMD)

	LGMD 2A	LGMD 2B	LGMD 2C	LGMD 2D	LGMD 2E	LGMD 2F	LGMD 2G	LGMD 2I
USA prevalence	4200	2850	675	1260	675	105		450
Inheritance	AR	AR	AR	AR	AR	AR	AR	AR
Gene location	4p21	2p12-14	13q12	17q21	4q12	5q33	17q12	19q13.3
Protein	Calpain-3	Dysferlin	γ-Sarcoglycan	α-Sarcoglycan (adhalin)	β-Sarcoglycan	δ-Sarcoglycan	Telethonin	Fukutin-related protein
Onset	Early <12 y Leyden-Möbius type: 13-29 y Late: >30 y	12-39 y Mean 19 ± 3 y	Mean 5-6 y C283Y mutation: <2 y	2-15 y	3 y-teens Intrafamilial variability	2-10 y	Mean 12.5 y Range 9-15 y	0.5-27 y 61% less than 5 y
Severity & course	Variable Mild phenotype in majority Early onset has more severe progression	Slow progression Mild weakness	Variable progression (some like DMD; others like BMD) Death common in second decade	Variable Absent adhalin: rapid progression Reduced adhalin: later onset & milder weakness	Moderate progression & severity	Rapid progression Death in second decade	Slow progression Mild weakness	Variable Early onset: nonambulant by teens Later onset: slowly progressive
Ambulation status	Loss of ambulation 10-30 y after onset	Loss of ambulation 10-30 y after onset; most walk until their fourth decade	Loss of ambulation: 10-37 y. (mean 16 y)	Early onset: loss of adhalin Later onset: reduced adhalin	Often in wheelchair by 10-15 y; usually by 25 y	Loss of ambulation: 9-16 y	40% nonambulatory in third to fourth decade	30% nonambulant by fourth to sixth decade
Weakness	Scapula pelvic girdle and trunk weakness Proximal legs > arms	Weakness in gastrocnemius, quadriceps & psoas Weakness in biceps after legs	Proximal > distal Patchy distribution with some mutations Quadriceps: spared	Proximal > distal Symmetric quadriceps weakness	Proximal	Proximal Symmetric	Arms: proximal Legs: proximal and distal (foot drop)	Proximal > distal Legs: proximal Arms: proximal Face: mild weakness in older patients
Cardiac	No involvement	No involvement	Occasional; especially late in disease course	Dilated cardiomyopathy	Occasional cardiomyopathy	Dilated cardiomyopathy described; may occur without myopathy	Cardiac involvement in 55% of patients	Dilated cardiomyopathy in 30%-50% of patients

Respiratory	Variable respiratory involvement; some severe	Variable respiratory involvement	Variable respiratory involvement	Variable respiratory involvement	Functional vital capacity ranges from normal to severe	Functional vital capacity ranges from normal to severe	Rarely involved	Rarely involved: PFTs rarely <80% of normal
Muscle size	Calf, tongue and thigh hypertrophy; Wasting in regions of weakness	Calf hypertrophy 50%; Calf atrophy 50%	Calf hypertrophy; Cramps	Prominent muscle hypertrophy	Calf hypertrophy in some patients	Hypertrophy of calf & tongue in some patients	Hypertrophy: uncommon	Limbs, pelvic & shoulder; Atrophy of posterior compartments
Musculoskeletal	Contractures in ankles (especially in nonambulant); Scoliosis		Scapular winging	Shoulders: scapular winging & muscle wasting	Scapular winging	Lumbar hyperlordosis; Scapular winging	Contractures: calf (toe walking may be presenting sign)	Contractures: calf (toe walking may be presenting sign)
CNS	No intellectual defect reported	No intellectual defect reported	No intellectual defect reported	No intellectual defect reported	No intellectual defect reported	No intellectual defect reported; Hearing loss	No intellectual defect reported	Intelligence: normal to mild mental retardation
Muscle pathology	Myopathic; Necrosis & degeneration; Variable fiber size; Connective tissue; Type 1 fiber predominance; ↓ Staining for adhalin	Myopathic; Fiber degeneration; Fiber regeneration; Rimmed vacuoles; Telethonin absent from muscle	Myopathic; Fiber degeneration; Fiber regeneration; δ-Sarcoglycan absent; Other sarcoglycans absent or reduced	Myopathic; Sarcoglycans: usually absent; Dystrophin: often reduced, but not absent	Myopathic; Degeneration & regeneration; Variable fiber size; ↑ Endomysial connective tissue; Myopathic grouping of fibers; Absent or reduced adhalin & α-sarcoglycan	Myopathic; Inflammation: occasional; Severe disease: absent; Slowly progressive; Reduced γ-sarcoglycan; Dystrophin: normal or reduced	Myopathic; Necrosis & degeneration with variable fiber size; ↑ Endomysial connective tissue; Absent or ↑ dysferlin staining; Normal dystrophin & sarcoglycan	Myopathic; Necrosis & regeneration with fiber size variability; Endomysial fibrosis; Type I predominance with increasing weakness; Normal dystrophin & sarcoglycan
Blood chemistry	CK: very high (1000–8000)	CK: 3–30 times normal	CK: 10–50 times normal	CK: very high (often >5000)	CK: very high (often >5000)	CK: very high	CK: 10–72 times normal	CK: 7–80 times normal

Abbreviations: AR, autosomal recessive; PFT, pulmonary function test.

adult life. The cardiomyopathy can progress to left ventricular myocardial dysfunction or 4-chamber dilated cardiomyopathy resulting from fibrosis with complete heart block and ventricular arrhythmias.[85,86] Atrial arrhythmia usually appears before complete heart block. Frank syncope can develop in the late second and early third decades, and patients often require a cardiac pacemaker by age 30 (with an indication being bradycardia with heart rate <50). Electrocardiograph (ECG) changes include slow heart rate, absent or small P waves, atrioventricular block, and atrial fibrillation/flutter.[85,86] Evidence of cardiac arrhythmia often requires 24-hour Holter monitoring. A significant percentage of female carriers have conduction defects and arrhythmias; therefore they warrant monitoring with annual ECGs.

Laboratory evaluation is usually done with molecular genetic studies and/or muscle biopsy. Serum CK is mildly elevated to less than 10 times normal, and levels decrease with age. Muscle biopsy reveals emerin loss by immunohistochemistry in more than 95% of patients.

Emery-Dreifuss muscular dystrophy 2

EMD2 is caused by a lamin A/C protein abnormality and has been linked to chromosome 1q21.2. Inheritance can be dominant or recessive, and lamin A/C mutations can be either frameshift or missense.[85] Those with missense mutations have childhood onset with a mean age of onset of 2.4 years. Weakness is in a scapuloperoneal distribution. Patients demonstrate paravertebral weakness or rigidity, and tendon contractures are common. Those with frameshift mutations producing a truncated protein have adult onset with mean age of 30.5 years, and cardiomyopathy is more frequent than weakness.[85] Contractures are rare, and weakness is in a limb girdle distribution. The disorder is allelic with autosomal dominant LGMD 1B.

Congenital Muscular Dystrophy

The term congenital muscular dystrophy has been widely used for a group of infants presenting with hypotonia, muscle weakness at birth or within the first few months of life, congenital contractures, and immunohistochemical findings of dystrophic changes on muscle biopsy: muscle fiber necrosis and regeneration, increased endomysial connective tissue, and replacement of muscle with fat tissue. The early contractures might include equinovarus deformities, knee flexion contractures, hip flexion contractures, and tightness of the wrist flexors and long finger flexors. The contractures can become more severe over time, with prolonged static positioning and lack of adequate passive range of motion and splinting/positioning. Classic congenital muscular dystrophies are clinically confined to the musculoskeletal system, but other congenital muscular dystrophies, including muscle-eye-brain disease and Walker-Warburg syndrome, are characterized by significant cerebral neuronal migration defects and eye abnormalities. Classic congenital muscular dystrophies are further subdivided according to the presence or absence of merosin (laminin 2).[16] An additional subgroup with collagen VI abnormalities has been identified and referred to as Ullrich congenital muscular dystrophy (see **Fig. 12**).

Congenital Myopathies

The term congenital myopathy is used to describe a group of heterogeneous disorders usually presenting with infantile hypotonia as a result of genetic defects causing primary myopathies.[87] There is an absence of any structural abnormality of the CNS or peripheral nerves. A specific diagnosis of each entity is made based on specific histologic and electron microscopic changes found on muscle biopsy. Molecular genetic studies are increasingly being used to confirm subtypes diagnostically.[87]

Although patients can be hypotonic during early infancy, they later develop muscle weakness that is generally nonprogressive and static. The weakness is predominantly proximal, symmetric, and in a limb girdle distribution. The serum CK values are frequently normal, and the EMG can be normal or might show mild, nonspecific changes, usually of a myopathic character (small amplitude polyphasic potentials). The only congenital myopathy consistently associated with spontaneous activity is myotubular (centronuclear) myopathy. In this disorder, the EMG reveals myopathic motor unit action potentials with frequent complex repetitive discharges and diffuse fibrillation potentials. These myopathies can be considered primarily structural in nature, and patients do not actively lose muscle fibers, as is the case in dystrophic myopathies. Examples include central core myopathy, nemaline myopathy, centronuclear (myotubular) myopathy (non X-linked), Severe X-linked centronuclear (myotubular) myopathy, and congenital fiber-type size disproportion.

Myotonic Disorders

Myotonic muscular dystrophy type 1

DM1 is an autosomal dominant multisystem muscular dystrophy with an incidence of 1 in 8000.[84] It represents the most common inherited NMD of adults. The disorder affects skeletal muscle, smooth muscle, myocardium, brain, and ocular structures. Associated findings include baldness and gonadal atrophy (in males), cataracts, and cardiac dysrhythmias. Insulin insensitivity can be present. The gene has been localized to the region of the myotonin-protein kinase (DMPK) gene at 19q13.3. Patients demonstrate expansion of an unstable CTG trinucleotide repeat within the region. Molecular genetic testing is available for diagnosis. Normal individuals generally have fewer than 37 repeats, which are transmitted from generation to generation. DM1 patients can have 50 to several thousand CTG repeats with remarkable instability. The age of onset is inversely correlated to the number of repeat links.[73] Mild, late-onset DM1 usually is associated with 50 to 150 repeats; classic adolescent or young adult-onset DM1 shows 100 to 1000 repeats; and congenital DM1 patients show more than 1000 repeats (see **Fig. 11**).

The expanded CTG repeat further expands as it is transmitted to successive generations, providing a molecular basis for genetic anticipation. Several characteristic facial features of DM1 can be noted on inspection. The adult with long-standing DM1 often has characteristic facial features. The long thin face shows temporal and masseter wasting. Adult males often exhibit frontal balding. Myotonia, which is a state of delayed relaxation or sustained contraction of skeletal muscle, is easily identified in school-aged children, adolescents, and adults with DM1. Grip myotonia can be demonstrated by delayed opening of the hand with difficult extension of the fingers after tight grip. Percussion myotonia can be elicited by percussion of the thenar eminence with a reflex hammer, giving an adduction and flexion of the thumb with slow return (see **Fig. 8**). Symptomatic myotonia can be treated with agents such as mexiletine or membrane stabilizers such as carbamazepine or phenytoin sodium, which have been shown to affect the symptoms. The treated patients, however, have shown little functional gain.[88,89]

DM1 is one of the few dystrophic myopathies with greater distal weakness than proximal weakness, and weakness initially is often most predominant in the ankle dorsiflexors, ankle everters and inverters, and hand muscles. Neck flexors, shoulder girdle musculature, and pelvic girdle musculature can become significantly involved over decades. As with other dystrophic myopathies, significant muscle wasting can occur over time. In DM1 patients with infantile onset, a congenital club foot or talipes equinovarus is a fairly common deformity. Many novel pharmacologic agents are on the horizon (eg, antisense oligonucleotides) to decrease organ system effects from the trinucleotide repeat expansion and resultant RNA toxicity.

Proximal myotonic myopathy (DM2)

Proximal myotonic myopathy, also referred to as MMD 2 (DM2), is a disorder with clinical similarities to DM1.[90] The abnormal protein in this autosomal dominant disorder is the zinc finger protein 9 with genetic loci at chromosome 3q21. Clinical severity is unrelated to variable size CCTG repeats. The prognosis is more benign than DM1, and there is not a severe congenital-onset form. Onset is 8 to 60 years of age, and there is intrafamilial variability. Patients present with muscle stiffness and pain. Weakness involves the proximal legs (hip flexors and extensors) more than the proximal arms. The distal arms (particularly the thumb and finger flexors) can also show involvement early in the course of the disease. Facial weakness is seen in a minority of patients. Respiratory muscles and distal legs are not clinically affected. A hallmark is the enlargement of calf muscles. Muscle pain is present in proximal muscle groups, is induced by palpation, occurs with exercise or at rest, and is unrelated to the myotonia. The myotonia is induced with grip or percussion in distal upper extremities, and is often asymmetric. The myotonia in DM2 increases with warmth and decreases with cold. Cataracts are noted on slit-lamp examination in all patients older than 20 years. Cardiac conduction defects are present in 20%, diabetes mellitus in 20%, and hearing loss in 20%. MRI shows white matter hyperintensity on T2-weighted images. CK is normal to less than 10 times elevated. EMG shows profound myotonia, and CMAP amplitudes increment by 60% with exercise and reduce by 40% with rest. No decrement is noted on short bouts of exercise or slow or rapid repetitive stimulation. Myopathic motor units are seen proximally. MRI shows selective muscle involvement of the erector spinae and gluteus maximus. Diagnosis is confirmed by molecular genetic studies. A comparison of DM1 with the less common DM2 subtype is shown in **Table 7**.

Myotonia congenita

Myotonia congenita (Thomsen disease) presents in infancy and is inherited as an autosomal dominant condition. An abnormality of the muscle chloride channel is observed, and the disease is linked to the 7q35 loci. There is variable penetrance. Symptoms can be present from birth but usually develop later. The myotonia is relatively mild, and can be manifest as difficulty in releasing objects or difficulty walking or climbing stairs. Most patients do not show overt weakness. Functional difficulties in climbing stairs can be present. The myotonia is exacerbated by prolonged rest or inactivity. A "warm-up" phenomenon with reduced myotonia is noted after repeated activity. The myotonia can be aggravated by cold, hunger, fatigue, and emotional upset. Patients can demonstrate grip myotonia or lid lag after upward gaze or squint, and diplopia after sustained conjugate movement of the eyes in one direction. Nearly all have electrical myotonia on EMG, but there is a warm-up phenomenon with the myotonia reduced after a period of maximal contraction. Half of individuals also have percussion myotonia. Patients can be symptom-free for weeks to months. The other common feature of myotonia congenita is muscle hypertrophy. Patients can exhibit a "Herculean" appearance. Patients have shown some benefit from treatment with quinine, mexiletine, phenytoin, procainamide, carbamazepine, and acetazolamide.

A recessive form of myotonia congenita (Becker form) also exists, with later onset (age 4–12 years), more marked myotonia, more striking hypertrophy of muscles, and associated weakness of muscles, particularly with short bouts of exercise. EMG shows myotonia in distal muscles and less myotonia after maximal contraction.

Table 7
Comparison of myotonic muscular dystrophy (DM) types 1 and 2

Feature	DM1	DM2
General		
Epidemiology	Widespread	European
Onset age	0 to Adult	8–60 y
Anticipation	+	Mild
Congenital form	+	Rare
Muscle		
Weakness		
Face	+	Mild
Ptosis	+	Mild
Sternomastoid	+	Variable
Proximal legs	Late	Early
Distal	+	Hands
Any location	+	+
Muscle pain	±	+
Myotonia	+	+
Calf hypertrophy	−	+
Systemic		
Cataracts	+	+
Balding	+	+
Cardiac arrhythmias	+	Variable
Gonadal failure	+	20%
Hypersomnia	+	Variable
Hyperhidrosis	Variable	+
Cognitive disorder	Mild to severe	Mild
Laboratory		
Hyperglycemia	+	20%
EMG: myotonia	+	+
Muscle		
Internal nuclei	Varied	Type 2 fibers
Chromosome	19q13.3	3q21
Mutated gene	DMPK	ZNF9
Mutation type	CTG repeats	CCTG repeats
Repeat size	100–4000	Mean ~5000
CNS MRI Δ	White & gray matter	White matter

Abbreviations: EMG, electromyography; MRI, magnetic resonance imaging.
From Pestronk A. Neuromuscular Disease Center Web site. St Louis (MO): Washington University; 2011. Available at: http://neuromuscular.wustl.edu.

On repetitive stimulation there is a decremental CMAP response at high stimulation frequency (30 Hz) and after exercise. The recessive form seems less prone to aggravation of the myotonia by cold. Diagnosis is suspected based on clinical information and the presence of classic myotonic discharges on EMG. Diagnosis is confirmed with molecular genetic testing.

Paramyotonia congenita

Paramyotonia congenita is an autosomal dominant myotonic condition with at least 2 distinct genetic causes. One involves the sodium channel α subunit located at chromosome 17q35, and the other a muscle chloride channel located at chromosome 7q35. The worsening of the myotonia with exercise is referred to as paradoxic myotonia. Weakness or stiffness can occur together or separately; there is cold and exercise aggravation, hypertrophy of musculature, and more severe involvement of hands and muscles of the face and neck. Myotonic episodes usually subside within a matter of hours but can last for days. Some patients become worse with a potassium load. On electrodiagnostic studies there is a drop in CMAP amplitude with cooling. Dense fibrillations disappear below 28°C; myotonic bursts disappear below 20°C; and electrical silence can occur below 20°C.

Treatment has involved mexiletine or tocainide.

Schwartz-Jampel syndrome (chondrodystrophic myotonia)

Schwartz-JAMPEL syndrome is an autosomal recessive disorder with myotonia, dwarfism, diffuse bone disease, narrow palpebral fissures, blepharospasm, micrognathia, and flattened facies. Onset is usually before age 3. Patients have respiratory and feeding difficulties with impaired swallowing. Limitation of joint movement can be present along with skeletal abnormalities, including short neck and kyphoscoliosis. Muscles are typically hypertrophic and clinically stiff. A characteristic facies with pursed lips, micrognathia, and small mouth is seen. Patients can be difficult to intubate. Ocular changes include myopia and cataracts. Hirsutism and small testes can also be seen. The symptoms are not progressive. The protein perlecan with gene loci at chromosome 1p34-p36 has been implicated.

Electrodiagnostic studies show continuous electrical activity with electrical silence being difficult to obtain. Relatively little waxing and waning in either amplitude or frequency of complex repetitive discharges is observed. Abnormal sodium-channel kinetics in the sarcolemma of muscle has been demonstrated. Some therapeutic benefit has been reported with procainamide and carbamazepine.

Inflammatory Myopathies

The hallmark of an inflammatory myopathy is the predominance of inflammatory cells on muscle biopsy. The 3 primary types are polymyositis, dermatomyositis, and IBM. Although each is distinct, this group of myopathies is thought to involve immune mediated processes possibly triggered by environmental factors in genetically susceptible individuals. Dermatomyositis and polymyositis can be associated with disorders of the heart and lung, as well as neoplasms. An inflammatory myopathy can also be present as part of a multisystem disorder in other connective tissue diseases, most commonly scleroderma, systemic lupus erythematosus, mixed connective tissue disease, and Sjögren syndrome. Overall, the age of onset for idiopathic inflammatory myopathies is bimodal, with peaks between 10 and 15 years of age in children and between 45 and 60 years in adults. Women are affected twice as often, with the exception of IBM, which is twice as common in men. It is important to diagnose accurately and in a timely fashion for both dermatomyositis and polymyositis, because treatment is available and the prognosis depends on early initiation of immunotherapy.

Dermatomyositis

Characteristic features of dermatomyositis include muscle weakness that can present acutely, subacutely, or insidiously, along with a characteristic rash. This violaceous, scaling rash typically involves the eyelids and occurs with periorbital edema, termed a heliotrope rash. Other common locations for the rash are the dorsum of the hands, extensor surfaces of the knees and elbows, and ankles. Myalgias might or might not be present. The weakness initially involves the proximal musculature and can progress to the distal muscles. Pharyngeal muscle involvement is evident from the frequent finding of dysphagia or dysphonia. Other manifestations include cardiac dysrhythmias and cardiomyopathy, joint arthralgias, and interstitial lung disease. There appears to be an association between dermatomyositis and occult carcinoma in adults, and a judicious workup for carcinoma is advisable in newly diagnosed adult patients. Childhood dermatomyositis differs somewhat from the adult version because of the higher incidence of vasculitis, ectopic calcification in the subcutaneous tissues or muscle, and lipodystrophy. Corticosteroids alone are often highly effective in both inducing a remission and preventing a recurrence, and can usually be gradually withdrawn. Adults with dermatomyositis do not respond to corticosteroids so predictably, and other immunosuppressive agents are often required. It can be difficult to fully discontinue pharmacologic treatment.

Polymyositis

The diagnosis of polymyositis is often more difficult to make than dermatomyositis because no distinctive rash is present. Polymyositis rarely occurs before age 20 years. Proximal limb and neck flexor muscle weakness presenting subacutely or insidiously should raise suspicion for polymyositis. Myalgias are present in as many as one-third of patients but are not generally the predominant symptom. CK elevation usually occurs at some point in the disease and is generally a reasonable indicator of disease severity. CK can be normal in advanced cases, with significant muscle atrophy. Needle EMG shows a classic triad of abnormal spontaneous rest activity, myopathic motor unit action potentials with early myopathic recruitment, and complex repetitive discharges. Increasingly MRI of affected muscles with both T2 and short-tau inversion recovery images is used diagnostically for polymyositis and dermatomyositis.[88] Muscle biopsies must be interpreted with caution because of the potential for sampling error. Potential cardiac and pulmonary manifestations are similar to those of dermatomyositis.

Underlying carcinoma might less commonly occur than with dermatomyositis in adults. Treatment is primarily with corticosteroids supplemented by other immunosuppressive medications.

Inclusion body myositis

A third type of inflammatory myopathy with a different pattern of involvement is termed IBM because of the presence of both inflammatory cells and vacuolated muscle fibers with nuclear and cytoplasmic fibrillary inclusions. IBM is now recognized as the most common myopathy in patients aged more than 50 years.[91] Males are affected more than females. IBM has distinctive involvement of both proximal and distal musculature. In particular, the wrist and finger flexors are often more affected than the extensors, and the quadriceps can be affected out of proportion to other muscle groups. About one-third have dysphagia, and the disease can be mistaken for ALS because age of onset is frequently after 50 years. IBM is relentlessly progressive in most cases, sometimes to the point of requiring a wheelchair for mobility. Unfortunately it is not responsive to immunosuppressive medications, and treatment primarily involves appropriate rehabilitation interventions such as provision of assistive devices. For sporadic nonhereditary IBM, clinical trials are on the horizon using small molecules that produce anabolic effects through varied approaches to induce inhibition of myostatin. In addition, follistatin gene therapy will also soon be evaluated in trials.

Metabolic Myopathies

Inborn errors of glycogen metabolism and fatty acid metabolism can result in neuro-muscular disorders. The major clinical presentations include fixed and progressive weakness, or exercise intolerance, cramps, myalgias, and myoglobinuria. Fixed and progressive weakness can be caused by glycogenoses (acid maltase deficiency or Pompe disease, debrancher deficiency, brancher deficiency, and aldolase A deficiency) or disorders of lipid metabolism (primary systemic carnitine deficiency, primary myopathic carnitine deficiency, secondary carnitine deficiency, short-chain acylcoenzyme A synthetase deficiency, medium-chain acylocoenzyme A synthetase dehydrogenase deficiency, and so forth). Exercise intolerance, cramps/myalgias, and myoglobinuria can be caused by glycogenoses (myophosphorylase deficiency or McArdle disease, phosphorylase kinase deficiency, phosphofructokinase deficiency, phosphoglycerate mutase deficiency, and so forth), disorders of lipid metabolism (CPT2 deficiency, VLCAD deficiency, TP deficiency, and so forth), and respiratory chain defects (coenzyme Q10 deficiency, complex I deficiency, complex III deficiency, and complex IV deficiency). Three prototypical metabolic myopathies, namely McArdle disease, Pompe disease, and CPT2 deficiency, deserve special mention.

Myophosphorylase deficiency (McArdle disease)

The most common glycogen storage disease is myophosphorylase deficiency, also known as McArdle disease or glycogenosis type 5. The autosomal recessive disorder has been linked to chromosome 11q13, and more than 65 different disease-causing mutations have been identified. Initial onset of symptoms often occurs during child-hood and consists of poor endurance, fatigue, and exercise-induced cramps and myalgia that mainly affect active muscle groups. Myoglobinuria can also be absent during childhood with prevalence of fixed muscle weakness increasing as the patient ages. Symptoms can be precipitated by activities such as lifting heavy weights or climbing long flights of stairs. The "second-wind" phenomenon is characteristic of this disorder. With the onset of myalgia, patients who rest briefly are then able to continue their physical activity with few or no symptoms. The normal function of muscle myophosphorylase is to catalyze the removal of 1,4-glycosyl residues from glycogen to produce glucose-1-phosphate.

This absence leads to decreased metabolic substrate for glycolysis to produce adenosine triphosphate. CK is persistently elevated between episodes of myoglobinu-ria. EMG is normal when patients are asymptomatic but can show myotonic discharges and fibrillation potentials during an acute attack. Nonischemic forearm exercise testing shows only an increase in ammonia and stable levels of lactic acid and pyruvate. The diagnosis is made by demonstrating absence of myophosphorylase on muscle biopsy or by genetic mutation analysis. Possible treatments include high-protein diet, pyridoxine, and creatine monohydrate.

Acid maltase deficiency (glycogenosis type 2, Pompe disease)

Acid maltase deficiency is also referred to as glycogenosis type 2 or Pompe disease. It is caused by a deficiency of acid α-1,4-glucosidase (GAA). Inheritance is autosomal recessive with linkage to chromosome 17q23. Disease incidence is 1 in 40,000 to 50,000 live births. The level of residual enzyme activity correlates with the severity of disease. The GAA activity is less than 1% for those with infantile onset (birth to 1 year), 2% to 6% for childhood and juvenile onset (1 year to teens), and 1% to 29% in those with adult onset (third decade or later). All patients have glycogen accu-mulation in tissues. In those with infantile onset, clinical symptoms and signs usually include hypotonia, weakness, cardiomegaly, congestive heart failure, and arrhythmia.

Liver and pulmonary involvement is also noted. Death occurs within the first year of life in 80% to 95% of untreated patients. In childhood onset there is mildly enlarged tongue, symmetric proximal weakness, and calf hypertrophy. Death occurs between 3 and 24 years as a result of respiratory failure. Glycogen accumulation is observed mainly in muscle. Patients with adult-onset Pompe disease present with proximal lower extremity weakness and restrictive lung disease. Sleep-disordered breathing is common. Expiration is more involved than inspiration because of chest wall muscle involvement. Nocturnal noninvasive ventilation is occasionally necessary. Atrophy of paraspinous muscles and scapular winging is seen. The disease course is one of slow progression over years. Pain, fatigue, and cramps are common complaints. There can be mild calf hypertrophy and diffuse muscle atrophy more proximally. Progressive disability is related to disease duration rather than age of onset. Eventually respiratory involvement is common, and many patients need wheelchairs or walking devices. Death is most often the result of respiratory failure.

This diagnosis is one the neuromuscular specialist, neurologist, or physiatrist does not want to miss, because it is a potentially treatable disorder. The diagnosis of Pompe disease is confirmed with either molecular genetic studies or biochemical analysis of acid maltase activity with muscle biopsy. New methods using blood samples to measure GAA activity, however, are rapidly becoming adopted because of their speed and convenience.[92,93] Typically serum CK is elevated (<10 times) in infants and is less elevated in adults. The EMG findings include an irritative myopathy with fibrillations, complex repetitive discharges, and myotonic discharges. Treatment now involves enzyme replacement with intravenous administration of recombinant α-glucosidase (Myozyme). Better outcomes are seen with earlier initiation of therapy. Myozyme has been shown to benefit infantile disease and possibly late-onset disease. Improvement is noted in strength of distal and proximal muscles, pulmonary function, cardiomyopathy, and increased survival.[88,94]

Carnitine palmitoyltransferase II deficiency

Carnitine palmitoyltransferase II (CPT2) is a rare autosomal recessive disorder of mitochondrial fatty acid oxidation and represents the most common metabolic cause of repeated myoglobinuria. The CPT2 protein mediates transport of fatty acid–CoA across the inner mitochondrial membrane and is involved in fatty acid β-oxidation. The metabolic defect promotes glycogen depletion in the adolescent and adult later-onset form of this recessive and semidominant disease (linked to chromosome 1p32.3). The disease is characterized by muscle stiffness, myalgia, cramps, and exercise intolerance. Rhabdomyolysis is triggered by activities requiring fatty acid oxidation, prolonged exercise, cold, a low-carbohydrate/high-fat diet, fasting, infections, and treatment with valproate. Other symptoms include malaise and asthenia. The attack frequency has been shown to be reduced by behavior modification. With regard to overt myopathy early in the disease course, patients show normal strength between attacks, but later in the disease course patients may show weakness on examination. Males are more commonly symptomatic than females (80% of presenting patients are typically males). Patients may develop renal failure with rhabdomyolysis episodes. Laboratory studies show the serum CK to be normal or mildly elevated (50%) between episodes and high with rhabdomyolysis. Serum long-chain acylcarnitine shows a high ratio of (palmitoylcarnitine (C16:0) + oleoylcarnitine (C18:1))/Acetylcarnitine (C2), and the serum carnitine is usually normal. When fasting there is a normal increase in ketone bodies and no myoglobinuria. Intravenous glucose administration improves exercise tolerance; however, oral glucose is not effective. The EMG is myopathic or normal. Muscle biopsy shows normal or varied fiber size (small type 1) and type 2 muscle-fiber predominance. Lipid is increased in muscle fibers (50% increased). The CPT activity is reduced by 80% to 90% in homozygotes.

Treatment emphasizes a low-fat, high-carbohydrate diet with frequent meals. In addition, patients should avoid exercise with fasting or infection. General anesthesia should provide intravenous glucose before and during procedures. For specific treatment a diet with triheptanoin (anaplerotic) at 30% to 35% of total daily caloric intake is recommended. In one study no one experienced rhabdomyolysis or hospitalizations while on the diet. All patients returned abnormal SF-36 physical composite scores and returned to normal levels, which persisted for the duration of the therapy in all symptomatic patients.[95] In a pilot study of 6 patients,[96] it was found that bezafibrate, a commonly used hypolipidemic drug, restored the capacity for normal fatty acid oxidation in muscle cells from patients with a mild form of CPT2 deficiency by stimulating the expression of the mutated gene. Bezafibrate was administered for 6 months (at a dose of 3 200-mg tablets per day) and the primary end point was the level of fatty acid oxidation in skeletal muscle biopsy. After bezafibrate treatment, the values of fatty acid oxidation increased significantly in the 6 patients (by 60%–284%), and CPT2 messenger RNA in skeletal muscle increased in all patients (by 20%–93%), as did the CPT2 protein level.[96] These findings were consistent with the increased oxidation levels. Patient-reported outcomes in physical function and bodily pain also improved.

Mitochondrial Encephalomyopathies

Mitochondrial encephalomyopathies, also referred to as mitochondrial cytopathy, represent a complex group of disorders that affect multiple organ systems. Mitochondria are essential cellular organelles that convert carbohydrates, lipids, and proteins into usable energy in the form of adenosine triphosphate via an aerobic metabolism. Although the human mitochondrial genome is only 16.5 kilobase pairs and encodes 13 proteins, many different clinical syndromes can result from mutations of these genes. Mutant mitochondrial DNA can be present in different proportions in various cell populations in a phenomenon known as heteroplasmy . The pathogenic effect of the mutation is only manifested when a critical level of mutation is reached. Mutant and normal mitochondrial DNA segregate randomly during cell division, changing the proportion of mutant DNA in different cells over time. All mitochondria and mitochondrial DNA are derived from the mother's oocyte. A family history compatible with maternal inheritance is strong evidence for a primary mitochondrial DNA mutation. Different family members in the maternal lineage can be asymptomatic or oligospermatic. Of the many clinical features of mitochondrial disorders that involve multiple organ systems, some are frequently present together and should alert the clinician to a mitochondrial etiology. Ptosis and PEO are hallmarks of Kearns-Sayre syndrome, which produces diplopia and blurred vision. Myopathy is common among patients with mitochondrial disorders. Neck flexors can be affected earlier and more severely than neck extensors. Progressive fixed proximal weakness is more common, and patients can develop decreased muscle bulk. Premature fatigue, exercise intolerance, myalgia, and recurrent myoglobinuria can be symptoms of mitochondrial disorders. Serum lactate and pyruvate often are elevated at rest, and these levels can increase significantly after moderate exercise. Sensorineural hearing loss is frequently associated with mitochondrial encephalomyopathies. The hearing loss can be asymmetric and fluctuating in severity. Maternally inherited deafness and diabetes is another phenotypic combination in patients with mitochondrial DNA mutations. Dementia can be a prominent feature in mitochondrial cytopathy.

The diagnostic workup of a mitochondrial disorder often includes a complete blood count, serum electrolytes (including calcium and phosphate), liver function tests, blood urea nitrogen, creatinine, blood lactate and pyruvate, ECG, lumbar puncture for CSF protein, glucose, lactate, and pyruvate, EMG and nerve conduction study, brain imaging with MRI, and muscle biopsy for histology and electron microscopy. Histochemical stains for mitochondrial enzymes (succinate dehydrogenase, NADH-tetrazolium reductase, and cyclooxygenase) can be obtained, and the activities of mitochondrial respiratory chain enzymes can be measured in muscle tissue. The identification of numerous mitochondrial DNA mutations provides specific genetic diagnoses, including duplications, deletions, multiple deletions, and more than 100 pathogenic point mutations. Treatment is symptomatic for seizures (with avoidance of valproic acid, which is contraindicated because of depletion of carnitine and direct inhibitory effects on the mitochondrial respiratory chain). Electrolyte disturbances related to hypoparathyroidism and diabetes mellitus are corrected. Thyroid replacement alleviates hypothyroidism, and cardiac pacemaker placement prolongs life in those with Kearns-Sayre syndrome with conduction defects. Impairments in the oxidative phosphorylation pathway can generate increased amounts of free radical; consequently, antioxidants are prescribed (which include β-carotene, vitamin C, vitamin E, and CoQ 10). CoQ 10 shuttles electrons from complex I and II to complex III and can stabilize the oxidative phosphorylation enzyme complexes within the inner mitochondrial membrane. The dose for CoQ 10 in adults is 50 to 100 mg, 3 times per day. L-Carnitine is also recommended. Dichloroacetate increases the pyruvate dehydrogenase complex and reduces lactate. Aerobic training is recommended for those with some mitochondrial conditions. Brief descriptions of common mitochondrial disorders follow.

Kearns-Sayre syndrome
These patients show progressive external ophthalmoplegia, retinitis pigmentosa on fundoscopic examination, and complete heart block. Onset is usually before 20 years of age. Cerebellar findings can be present on physical examination, and patients can show limb weakness, hearing loss, diabetes mellitus, hypoparathyroidism, irregular menses, and growth hormone deficiency. Dementia can be progressive. CSF protein is frequently greater than 100 mg/dL.

Myoclonus epilepsy with ragged-red fibers
This clinical syndrome is defined by the presence of myoclonus, generalized seizures, ataxia, and ragged-red fibers on muscle biopsy. Symptoms usually begin in childhood. Other common clinical manifestations include hearing loss, dementia, exercise intolerance, and lactic acidosis. Multiple lipomatosis is common. Multiple members of a pedigree usually show the full syndrome.

Mitochondrial encephalopathy, lactic acidosis, and strokelike episodes
One particular mitochondrial cytopathy the clinician does not want to miss is mitochondrial encephalopathy, lactic acidosis, and strokelike episodes (MELAS). This clinical syndrome is characterized by strokelike episodes at a young age (typically before 40 years), lactic acidosis, and encephalopathy evident as seizures, dementia, or both. Muscle biopsy shows ragged-red fibers as a result of respiratory chain defects. Other frequent clinical features include normal early development, limb weakness, ataxia, myoclonus, migraine-like headaches, recurrent nausea and vomiting, and hearing loss. The abrupt-onset strokes often affect the occipital cortex but can involve other regions of the brain. These patients often describe an antecedent history of migraine headaches that often occur before the strokelike event. Patients can experience improvement over weeks to months, but these events virtually always recur. The lesions do not conform to territories of large vessels, a finding that favors the term strokelike episodes. Based on the hypothesis that MELAS is caused by impaired

vasodilation in an intracerebral artery, oral L-arginine, a nitric oxide precursor, has been administered acutely within 30 minutes of a stroke, and this treatment was shown to significantly decrease the frequency and severity of strokelike episodes.[19]

Neuropathy, ataxia, and retinitis pigmentosa (NARP)

This disorder consists of the variable combinations of proximal neurogenic limb weakness, sensory neuropathy, ataxia, pigmentary retinopathy, developmental delay, dementia, and seizures. The onset occurs in teens and young adults, and the course is gradually progressive.

Mitochondrial neurogastrointestinal encephalomyopathy

This syndrome is clinically recognized by the unusual combination of 6 features: PEO, severe gastrointestinal dysmotility, cachexia, peripheral neuropathy, diffuse leukoencephalopathy on MRI, and evidence of mitochondrial dysfunction (histologic, biochemical, or genetic). The peripheral neuropathy and the prominent gastrointestinal dysmotility are defining features. Lactic acidosis at rest is present in two-thirds of patients. Both axonal and demyelinating polyneuropathy is frequent. Muscle biopsy reveals ragged-red fibers and neurogenic changes.

SUMMARY

This article reviews the clinical approach to the diagnostic evaluation of progressive NMDs with an emphasis on relevant neuromuscular history, family history, clinical examination findings, laboratory studies, and a brief discussion of the role of muscle biopsy. Molecular genetic and immunocytochemistry studies of muscle have been major advances in the diagnostic evaluation of the NMD patient; however, all diagnostic information needs to be interpreted within the context of relevant clinical information. In some instances, a precise diagnosis is not medically possible; however, the accurate characterization of an individual patient within the most appropriate NMD clinical syndrome often allows the clinician to provide the patient and family with accurate prognostic information and anticipatory guidance for the future. After synthesizing all available clinical and diagnostic information, the physiatrist or neurologist may at times determine that an NMD patient has an inappropriate diagnosis warranting further diagnostic evaluation.

The current and subsequent issues focus on the management and rehabilitation of progressive NMDs with an emphasis on optimization of health, prevention or minimization of complications, and enhancement of quality of life. Appropriate rehabilitation approaches and novel therapeutics require an accurate and timely diagnosis. In addition, patient education in NMD is dependent on access to current and accurate diagnostic information. The first step in providing accurate information and appropriate treatment is constantly ensuring that all NMD patients have appropriate diagnoses based on a thorough evaluation of clinical information and physical examination, and appropriate application of current medical science and available diagnostic technology. Thorough discussions of these diagnostic technologies are reviewed in the following 3 articles.[1,39,51]

REFERENCES

1. Neuromuscular disorders: gene location. Neuromuscul Disord 2006;16(1):64–90.
2. Gospe SM, Lozaro RP, Lava NS, et al. Familial X-linked myalgia and cramps: a non-progressive myopathy associated with a deletion in the dystrophin gene. Neurology 1989;39:1277–80.

3. Mills KR, Edwards RH. Investigative strategies for muscle pain. J Neurol Sci 1983; 58:73.
4. Cros D, Harnden P, Pellisier JF, et al. Muscle hypertrophy in Duchenne muscular dystrophy: a pathological and morphometric study. J Neurol 1989;236:43–7.
5. Reimers CD, Schlotter B, Eicke BM, et al. Calf enlargement in neuromuscular diseases: a quantitative ultrasound study in 350 patients and review of the literature. J Neurol Sci 1996;143(1–2):46–56.
6. Pradhan S. New clinical sign in Duchenne muscular dystrophy. Pediatr Neurol 1994;11:298–300.
7. Ianassecu V. Charcot-Marie-Tooth neuropathies: from clinical description to molecular genetics. Muscle Nerve 1995;18:267–75.
8. Sigford B. Psychosocial, cognitive and educational issues in neuromuscular disease. Phys Med Rehabil Clin N Am 1998;9(1):249–70.
9. Meyerson MD, Lewis E, ILL K. Facioscapulohumeral muscular dystrophy and accompanying hearing loss. Arch Otolaryngol 1984;110(4):261–6.
10. Padberg GW, Brouwer OF, deKeizer RJ, et al. On the significance of retinal vascular disease and hearing loss in facioscapulohumeral muscular dystrophy. Muscle Nerve 1995;2:S73–80.
11. Verhagen WI, Huygen PL, Padberg GW. The auditory, vestibular and oculomotor system in facioscapulohumeral dystrophy. Acta Otolaryngol Suppl 1995;520(Pt 1): 140–2.
12. Guenther UP, Handoko L, Laggerbauer B, et al. IGHMBP2 is a ribosome-associated helicase inactive in the neuromuscular disorder distal SMA type 1 (DSMA1). Hum Mol Genet 2009;18(7):1288–300.
13. Young ID, Harper PS. Hereditary distal spinal muscular atrophy with vocal cord paralysis. J Neurol Neurosurg Psychiatry 1980;43:413–8.
14. Innaccone ST, Browne RH, Samaha FJ, et al. DCN/SMA Group: prospective study of spinal muscular atrophy before age 6 years. Pediatr Neurol 1993;9:187–93.
15. Munsat TL, Davies KE. Meeting report: international SMA consortium meeting. Neuromuscul Disord 1992;2:423–8.
16. Muntoni F, Valero de Bernabe B, Bittner R, et al. 114th ENMC International Workshop on Congenital Muscular Dystrophy (CMD) 17-19 January 2003, Naarden, The Netherlands: (8th Workshop of the International Consortium on CMD; 3rd Workshop of the MYO-CLUSTER project GENRE). Neuromuscul Disord 2003; 13(7–8):579–88.
17. Parano E, Fiumara A, Falsaperla R, et al. A clinical study of childhood spinal muscular atrophy in Sicily: a review of 75 cases. Brain Dev 1994;16(2):104–7.
18. Bach JR, Want TG. Noninvasive long-term ventilatory support for individuals with spinal muscular atrophy and functional bulbar musculature. Arch Phys Med Rehabil 1995;76:213.
19. Koga Y, Akita Y, Nishioka J, et al. L-arginine improves the symptoms of strokelike episodes in MELAS. Neurology 2005;64(4):710–2.
20. Arkin AM. Absolute muscle power: the internal kinesiology of muscle, thesis. Ames, (IA): Department of Orthopedic Surgery. State University of Iowa; 1939.
21. Von Recklinghausen H. Gliedermechanik and Lahmungsprothesen. Berlin: Springer-Verlag; 1920.
22. Kilmer DD, McCrory MA, Wright NC, et al. The effect of high resistance exercise program in slowly progressive neuromuscular disease. Arch Phys Med Rehabil 1994;75:560–3.
23. Aitkens S, Lord J, Bernauer E, et al. Relationship of manual muscle testing to objective strength measurements. Muscle Nerve 1989;12:173–7.

24. Lord JP, Aitkens S, McCrory M, et al. Isometric and isokinetic measurement of hamstring and quadriceps strength. Arch Phys Med Rehabil 1992;73:324–30.
25. Aitkens SG, McCrory MA, Kilmer DD, et al. Moderate resistance exercise program: its effect in slowly progressive neuromuscular disease. Arch Phys Med Rehabil 1993;74:711–5.
26. Carter GT, Abresch RT, Fowler WM Jr, et al. Profiles of neuromuscular diseases: hereditary motor and sensory neuropathy, types I and II. Am J Phys Med Rehabil 1995;749(Suppl):S140–9.
27. Fowler WM Jr, Abresch RT, Aitkens S, et al. Profiles of neuromuscular diseases: design of the protocol. Am J Phys Med Rehabil 1995;74(Suppl):S62–9.
28. Fowler WM, Gardner GW. Quantitative strength measurements in muscular dystrophy. Arch Phys Med Rehabil 1968;48:629–44.
29. Johnson ER, Abresch RT, Carter GT, et al. Profiles of neuromuscular diseases: myotonic dystrophy. Am J Phys Med Rehabil 1995;74(Suppl):S104–16.
30. Kilmer DD, Abresch RT, McCrory MA, et al. Profiles of neuromuscular diseases: facioscapulohumeral muscular dystrophy. Am J Phys Med Rehabil 1995;74:S131–9.
31. McDonald CM, Abresch RT, Carter GT, et al. Profiles of neuromuscular diseases: Becker's muscular dystrophy. Am J Phys Med Rehabil 1995;74(Suppl):S70–92 S93–103.
32. McDonald CM, Abresch RT, Carter GT, et al. Profiles of neuromuscular diseases: Duchenne muscular dystrophy. Am J Phys Med Rehabil 1995;74(Suppl):S70–92.
33. McDonald CM, Jaffe KM, Shurtleff DB. Clinical assessment of muscle strength in children with meningomyelocele: accuracy and stability of measurements over time. Arch Phys Med Rehabil 1986;67:855–61.
34. Eng GD, Binder H, Koch B. Spinal muscular atrophy: experience in diagnosis and rehabilitation in management of 60 patients. Arch Phys Med Rehabil 1984;65: 549–53.
35. Munsat TL. Standardized forearm ischemic exercise test. Neurology 1970;20:1171.
36. Munsat TL. Workshop report: international SMA collaboration. Neuromuscul Disord 1991;1:81.
37. de Greef JC, Lemmers RJLF, Camaño P, et al. Clinical features of facioscapulo-humeral muscular dystrophy 2. Neurology 2010;75:1548–54.
38. Coleman RA, Stajich JM, Pact VW, et al. The ischemic exercise test in normal adults and in patients with weakness and cramps. Muscle Nerve 1986;9:216.
39. Sinkeler SP, Daanen HA, Wevers RA, et al. The relation between blood lactate and ammonia in ischemic handgrip exercise. Muscle Nerve 1985;8:523.
40. Fischer AQ, Carpenter DW, Hartlage PL, et al. Muscle imaging in neuromuscular disease using computerized real-time sonography. Muscle Nerve 1988;11:270–5.
41. Heckmatt JZ, Dubowitz V. Ultrasound imaging and directed needle biopsy in the diagnosis of selective involvement in neuromuscular disease. J Child Neurol 1987;2:205–13.
42. Heckmatt JZ, Leeman S, Dubowitz V. Ultrasound imaging in the diagnosis of muscle disease. J Pediatr 1982;101:656–60.
43. Heckmatt JZ, Pier N, Dubowitz V. Real-time ultrasound imaging of muscles. Muscle Nerve 1988;11:56–65.
44. Zaidman CM, Connolly AM, Malkus EC, et al. Quantitative ultrasound using backscatter analysis in Duchenne and Becker muscular dystrophy. Neuromuscul Disord 2010;20(12):805–9.
45. Finanger EL, Russman B, Forbes SC, et al. Use of skeletal muscle MRI in diagnosis and monitoring disease progression in Duchenne muscular dystrophy. Phys Med Rehabil Clin N Am 2012;23:1–10.

46. Huang Y, Majumdar S, Genant HK, et al. Quantitative MR relaxometry study of muscle composition and function in Duchenne muscular dystrophy. J Magn Reson Imaging 1994;4(1):59–64.

47. Liu GC, Jong YJ, Chiang CH, et al. Duchenne muscular dystrophy: MR grading system with functional correlation. Radiology 1993;186(2):475–80.

48. Liu M, Chino N, Ishihara T. Muscle damage progression in Duchenne muscular dystrophy evaluated by a new quantitative computed tomography method. Arch Phys Med Rehabil 1993;74(5):507–14.

49. Tomasová Studynková J, Charvát F, Jarosová K, et al. The role of MRI in the assessment of polymyositis and dermatomyositis. Rheumatology (Oxford) 2007;46(7):1174–9.

50. Topalogu H, Gucuyener K, Yalaz K, et al. Selective involvement of the quadriceps muscle in congenital muscular dystrophies: an ultrasonographic study. Brain Dev 1992;14:84–7.

51. Skalsky AJ, Han JJ, Abresch RT, et al. Regional and whole-body dual-energy X-ray absorptiometry to guide treatment and monitor disease progression in neuromuscular disease. Phys Med Rehabil Clin N Am 2012;23(1):67–73 x. Review.

52. Carter GT, Abresch RT, Fowler WM Jr, et al. Profiles of neuromuscular diseases: spinal muscular atrophy. Am J Phys Med Rehabil 1995;74(Suppl):S150–9.

53. McDonald CM, Johnson ER, Abresch RT, et al. Profiles of neuromuscular diseases: limb-girdle syndromes. Am J Phys Med Rehabil 1995;74(Suppl):S117–30.

54. Norris F, Sheperd R, Denys E, et al. Onset, natural history and outcome in idiopathic adult motor neuron disease. J Neurol Sci 1993;118(1):48–55.

55. Pradas J, Finison L, Andres PL, et al. The natural history of amyotrophic lateral sclerosis and the use of natural history controls in therapeutic trials. Neurology 1993;43(4):751–5.

56. Ringel SP, Murphy JR, Alderson MK, et al. The natural history of amyotrophic lateral sclerosis. Neurology 1993;43(7):1316–22.

57. Sharma KR, Miller RG. Electrical and mechanical properties of skeletal muscle underlying increased fatigue in patients with amyotrophic lateral sclerosis. Muscle Nerve 1996;19:1391–400.

58. Pasinelli P, Brown RH. Molecular biology of amyotrophic lateral sclerosis: insights from genetics. Nat Genet 2006;7:710–23.

59. Phoenix J, Betal D, Roberts N, et al. Objective quantification of muscle and fat in human dystrophic muscle by magnetic resonance image analysis. Muscle Nerve 1996;19(3):302–10.

60. Shaw CE, Al-Chalabi A. Susceptibility genes in sporadic ALS: separating the wheat from the chaff by international collaboration. Neurology 2006;67:738–9.

61. Sobue I, Saito N, Iida M, et al. Juvenile type of distal and segmental muscular atrophy of the upper extremities. Ann Neurol 1978;3:429–32.

62. Suput D, Zupan A, Sepe A, et al. Discrimination between neuropathy and myopathy by use of magnetic resonance imaging. Acta Neurol Scand 1993;87(2):118–23.

63. Andersen PM, Nilsson P, Keranen M-L, et al. Phenotypic heterogeneity in motor neuron disease patients with CuZn-superoxide dismutase mutations in Scandinavia. Brain 1997;120:1723–37.

64. Rosen DR, Siddique T, Patterson D, et al. Mutations in Cu/Zn superoxide dismutase gene are associated with familial amyotrophic lateral sclerosis. Nature 1993;362:59–62.

65. Wijesekera LC, Leigh PN. Amyotrophic lateral sclerosis. Orphanet J Rare Dis 2009;4:3.

66. Zerres K, Rudnik-Schoneborn S. Natural history in proximal spinal muscular atrophy. Arch Neurol 1995;52:518.
67. Parsons DW, McAndrew PE, Iannaccone ST, et al. Intragenic telSMN mutations: frequency, distribution, evidence of a founder effect, and modification of the spinal muscular atrophy phenotype by cenSMN copy number. Am J Hum Genet 1998;63(6):1712–23.
68. Swoboda KJ, Prior TW, Scott CB, et al. Natural history of denervation in SMA: relation to age, SMN2 copy number, and function. Ann Neurol 2005;57(5):704–12.
69. Swash M, Brown MM, Thakkar C. CT muscle imaging and the clinical assessment of neuromuscular disease. Muscle Nerve 1995;18(7):708–14.
70. Zerres K, Wirth B, Rudnik-Schöneborn S. Spinal muscular atrophy—clinical and genetic correlations. Neuromuscul Disord 1997;7(3):202–7.
71. Pineda M, Arpa J, Montero R, et al. Idebenone treatment in paediatric and adult patients with Friedreich ataxia: long-term follow-up. Eur J Paediatr Neurol 2008; 12(6):470–5.
72. Jones HR Jr, Bradshaw DY. Guillain-Barré syndrome and plasmapheresis in childhood. Ann Neurol 1991;29:688.
73. Ouvrier RA, McLeod JG, Pollard JD. Acute inflammatory demyelinating polyradiculoneuropathy. In: Peripheral neuropathy in childhood. International Review of Child Neurology Series. London: Mac Keith Press; 1999.
74. Bradshaw DY, Jones HR Jr. Guillain-Barré syndrome in children: clinical course, electrodiagnosis and prognosis. Muscle Nerve 1992;15(4):500.
75. Brooke MH, Fenichel GM, Griggs RC, et al. Clinical investigation in Duchenne dystrophy. 2. Determination of the "power" of therapeutic trials based on the natural history. Muscle Nerve 1983;6:91–103.
76. Epstein MA, Sladky JT. The role of plasmapheresis in childhood Guillain-Barré syndrome. Ann Neurol 1990;28:65.
77. Lamont PJ, Johnston HM, Berdoukas VA. Plasmapheresis in children with Guillain-Barré syndrome. Neurology 1991;41(12):1928.
78. Lavenstein BL, Shin W, Watkin T, et al. Four-year followup study of use of IVIG in childhood acute inflammatory demyelinating polyneuropathy (GBS). Neurology 1994;44:A169.
79. Shahar E, Murphy EG, Roifman CM. Benefit of intravenously administered immune serum globulin in patients with Guillain-Barré syndrome. J Pediatr 1990;116(1):141.
80. Tekgul H, Serdaroglu G, Tutuncuoglu S. Outcome of axonal and demyelinating forms of Guillain-Barré syndrome in children. Pediatr Neurol 2003;28(4):295–9.
81. Barisic N, Claeys KG, Sirotković-Skerlev M, et al. Charcot-Marie-Tooth disease: a clinico-genetic confrontation. Ann Hum Genet 2008;72(Pt 3):416–41 Review.
82. Carter GT, Weiss MD, Han JJ, et al. Charcot-Marie-Tooth disease. Curr Treat Options Neurol 2008;10(2):94–102.
83. Hoffman WH, Hat ZH, Frank RN. Correlates of delayed motor nerve conduction and retinopathy in juvenile-onset diabetes mellitus. J Pediatr 1983;102:351.
84. Emery AE. Population frequencies of inherited neuromuscular diseases—a world survey. Neuromuscul Disord 1991;1:19.
85. Muchir A, Worman HJ. Emery-Dreifuss muscular dystrophy. Curr Neurol Neurosci Rep 2007;7(1):78–83.
86. Voit T, Krogmann O, Lennard HG, et al. Emery-Dreifuss muscular dystrophy: disease spectrum and differential diagnosis. Neuropediatrics 1988;19:62.
87. D'Amico A, Bertini E. Congenital myopathies. Curr Neurol Neurosci Rep 2008; 8(1):73–9 Review.

88. Van den Hout JM, Kamphoven JH, Winkel LP, et al. Long-term intravenous treatment of Pompe disease with recombinant human alpha-glucosidase from milk. Pediatrics 2004;113(5):e448-57.
89. van Engelen BG, Eymard B, Wilcox D. 123rd ENMC International Workshop: management and therapy in myotonic dystrophy, 6-8 February 2004, Naarden, The Netherlands. Neuromuscul Disord 2005;15(5):389-94.
90. Udd B, Meola G, Krahe R, et al. 140th ENMC International Workshop: Myotonic Dystrophy DM2/PROMM and other myotonic dystrophies with guidelines on management. Neuromuscul Disord 2006;16(6):403-13.
91. Askanas V, Engel WK. Inclusion body myositis, a multifactorial muscle disease associated with aging: current concepts of pathogenesis. Curr Opin Rheumatol 2007;19(6):550-9.
92. Okumiya T, Keulemans JL, Kroos MA, et al. A new diagnostic assay for glycogen storage disease type II in mixed leukocytes. Mol Genet Metab 2006;88(1):22-8.
93. Pompe Disease Diagnostic Working Group, Winchester B, Bali D, et al. Methods for a prompt and reliable laboratory diagnosis of Pompe disease: report from an international consensus meeting. J Mol Genet Metab 2008;93(3):275-81.
94. Winkel LP, Van den Hout JM, Kamphoven JH, et al. Enzyme replacement therapy in late-onset Pompe's disease: a three-year follow-up. Ann Neurol 2004;55(4):495-502.
95. Roe CR, Yang BZ, Brunengraber H, et al. Carnitine palmitoyltransferase II deficiency: successful anaplerotic diet therapy. Neurology 2008;71(4):260-4.
96. Bonnefont JP, Bastin J, Behin A, et al. Bezafibrate for an inborn mitochondrial beta-oxidation defect. N Engl J Med 2009;360(8):838-40.

Electrodiagnosis in Neuromuscular Disease

Bethany M. Lipa, MD[a,c,*], Jay J. Han, MD[a,b,c]

KEYWORDS

- Electrodiagnosis • Neuromuscular disease • Peripheral neuropathy
- Motor neuron disease • Neuromuscular junction • Myopathy

KEY POINTS

- The electrodiagnostic examination (EDX) remains an important diagnostic tool to assist in the diagnosis of many neuromuscular diseases despite the increasing availability of molecular genetic testing.
- Peripheral neuropathies may be classified by cause, acquired and inherited, or through electrophysiologic findings.
- Various forms of motor neuron disease, including the spinal muscular atrophies, amyotrophic lateral sclerosis, and polio, share several electrodiagnostic features but differ clinically, particularly with respect to disease progression.
- Special tests, such as repetitive nerve stimulation and single fiber electromyography, are available for the evaluation of neuromuscular junction disorders.
- The EDX examination is less sensitive for detecting myopathies compared with other groups of neuromuscular diseases and is rarely helpful in differentiating between the various myopathic disorders.

The electrodiagnostic examination (EDX) remains an important diagnostic tool to assist in the diagnosis of many neuromuscular diseases despite the increasing availability of molecular genetic testing. Challenges exist when conducting an EDX in the setting of neuromuscular disease. The distribution of abnormalities may be patchy, findings may be subtle (especially with myopathies), and the use of special techniques, such

Funding sources: Dr Lipa, RRTC; Dr Han, NIDRR.
Conflict of interest: Dr Lipa, none; Dr Han, Genzyme.
[a] Department of Physical Medicine and Rehabilitation, University of California Davis School of Medicine, 4860 Y Street, Suite 1700, Sacramento, CA 95817, USA; [b] Muscular Dystrophy Association (MDA), Neuromuscular Disease Clinic, Department of Physical Medicine and Rehabilitation, University of California Davis School of Medicine, Sacramento, CA, USA; [c] Lawrence J. Ellison Ambulatory Care Center, Department of Physical Medicine and Rehabilitation, University of California Davis School of Medicine, 4860 Y Street, Suite 1700, Sacramento, CA 95817, USA
* Corresponding author. Lawrence J. Ellison Ambulatory Care Center, 4860 Y Street, Suite 1700, Sacramento, CA 95817.
E-mail address: Bethany.lipa@ucdmc.ucdavis.edu

Phys Med Rehabil Clin N Am 23 (2012) 565–587
http://dx.doi.org/10.1016/j.pmr.2012.06.007
1047-9651/12/$ – see front matter © 2012 Elsevier Inc. All rights reserved.

as repetitive stimulation studies and single fiber electromyography (SFEMG), may be required. This article presumes a basic knowledge of EDX and presents a general approach to the electrodiagnosis of patients with neuromuscular diseases followed by a description of the unique EDX features of polyneuropathies, motor neuron disease, neuromuscular junction disorders, and myopathies.

A GENERAL APPROACH TO THE ELECTRODIAGNOSTIC EVALUATION OF PATIENTS WITH NEUROMUSCULAR DISEASES

Before undergoing the EDX, a detailed history and physical examination should be performed. The electromyographer should then have an idea of whether the disease process is primarily neuropathic, myopathic, or of neuromuscular junction to help focus the ensuing EDX studies. Knowledge of clinically weak muscles based on the physical examination will also increase the diagnostic yield.

The evaluation of patients suspected of having peripheral neuropathy or motor neuron disease can typically begin with nerve conduction studies (NCS) in the bilateral lower limbs and one upper limb, generally beginning the EDX on the side of the body that is most affected if the process is asymmetric. Motor NCS typically include the peroneal, tibial, and ulnar nerves. Sensory NCS include the sural, ulnar, and radial nerves. If the sural response is present, the electromyographer may attempt to elicit a medial plantar mixed nerve or sensory response; loss of the medial plantar response can be an early sign of peripheral neuropathy.[1] NCS may also include at least one upper and one lower extremity F wave and an H reflex. F waves are useful in detecting demyelinating neuropathies. Any abnormalities detected by NCS that seem inconsistent with the overall findings should prompt a comparison in the contralateral limb. For example, finding a low amplitude ulnar compound muscle action potential (CMAP) in a mild generalized sensorimotor polyneuropathy suggests a concomitant focal ulnar nerve lesion. Comparison with the contralateral ulnar nerve may help clarify the situation.

The needle electrode examination (NEE) in the evaluation of a neuropathic process should focus on distal muscles, especially in the lower extremities. In most generalized peripheral polyneuropathies, distal lower limb muscles are affected first. Typical lower limb muscles for evaluation can include the extensor digitorum brevis, tibialis posterior, medial gastrocnemius, tibialis anterior, vastus lateralis, and gluteus medius muscles in the distal to proximal direction. Additional muscles can then be examined depending on the areas of weakness noted on the examination and EDX abnormalities of the aforementioned muscles. For mild generalized polyneuropathies, proximal upper limb muscles need not be studied if the intrinsic muscles of the hand are normal. If the hand intrinsic muscles are abnormal, the remainder of the upper limb should be studied. As an upper extremity screen, typical muscles for examination include the first dorsal interosseous, extensor indices proprius, pronator teres, biceps, triceps, and deltoid muscles, with lower cervical paraspinals when needed. In cases of suspected motor neuron disease, proximal and distal muscles in both the upper and lower limbs should be examined.

In general, fewer NCS are needed for the evaluation of a myopathic process. In most myopathies, the NCS are normal unless significant distal atrophy has occurred. An NCS screen should include at least one upper and one lower limb motor and sensory nerve. The choice of specific nerves may vary; at a minimum, the authors typically perform sural sensory, peroneal motor, ulnar sensory, and ulnar motor NCS. If a very low CMAP is obtained, the study should be repeated after a 10-second maximal isometric contraction of the target muscle to look for facilitation, as in seen in Lambert-Eaton myasthenic syndrome. An abnormal result in only one nerve should prompt a comparison with the contralateral NCS.

In suspected myopathy, the NEE should generally focus on proximal muscles and muscles that are weak. Other muscles for examination should include the paraspinals and a few targeted distal muscles. The initial examination includes the supraspinatus, deltoid, triceps, biceps, brachioradialis, pronator teres, first dorsal interosseous, gluteus medius, iliopsoas, vastus lateralis, adductor longus, short head of biceps femoris, tibialis anterior, medial gastrocnemius, and cervical and lumbar paraspinals. Any clinically weak muscle should be examined. If no abnormalities are seen in a clinically weak muscle, a second or third needle insertion at another site within the same muscle may reveal abnormalities. Inflammatory myopathies have patchy involvement, even within the same muscle. If a needle biopsy is anticipated in the near future, the limb to be biopsied should not undergo NEE.

NEUROPATHIES

Peripheral neuropathies may be classified by cause, acquired and inherited, or through electrophysiologic findings. Electrophysiologically, neuropathies may be divided into 6 major categories: (1) uniform demyelinating; (2) segmental demyelinating; (3) axonal, sensorimotor; (4) axonal, motor, sensory; (5) axonal, sensory; and (6) combined axonal and demyelinating. The EDX helps to categorize neuropathic disorders into one of these 6 categories, suggesting a limited differential diagnosis but seldom can identify the exact underlying cause. Within each of the 6 categories, the differential diagnosis requires knowledge of the history, physical examination, laboratory testing, molecular genetic testing, and occasionally nerve biopsy. Electrodiagnostic findings of the 6 categories of peripheral neuropathies are further described.

Uniform Demyelinating Neuropathies

The uniform demyelinating neuropathies are all hereditary and are characterized by conduction velocity slowing, prolonged distal latencies, prolonged F waves, absent or reduced sensory nerve action potential (SNAP), and absent or reduced CMAPs when recording over distal muscles. Temporal dispersion and conduction block (CB) are not seen because the demyelination is uniform. This characteristic differentiates hereditary from acquired demyelinating neuropathies. NEE shows characteristic neuropathic findings, such as decreased recruitment, motor unit action potentials (MUAPs) of increased duration and amplitude, and fibrillation potentials and positive sharp waves (PSWs) in distal muscles.

Charcot-Marie-Tooth (CMT) disease subtypes are many and as a group represent the most common and well known of the hereditary neuropathies (**Table 1**). CMT is also referred to as hereditary motor sensory neuropathies (HMSN). **Table 2** shows some common and typical electrodiagnostic characteristics for different CMT subtypes and acquired forms of neuropathies for comparison. In the demyelinating form of CMT, velocity slowing is symmetric and nearly identical in both proximal and distal nerve segments.[2] Conduction blocks are rare in CMT1A (the most common form) but are seen in CMT1 types B and C and acquired demyelinating neuropathies.[3] SNAPs are usually absent after 10 years of age. Nerve conduction velocities generally reach their nadir by 5 years of age and distal latencies by 10 years of age, but CMAP amplitudes may continue to decline throughout life and are often unrecordable in the distal lower limb muscles of adults. Motor conduction velocities are 20 to 25 m/s but may drop as low as 10 to 15 m/s in the lower limbs. As in all demyelinating neuropathies, clinical weakness correlates with the degree of reduction in CMAP amplitude but not with the extent of conduction velocity slowing. Low nerve conduction velocities (NCVs) can even be detected in asymptomatic individuals and as early

Table 1
Summary of the genetic basis for Charcot-Marie-Tooth disease

	Chromosome	Gene Locus	Inheritance	Gene Abnormality
Charcot-Marie-Tooth I				
CMT 1A	17p11.2-12	PMP22	AD	Duplication/point mutation
CMT 1B	1q22-23	P_0	AD	Point mutation
CMT 1C	16p12-p13	SIMPLE	AD	Point mutation
CMT 1D	10q21-q22	EGR2	AD/AR	Point mutation
Charcot-Marie-Tooth 2				
CMT 2A	1p35-36	MFN2	AD	Point mutation
CMT 2B	3q13-q22	RAB7	AD	Point mutation
CMT 2C	12q23-q24	Unknown	AD	Unknown
CMT 2D	7p14	GARS	AD	Point mutation
CMT 2E	8p21	NF-L	AD	Point mutation
Dejerine-Sottas disease				
DSDA	17p11.2-12	PMP22	AD	Point mutation
DSDB	1q22-23	P_0	AD	Point mutation
DSDC	10q21-q22	EGR2	AD	Point mutation
DSDD	19q13	PRX	AD	Point mutation
Charcot-Marie-Tooth 4				
CMT4A	8q13-q21	GDAP1	AR	Point mutation
CMT4B1	11q22	MTMR2	AR	Point mutation
CMT4B2	11p15	SBF2	AR	Point mutation
CMT4D (HMSN-Lom)	8q24	NDRG1	AR	Point mutation
CMT4F	19q13	PRX	AR	Point mutation
Charcot-Marie-Tooth X				
CMTX	Xq13.1	Connexin 32	XD	Point mutation
HNPP				
HNPP	17p11.2	PMP22	AD	Deletion/point mutation

Genetic spectrum of inherited neuropathies.

Abbreviations: AD, autosomal dominant; AR, autosomal recessive; Cx32, connexin32; EGR2 or Krox-20, early growth response 2 gene; GARS, glycyl tRNA synthase; GDAP1, ganglioside-induced differentiation-associated protein-1; HMSN, hereditary motor sensory neuropathies; HNPP, hereditary neuropathy with liability to pressure palsies; Inheritance: LAMN, lamin A/C; MFN2, Mitofusin; MTMR2, myotubularin-related protein-2; NDRG1, N-myc-downstream regulated gene 1; NEF-L, neurofilament; P_0, myelin protein zero; PMP22, peripheral myelin protein 22; PRX, periaxin; RAB7, small GTP-ase late endosomal protein gene 7, light chain; SBF2, set binding factor 2; SIMPLE, small integral membrane protein of late endosome; XD, X-linked dominant.

Data from Carter GT, Weiss MD, Han JJ, et al. Charcot Marie Tooth Disease. Curr Treat Options Neurol 2008 Mar;10(2):94–102.

as 1 year of age.[4] Fibrillation potentials and PSWs are common in distal muscles of the upper and lower limbs. Dejerine-Sottas syndrome (HMSN III) is the most severe form of demyelinating neuropathy and is characterized by conduction velocities less than 10 m/s and often as low as 2 to 3 m/s.[5,6] SNAPs cannot be recorded, and CMAP amplitudes are very low. Fibrillation potentials and PSWs are seen in proximal and distal muscles. Nerves have elevated electrical thresholds and, therefore, require

Table 2
Electrodiagnostic characteristics of the hereditary and acquired motor and sensory neuropathies

Neuropathy Form	Conduction Velocity Characteristics	Axonal Loss	Conduction Block	Temporal Dispersion	Focal Slowing
CMT 1	Uniform slowing, usually <38 m/s but may be faster	Yes	No	No	No
CMT 2	Minimal slowing to normal	Yes (primary)	No	No	No
CMT X1	Heterogeneous slowing (30–40 m/s); temporal dispersion	Yes	No	Occasionally	Occasionally
HNPP	Nonuniform, intermediate slowing, distal >proximal	Yes	Yes	Yes	Yes
Dejerine-Sottas	Uniform, severe Slowing (<20 m/s)	Yes	No	Yes	No
Diabetic Neuropathy	Nonuniform, intermediate to severe slowing	Yes	Maybe[a]	Maybe[a]	Yes
CIDP	Nonuniform, multifocal, asymmetric, intermediate to severe slowing	Yes	Often	Often	Yes
AIDP	Nonuniform, segmental slowing	No	Yes	Yes	Yes

Abbreviations: CIDP, chronic inflammatory demyelinating neuropathy; HNPP, hereditary neuropathy with liability to pressure palsies; m/s, meters per second.

[a] If superimposed focal compression or entrapment present (compression can occur in the absence of entrapment).

Data from Carter GT, Weiss MD, Han JJ, et al. Charcot Marie Tooth Disease. Curr Treat Options Neurol.

a long stimulus duration in attempts to achieve supramaximal stimulation (see **Tables 1** and **2**).

Segmental Demyelinating Neuropathies

All of the segmental demyelinating neuropathies, with the exception of hereditary neuropathy with liability to pressure palsies (HNPP), are acquired. HNPP typically presents as a mononeuropathy involving a nerve at a common entrapment site or as a multiple mononeuropathies, often following an episode of minor trauma. Conduction velocity is slowed to 10% to 70% of normal across the injured nerve segment. CB and temporal dispersion can also be demonstrated across sites of compression. In addition to findings associated with the focal nerve injury, there is a distinctive mild generalized sensorimotor peripheral neuropathy.[7] It is characterized by diffuse sensory NCV slowing and prolongation of distal motor latencies with an infrequent and minor reduction of motor nerve conduction velocities. The amplitudes of CMAPs are normal or only slightly reduced.[8]

Three subtypes of Guillain-Barré syndrome (GBS) have been described: acute inflammatory demyelinating polyradiculoneuropathy (AIDP), acute motor axonal neuropathy, and acute motor and sensory axonal neuropathy. In North America and Europe, typical patients with GBS usually have AIDP as the underlying subtype and about 5% of patients have axonal subtypes. Large studies in Northern China, Japan, Central America, and South America show that axonal forms of the syndrome constitute 30% to 47% of cases. AIDP and the 2 axonal subtypes usually affect all 4 limbs and can involve the cranial nerves and respiration.[9]

AIDP is the classic example of an acquired segmental demyelinating neuropathy. Motor nerve conduction abnormalities occur before sensory nerve abnormalities, with a nadir of abnormality occurring at week 3. Sensory nerve conduction abnormalities peak during week 4.[10] Electrodiagnostic criteria for AIDP is summarized in **Box 1**.

At initial presentation, too few EDX criteria of demyelination may be present for a definite diagnosis of AIDP. Repeating the examination in 7 to 10 days may be helpful in these cases. The most common electrophysiological findings in early GBS include decreased CMAP amplitudes, abnormal F waves, and abnormal H reflexes. In equivocal cases, observed disintegration of the CMAP over time strongly suggests a demyelinating disorder. The most sensitive EDX parameter in patients with early GBS is CB in the most proximal segments of the peripheral nervous system, directly determined in the Erb-to-axilla segment or indirectly as an absent H reflex.[11] The lowest mean distal CMAP amplitude recorded within the first 30 days of onset is the best single electrodiagnostic predictor of prognosis. A value less than 20% of the lower limit of normal is associated with a poor functional outcome.[9]

SNAP amplitude abnormalities are much more common than sensory distal latency or sensory conduction velocity abnormalities.[12] Unlike the pattern in most other neuropathies, the median nerve tends to be affected earlier and more severely than

---

Box 1
Electrodiagnostic criteria for AIDP

1. At least 1 of the following in 2 nerves:

   a. Motor conduction velocity less than 90% of the lower limit of normal (LLN) (85% if distal CMAP amplitude <50% LLN)

   b. Distal motor latency greater than 110% of the upper limit of normal (>120% if distal CMAP amplitude <100% LLN)

   c. Proximal CMAP amplitude/distal CMAP amplitude ratio less than 0.5 and distal CMAP amplitude greater than 20% LLN

   d. F-response latency greater than 120% of the upper limit of normal

or

2. At least 2 of the following in 1 nerve if all others are unexcitable and distal CMAP amplitude is greater than 10% LLN:

   a. Motor conduction velocity less than 90% LLN (85% if distal CMAP amplitude <50% LLN)

   b. Distal motor latency greater than 110% of the upper limit of normal (>120% if distal CMAP amplitude <100% LLN)

   c. Proximal CMAP amplitude/distal CMAP amplitude ratio less than 0.5 and distal CMAP amplitude greater than 20% of the LLN

   d. F-response latency greater than 120% of the upper limit of normal

Data from Hughes RA, Cornblath DR. Guillain-Barré syndrome. Lancet 2005;366(9497):1653–66.

the sural nerve. Approximately half of patients have a normal sural sensory study with abnormal median sensory study,[13] which is referred to as the normal sural-abnormal median pattern.[9]

In early AIDP, NEE typically shows decreased recruitment that is most prominent distally. Despite the primary and initial demyelinating process, fibrillation potentials and PSWs can appear 2 to 4 weeks after the onset of symptoms and are most prominent between weeks 6 to 10. Polyphasic MUAPs are most prominent between weeks 9 and 15.[10]

The time course and evolution of symptoms as well as the electrophysiologic abnormalities distinguishes chronic inflammatory demyelinating polyradiculoneuropathy (CIDP) from AIDP. In general, the prevalence of CIDP may be underestimated because of the limitations in clinical, serologic, and electrophysiologic diagnostic criteria. There is a range of diagnostic criteria for CIDP. There are stringent diagnostic criteria for research purposes and more sensitive criteria that can identify a broader range of patients with CIDP who may benefit from treatment.[14] There is no consensus on one criterion standard for making the diagnosis.[15] Early in the course of CIDP, sensory abnormalities may appear in the median nerve before the sural nerve. In long-standing CIDP, all sensory responses may be absent. The combination of absent or abnormal SNAPS with normal sural responses occurs but is uncommon in CIDP compared with AIDP. Motor conduction velocities may be markedly reduced, F response latencies are very prolonged (or absent), and temporal dispersion is more prominent than observed in AIDP.[13] Although motor conduction velocities are reduced by a greater percentage in the upper limb than in the lower limb, CMAP amplitudes tend to be more severely reduced in the lower limbs.[16] NEE may show fibrillation potentials and PSWs in distal and proximal muscles, including the paraspinals, depending on disease severity **Box 2**.

POEMS syndrome (polyneuropathy, organomegaly, endocrinopathy, monoclonal protein and skin changes) is a paraneoplastic disorder with a demyelinating peripheral neuropathy that is often mistaken for CIDP. Compared with CIDP, there is greater axonal loss (reduction of motor amplitudes and increased fibrillation potentials), greater slowing of the intermediate nerve segments, less common temporal dispersion and conduction block, and absent sural sparing.[17]

There are several variants of CIDP that may also respond to treatment and are, therefore, important to recognize.[14] One variant is multifocal motor neuropathy (MMN) with CB. An EDX evaluation shows motor CB at sites other than those of

---

Box 2
Criteria suggestive of demyelination in the electrodiagnostic evaluation of CIDP

Evaluation should satisfy at least 3 of the following in motor nerves (exceptions noted later):

1. Conduction velocity less than 75% of the lower limit of normal (2 or more nerves)[a]

2. Distal latency exceeding 130% of the upper limit of normal (2 or more nerves)[b]

3. Evidence of unequivocal temporal dispersion or CB on proximal stimulation consisting of a proximal-to-distal amplitude ratio less than 0.7 (1 or more nerves)[b,c]

4. F-response latency exceeding 130% of the upper limit of normal (1 or more nerves)[a,b]

[a] Excluding isolated ulnar or peroneal nerve abnormalities at the elbow or knee, respectively.
[b] Excluding isolated median nerve abnormality at the wrist.
[c] Excluding the presence of anomalous innervation (eg, median to ulnar nerve crossover).
Data from Albers JW, et al. Acquired inflammatory demyelinating polyneuropathies: clinical and electrodiagnostic features. Muscle Nerve 1989;12:435–51.

common entrapment, absence of temporal dispersion, normal distal motor latencies, and normal or mildly slow motor conduction velocities. Sensory-nerve-conduction studies are needed to exclude sensory abnormalities at the sites of CB in MMN and can help to differentiate MMN from CIDP.[18] CB is not present in sensory nerves. Fasciculations are common on NEE, and MMN occasionally is misdiagnosed as motor neuron disease.

Axonal Mixed Sensorimotor Neuropathies

The axonal mixed sensorimotor neuropathies encompass the category of neuropathies with the longest differential diagnosis and include nutritional, toxic, and connective tissue disease–related neuropathies. They are electrodiagnostically indistinguishable and findings are typically symmetric. Sensory nerves are affected earlier than motor nerves, and distal lower limb nerves are affected before upper limb nerves. The earliest abnormality is a decrease in sural SNAP amplitude followed by the disappearance of the sural SNAP and H reflex. Subsequent abnormalities include decreased ulnar and median SNAPs along with decreased CMAP amplitude recording from the intrinsic foot muscles. There may be a slight prolongation of distal latencies and slowing of conduction velocities caused by the loss of the fastest conducting fibers but these changes do not overlap with criteria for demyelination. On NEE, fibrillation potentials, PSWs, and decreased recruitment appear first in the most distal lower limb muscles and much later in the distal upper limb muscles. Fibrillation potentials usually are not seen in the upper limb until after they are found in the tibialis anterior and gastrocnemius muscles. Motor unit remodeling occurs to varying degrees depending on the time course and severity of the disease and results in MUAP changes.

Axonal Neuropathies with Predominant Motor Involvement

Axonal neuropathies with predominant motor involvement may be hereditary or acquired. The hereditary neuropathies in this group are distal hereditary motor neuropathies (dHMN) and porphyria.

The dHMN compose a heterogeneous group of diseases that share the common feature of a length-dependent, predominantly motor neuropathy and present as a slowly progressive, length-dependent condition often starting in the first 2 decades. Several forms of dHMN have minor sensory abnormalities and may also have a significant upper-motor-neuron component. Overlap with the axonal forms of CMT disease (CMT2), juvenile forms of amyotrophic lateral sclerosis (ALS), and hereditary spastic paraplegia (HSP) exist.[18] The CMAP from the extensor digitorum brevis muscle usually is low, but the CMAP recorded from more proximal muscles usually is normal or slightly slowed. NEE shows evidence of denervation in intrinsic foot and distal leg muscles.

DHMN types I and II are typical distal motor neuropathies beginning in the lower limbs and presenting in either childhood or adulthood respectively. If there is sensory involvement, the disease is termed CMT2F if it is caused by mutations in HSPB1 and CMT2L if the mutation is in HSPB8. Type V is characterized by upper limb onset and can be caused by mutations in BSCL2 or GARS. If it is caused by a mutation in GARS and there is sensory involvement, it is termed CMT2D. Types III and IV have been linked to the same loci and are chronic forms of dHMN. They are differentiated by the presence of diaphragmatic palsy in type IV. Type VI occurs in infancy and is characterized by distal weakness and respiratory failure.[19]

Porphyria presents with acute abdominal pain, agitation, and restlessness. Within 48 to 72 hours, weakness can develop. Weakness can occur distally or proximally and may start in either the upper or lower limb. The primary abnormality on NCS is reduction of

CMAP amplitudes. SNAPs are reduced in approximately 50% of patients. NEE during the acute attack may show reduced recruitment. Fibrillation potentials and PSWs in affected muscles typically occur 4 to 6 weeks after the onset of an attack. Abnormal spontaneous activity can be present in both distal and proximal muscles, including the paraspinal muscles. Patients who have had multiple attacks may develop complex repetitive discharges (CRDs) and evidence of motor unit remodeling.[8]

Axonal Sensory Neuropathies

Axonal sensory neuropathies may be hereditary or acquired. They are characterized by absent or decreased SNAPs with normal motor NCS. Minor NEE abnormalities in the intrinsic foot muscle, such as a few fibrillation potentials or chronic neurogenic MUAP changes, may be seen in long-standing cases. In one series of 35 patients found to have sensory neuropathy, nearly 50% of were categorized as idiopathic, with only 6% being hereditary and 11% paraneoplastic. A marked female predominance was also noted.[20] In Friedreich ataxia (FA), antidromic SNAPs may be absent by 6 years of age, whereas CMAPs are preserved even in adulthood. In patients with FA followed over many years, NCS findings do not change significantly despite increasing functional impairment. H reflexes are generally absent, but blink reflexes are present. Mild recruitment abnormalities may be seen on NEE in long-standing disease. Patients with spinocerebellar ataxias (SCA) may also present with a concomitant predominantly sensory neuropathy (SCA1, SCA2, SCA3, SCA4, SCA18, SCA25, SCA27) but the abnormalities are not as severe as those seen in Friedreich ataxia.[21,22] The hereditary sensory and autonomic neuropathies (HSAN 1-V) are rare and have been classified into 5 types by mode of inheritance, age of onset, and clinical features. HSAN I is the most common type. The typical electrodiagnostic finding in HSAN I and II is complete absence of SNAPs in upper and lower extremities with normal motor NCS and NEE.[8] In HSAN IV, NCS are normal but sympathetic skin responses are absent.[23]

Combined Axon Loss and Demyelinating Neuropathies

Combined axon loss and demyelination are seen in diabetes mellitus and uremia.

Diabetic polyneuropathy presents in many forms, including distal symmetric form, cranial diabetic neuropathy, and focal and multifocal limb neuropathies.[24] A unique feature of uremic neuropathy is that motor and sensory involvement occurs simultaneously rather than the sensory involvement preceding motor involvement.[16] Abnormalities of sural nerve conduction and of late responses are present in all patients. Motor nerve conduction velocities may be slowed to 60% to 70% of the lower limit of normal, and F waves are prolonged early in the course of the neuropathy, indicating both proximal and distal demyelination.[25] Findings on NEE are similar to those seen in other axonal peripheral neuropathies, with fibrillation potentials appearing in the distal upper limb muscles after denervation has reached the tibialis anterior and gastrocnemius in the lower extremity.

Motor Neuron Disease

The various forms of motor neuron disease, including the spinal muscular atrophies (SMA), ALS, and polio, share several electrodiagnostic features but differ clinically particularly with respect to disease progression. General EDX characteristics of motor neuron disease include normal sensory NCS, low motor amplitudes, and normal distal motor latencies and conduction velocities. With profound loss of motor amplitude, conduction velocities may drop because of the loss of the fastest conduction fibers.[26] The NEE reveals a decreased recruitment pattern, either small or large MUAPs (depending on degree of anterior horn cell loss) with or without evidence of remodeling depending on the specific disease process, and spontaneous activity, including positive sharp waves, fibrillation potentials, fasciculations, and CRDs.

SMA

The EDX features of the proximal SMAs I to IV, as classified by Dubowitz,[27] are determined by the rate of anterior horn cell degeneration and the stage in the course of the disease. SMA I, or Werdnig-Hoffmann disease, presents in utero or in infancy, is rapidly progressive and generally leads to death before 2 years of age if ventilatory support and manual or mechanical airway clearance (ie, cough assist) is not provided. SMA II has an age of onset between 6 and 18 months. Children usually achieve independent sitting but not independent ambulation and often survive into adulthood. Cranial nerve innervated muscles are less likely to be involved in SMA II. SMA III, or Kugelberg-Welander disease, has an insidious onset between 3 and 30 years of age and is slowly progressive, with ambulation possible for 10 to 30 years after disease onset.

Sensory NCS are normal in all forms of SMA. CMAPs are decreased in proportion to the degree of muscle atrophy. Motor velocities are most likely to be abnormally slow in SMA I because of the extensive loss of large myelinated axons and slower baseline conduction velocities in children younger than 5 years. Motor conduction velocity slowing is usually no more than 25% less than the lower limit of normal.[26]

The most profound loss of MUAPs is seen in SMA I. With maximal effort, only a few MUAPs may fire at a rapid rate. Small MUAPs are common because reinnervation cannot compensate for the rapid loss of anterior horn cells. Myopathic-appearing, low-amplitude, polyphasic, short-duration MUAPs also may be seen because of muscle fiber degeneration. In the other types of SMA, large-amplitude MUAPs (up to 10–15 mV) may be observed because the number of muscle fibers per motor unit increases as reinnervation occurs. These large units may be polyphasic with increased duration. Satellite potentials appear as remodeling occurs.

On NEE in SMA I, fibrillation potentials and PSWs are diffuse and seen in many muscles, including the paraspinals. Fasciculation potentials are uncommon and are found in less than 35% of children with SMA1.[28] Spontaneously firing MUAPs at 5 to 15 Hz, even during sleep, are a unique EDX feature of both SMA I and II.[29] In more chronic forms of SMA, fibrillation potentials and PSWs are even more common and increase in frequency as age increases. CRDs are often seen in SMA II and III, and fasciculations are more common than in SMA I.[30]

Kennedy disease

Kennedy disease, also known as X-linked bulbospinal muscular atrophy, is a slowly progressive X-linked recessive motor neuron disease characterized by proximal limb and bulbar weakness, tongue atrophy, and prominent muscle cramping and fasciculations. In addition, it is associated with diabetes, gynecomastia, and testicular atrophy because of an androgen receptor defect. Although patients generally do not have sensory complaints, absence or reduction of SNAPs is a common finding.[31] Motor NCS are normal or may show a reduction in amplitude. NEE shows large-amplitude and long-duration MUAPs consistent with an indolent neurogenic disease course. Fibrillation potentials and PSWs may be prominent and present in all muscles examined. Fasciculation potentials are also abundant in limb, facial, and tongue muscles.[26]

Adult nonhereditary motor neuron disease

The most common form of adult nonhereditary motor neuron disease is ALS. Less common forms of adult nonhereditary motor neuron disease include progressive muscular atrophy (PMA) with lower motor neuron findings only, progressive lateral sclerosis (PLS) with upper motor neuron findings only, and progressive bulbar palsy (PBP) with only lower motor neuron bulbar muscle involvement. Over time, individuals initially diagnosed with PMA, PLS, or PBP often develop ALS. Approximately 10% of patients with ALS have familial ALS that can be inherited either as an autosomal dominant or recessive trait.[32] Clinical and electrodiagnostic features of these patients are no different from those with sporadic ALS.

For years, Lambert's criteria were the standard for the electromyographic diagnosis of ALS. The following 4 criteria must be met to make a definite diagnosis of ALS[25]: (1) positive sharp waves or fibrillation potentials in 3 of 5 limbs, counting the head as a limb (For a limb to be considered affected, at least 2 muscles innervated by different peripheral nerves and roots should show active denervation.[10]); (2) normal sensory nerve conduction studies[13]; (3) normal motor conduction studies (However, if the CMAP amplitude is very low, the conduction velocity may decrease as low as 70% of the lower limit of normal.[7]); and (4) reduced recruitment of MUAPs on needle examination. The EDX findings in PMA are identical to those in ALS; the distinction between the two diagnoses is made by the presence or absence of upper motor neuron signs on physical examination. By definition, the EDX examination is normal in PLS. In PBP, active denervation is found only in the muscles of the head and neck.

In 1990, a special task force of the World Federation of Neurology developed the El Escorial Criteria for diagnosing ALS in response to the stringency of the Lambert criteria.[33] The EDX portion of the criteria differs somewhat from Lambert's criteria. The criteria stated that electrodiagnostic findings must be present in at least 2 of 4 regions (bulbar, cervical, thoracic, and lumbar) for a diagnosis of ALS. Electrophysiologic features required to define clinically definite disease include the following: (1) reduced recruitment, (2) large MUAPs, and (3) fibrillations potentials.[33] The revised El Escorial Criteria was developed in 2000 and categorizes patients into 4 levels of certainty[25]: clinically definite ALS,[10] clinically probable ALS,[13] clinically probable laboratory–supported ALS, and[7] clinically possible ALS. For electromyogram (EMG) findings to support a diagnosis of ALS, there must be signs of chronic and active denervation in at least 2 muscles in the cervical and lumbosacral regions and 1 muscle in the brainstem and thoracic regions.

In December 2006, an International Federation of Clinical Neurophysiology-sponsored consensus conference was convened on Awaji Island, Japan to consider how clinical neurophysiology could be used more effectively to facilitate early diagnosis. An evidence-based approach was used and consensus recommendations were made (**Box 3**). They concluded that because needle EMG is essentially an extension of the clinical examination in detecting features of denervation and reinnervation, the finding of neurogenic EMG changes in a muscle should have the same diagnostic significance as clinical features of neurogenic change in an individual muscle. Specific EMG features suggestive of ALS were found to be the following: (1) chronic neurogenic change (MUAPs of increased amplitude and duration, usually with an increased number of phases, as assessed by qualitative or quantitative studies); (2) decreased motor unit recruitment, defined by rapid firing of a reduced number of motor units; (3) presence of unstable and complex MUAPs using a narrow band pass filter (500 Hz to 5 kHz); (4) fibrillations and PSWs recorded in strong, nonwasted muscles; and (5) fasciculation potentials (preferably of complex morphology) are equivalent to fibrillations and PSWs in their clinical significance (see **Box 3**).[34]

Early in the progression of ALS, many patients with a suspected clinical diagnosis of ALS do not meet the electrodiagnostic criteria for a definite diagnosis. A repeat study several months later will often fulfill the EDX criteria for diagnosis. On the other hand,

Box 3
Awaji-shima consensus recommendations for the application of electrophysiological tests to the diagnosis of ALS, as applied to the revised El Escorial Criteria (Airlie House 1998)

1. Principles (from the Airlie House criteria)

The diagnosis of ALS requires

1. The presence of
   a. Evidence of *lower motor neuron (LMN) degeneration* by clinical, electrophysiological, or neuropathological examination
   b. Evidence of *upper motor neuron (UMN) degeneration* by clinical examination
   c. *Progressive spread of symptoms or signs* within a region or to other regions, as determined by history, physical examination, or electrophysiological tests
2. The absence of
   a. Electrophysiological or pathologic evidence of other disease processes that might explain the signs of LMN or UMN degeneration
   b. Neuroimaging evidence of other disease processes that might explain the observed clinical and electrophysiological signs

2. Diagnostic categories

Clinically definite ALS is defined by clinical or electrophysiological evidence by the presence of LMN and UMN signs in the bulbar region and at least 2 spinal regions or the presence of LMN and UMN signs in 3 spinal regions.

Clinically probable ALS is defined on clinical or electrophysiological evidence by LMN and UMN signs in at least 2 regions, with some UMN signs necessarily rostral to (above) the LMN signs.

Clinically possible ALS is defined when clinical or electrophysiological signs of UMN and LMN dysfunction are found in only one region, or UMN signs are found alone in 2 or more regions, or LMN signs are found rostral to UMN signs. Neuroimaging and clinical laboratory studies will have been performed and other diagnoses must have been excluded.

These recommendations emphasize the equivalence of clinical and electrophysiological tests in establishing neurogenic change in bodily regions. The category of clinically probable laboratory-supported ALS is redundant.

Data from de Carvalho M, et al. Electrodiagnostic criteria for diagnosis of ALS. Clin Neurophysiol 2008;119:497–503.

some patients who do not fulfill the clinical criteria for diagnosis because of the limited distribution of muscle weakness may have evidence of widespread denervation on EDX, allowing a diagnosis of ALS to be made based on the Awaji-shima consensus. This diagnosis is important when determining eligibility for clinical trial participation.

NCS changes in ALS are characterized by decreased CMAP amplitudes. The mild slowing of motor conduction velocity and the prolongation of F-wave latencies is attributed to the loss of the fastest conducting fibers. An interesting phenomenon observed in many patients is that of the split hand whereby CMAP amplitudes are decreased to a greater degree on the radial side of the hand than on the ulnar side. CMAPs obtained from the abductor pollicis brevis and first dorsal interosseous are much lower than those obtained from the abductor digit minimi.[35] More than 2 stimulation sites should be used in the evaluation of motor nerves to exclude the presence of CB because MMN with CB occasionally can be misdiagnosed as ALS. The ulnar nerve can be stimulated easily at the wrist, below and above the elbow, in the axilla and in the supraclavicular fossa. In limbs with upper motor neuron signs, H reflexes may be elicited from muscles in which they normally cannot be obtained. SNAP amplitudes may be abnormal in a small percentage of patients with otherwise typical ALS.[36] There have been case reports of concomitant sporadic ALS and a sensory neuropathy for which alternative causes could not be identified.[37] Repetitive stimulation studies may show decrement in CMAP with stimulation at 3 Hz. This decrement is caused by the instability of neuromuscular transmission in collateral nerve terminal sprouts. Some degree of decrement occurs in more than half of patients with ALS, and the amplitude decrement is usually less than 10%.[28]

The NEE is the most important part of the EDX in suspected ALS. Fasciculation potentials are seen in most patients with ALS but they are not necessary to meet diagnostic criteria. The significance of fasciculations depends on the company they keep and are pathologic only when accompanied by fibrillation potentials, PSWs, or the appropriate neurogenic MUAP changes. In patients with advanced disease, fibrillations potentials and PSWs are prominent in most muscles but they may be sparse early in the course of the disease when collateral sprouting can keep up with denervation.[28] Occasionally, CRDs and doublets or triplets are seen in patients with ALS but these are not typical findings. The thoracic paraspinals should be examined on NEE because they are typically spared in cervical and lumbar spinal stenosis. The primary NEE finding in ALS in involved muscles is decreased recruitment. If the disease is progressing slowly, MUAP amplitudes and durations become increased as a result of collateral sprouting. If the disease course is rapid, denervation outpaces reinnervation and enlarged MUAPs do not develop. The density and distribution of fasciculations and fibrillations does not correlate with the disease course or prognosis. Serial EDX are not useful for monitoring disease progression once a definite diagnosis has been made.

Polio

Acute poliomyelitis is an acquired disease of the anterior horn cells that most electromyographers likely will not encounter. However, the sequelae of previous polio frequently are encountered in the EMG laboratory and make the diagnosis of any superimposed neuromuscular problem difficult. In both acute and old polio, the NCS findings are similar to those of other motor neuron diseases: normal sensory studies, normal motor conduction velocities, and low CMAP amplitudes in atrophic muscles. Patients with postpolio frequently have superimposed entrapment neuropathies, such as median or ulnar mononeuropathies, from years of using assistive ambulatory devices.[1,38,39]

The NEE in acute polio will begin to show fibrillation potentials and PSWs in affected muscles 2 to 3 weeks after the onset of weakness. Fasciculation potentials may appear before fibrillation potentials. Initially, the recruitment pattern is decreased, but MUAP size is normal because remodeling of the motor units has not yet had time to occur. As time passes, collateral sprouting and motor unit remodeling occur, creating giant MUAPs with amplitudes up to 20 mV. Fibrillation potentials may persist indefinitely but are small (<100 uV) in chronic polio.

When patients with a history of polio are examined 20 to 30 years later, reduced recruitment, giant MUAPs, and fibrillation potentials may be seen diffusely, not just in muscles clinically involved in the acute polio episode. For this reason, superimposed neuromuscular disorders can be impossible to diagnose by EDX. A superimposed neuropathy may be diagnosed if sensory conduction studies are abnormal, but one cannot distinguish accurately between a pure sensory and a sensorimotor neuropathy. SFEMG studies in patients with chronic polio show increased jitter, blocking, and fiber density.[40]

Fifteen percent to 80% of patients with a history of polio develop postpolio syndrome years after their acute illness. Halstead's criteria for a diagnosis of postpolio syndrome include: (1) history of acute polio; (2) a period of at least 15 years of neurologic and functional stability before the onset of new problems; (3) gradual or abrupt onset of new neurogenic weakness; and (4) no apparent medical, orthopedic, or neurologic cause for the new weakness.[41] EDX is not useful in differentiating between chronic polio with and without postpolio syndrome because both groups have similar findings of NEE and SFEMG studies. The only useful role of EDX in diagnosing postpolio syndrome is to confirm that patients did indeed have polio in the past.

Neuromuscular junction disorders

Disorders of the neuromuscular junction (NMJ) may be classified as presynaptic (Lambert-Eaton myasthenic syndrome [LEMS] and botulism) or postsynaptic (myasthenia gravis [MG]) depending on the location of the defect. NMJ transmission disorders may also be acquired or inherited (congenital myasthenic syndromes). Presynaptic or postsynaptic dysfunction influences the electrophysiologic response to repetitive nerve stimulation (RNS), a technique developed to assist in the EDX of NMJ disorders. In general, findings on routine NCS and NEE in the NMJ disorders are similar to the findings in myopathies. Motor and sensory NCS are normal, with the exception of reduced CMAP amplitudes in presynaptic disorders. MUAPs in affected muscles are either normal or polyphasic with low amplitudes or decreased duration. Small MUAPs are caused by decreased neuromuscular transmission and are not truly myopathic. A unique feature of NMJ disorders is that cooling the muscle may minimize abnormalities seen with RNS and may cause an increase in duration and amplitude in myopathic-appearing MUAPs.[42] Recruitment pattern is full with a submaximal muscle contraction. Moment-to-moment amplitude variation, unstable motor unit, is seen on NEE when a single MUAP is isolated. Fibrillation potentials are seen only in severe disease with complete disintegration of the NMJ. **Table 3** outlines the EDX findings in various disorders of the NMJ transmission.

RNS studies are a technique for evaluating the safety factor of the NMJ. The safety factor refers to the number of acetylcholine receptors (AChRs) that must be opened to generate an end plate potential large enough to depolarize the muscle membrane and produce muscle contraction.[43] In healthy individuals, the safety factor can be reduced by exercise or repetitive nerve activation but not to a degree large enough to prevent the generation of an endplate potential. In presynaptic disorders, acetylcholine release is diminished, resulting in too few postsynaptic AChRs opening, thus decreasing the safety factor. In postsynaptic disorders, a normal amount of acetylcholine is released but too few AChRs are available for binding and the safety factor is again reduced.

RNS studies generally are performed at 2 stimulation rates: slow (2–3 Hz) and fast (20–30 Hz). With slow stimulation, each successive stimulus results in fewer vesicles of acetylcholine being released. In individuals with NMJ disorders, the safety factor is reduced. In patients with a baseline low safety factor, the safety factor is reduced to the extent that NMJ block occurs in some single muscle fibers so that fewer fibers contribute to the overall CMAP, thus reducing the CMAP amplitude. To perform slow RNS, a train of 5 supramaximal stimuli is delivered. A decrement in CMAP amplitude of greater than 10% is abnormal. When a decrement occurs, it should be greatest between the first and second recorded stimuli. The patient is then asked to exercise or maximally contract the target muscle for 10 to 20 seconds in the setting of a decrement and 30 to 60 seconds in the setting of no decrement. The normal response is up to a 15% increase in CMAP amplitude immediately following exercise. The train of 5 supramaximal stimuli is repeated immediately after exercise, at 30 seconds and at

Table 3
Electrodiagnostic findings in NMJ transmission disorders

Parameter	MG	LEMS	Botulism
Distal latency	nL	nL	nL
Conduction velocity	nL	nL	nL
SNAP amplitude	nL	nL	nL
CMAP amplitude	Usually nL	Decreased	nL or decreased
Slow RNS	Decrement	Decrement	± Decrement
Fast RNS or brief exercise	± Mild increment	Large increment (lasting 20–30 s)	Intermediate increment (lasting up to 4 min)
Postactivation exhaustion	Yes	Yes	No
MUAP configuration	Unstable motor unit (weak muscles) ± dec amplitude & duration	Unstable motor unit (all muscles), dec amplitude & duration, inc polyphasics	Unstable motor unit (weak muscles), dec amplitude & duration, inc polyphasics
Recruitment	nL or early	Early	Early
Spontaneous activity	Fibrillation in severe disease	None	Fibrillation in severe disease
SFEMG	inc jitter & blocking (increases with inc firing rate)	inc jitter & blocking (decreases with inc firing rate)	inc jitter & blocking (decreases with inc firing rate)

Abbreviations: dec, decreased; inc, increased; nL, normal.
Data from Krivickas LS. Electrodiagnosis in neuromuscular diseases. Phys Med Rehabil Clin N Am 1998;9:99.

1, 2, 3, and 4 minutes after exercise. Patients with defects in NMJ transmission may demonstrate complete or partial repair of the decrement immediately after exercise (postexercise facilitation); after 3 to 4 minutes, the decrement worsens (postactivation exhaustion). If the patient is too weak to exercise or is unable to follow directions concerning exercise, fast repetitive stimulation (20–30 Hz) of 1 or 2 seconds may be substituted for the exercise to produce the same result.[43]

SFEMG is the gold standard for the electrodiagnosis of disorders involving the NMJ when repetitive stimulation studies are negative or nonrevealing. Jitter is increased in both presynaptic and postsynaptic NMJ disorders but is nonspecific because it is also increased in motor neuron diseases, myopathies, and neuropathies in which immature NMJs are present. An SFEMG is most commonly performed in the extensor digitorum communis muscle because it is easy to isolate single MUAPs in this muscle. Twenty pairs of MUAPs are recorded, and the study is considered abnormal if the mean jitter of all pairs is increased, if 2 or more individual pairs have jitter greater than a given parameter (based on age), or if frequent blocking occurs. Blocking of neuromuscular transmission begins to occur when jitter reaches 80 microseconds.[44]

MG

MG is the most commonly encountered NMJ disorder and is a model for the electrophysiologic findings of all postsynaptic NMJ disorders. Other postsynaptic disorders include a subset of postsynaptic congenital myasthenic syndromes, organophosphate poisoning, and poisoning with curarelike compounds. Routine sensory and motor NCS are normal, with the exception of low CMAPs from the most severely weak muscles. When weakness is fairly severe in the muscle from which a CMAP is being recorded, a strong initial stimulus should be delivered to the nerve to avoid the necessity of multiple stimuli, which may result in NMJ fatigue and an even lower CMAP than would be recorded otherwise. A motor NCS should be conducted for every planned repetitive stimulation study. The abductor pollicis brevis and abductor digit minimi are the easiest to study with repetitive stimulation because they can be immobilized more easily than proximal muscles. However, in mild disease, proximal muscles are more likely to show an abnormal response to repetitive stimulation. The slow repetitive stimulation protocol outlined previously is used in an attempt to elicit the classic triad of findings characteristic of MG: (1) CMAP decrement with slow repetitive stimulation, (2) repair of decrement immediately after exercise, and (3) worsening of the decrement 2 to 4 minutes after exercise. If the RNS study of a distal muscle is negative, a proximal muscle should be evaluated; the nasalis and trapezius are commonly used proximal muscles. In patients with ocular myasthenia, it may be necessary to perform repetitive stimulation of the orbicularis oculi muscle. The most significant finding on NEE is MUAP moment-to-moment amplitude variation. This variation must be studied by isolating a single MUAP and observing its morphology over time. Amplitude variation is the needle electrode equivalent of the decrement seen on RNS studies. A small number of patients with severe, chronic disease have fibrillation potentials and PSWs in the weakest muscles because the muscles are functionally denervated at the NMJ. The dropout of single muscle fibers can decrease the amplitude and duration of MUAPs, giving them a myopathic appearance, which occurs more frequently than the presence of fibrillation potentials and PSWs.[45]

Single fiber EMG is necessary only when repetitive nerve stimulation studies fail to show a decrement, NEE does not show moment-to-moment amplitude variation in affected muscles and AChR antibody testing is negative. Generally, the extensor digitorum communis is examined first. If this study is normal, then a single fiber EMG is performed in the frontalis muscle. Single fiber EMG may be performed without stopping anticholinesterase medications because jitter is usually abnormal even while taking medication. Anticholinesterase medication must be discontinued 12 hours before repetitive nerve stimulation studies in order for accurate and valid assessment of obtained results.

LEMS

LEMS is the most commonly encountered presynaptic disorder of neuromuscular transmission. Botulism, tetanus, and some forms of congenital myasthenia are also presynaptic disorders. Sensory NCS are normal in pure LEMS. Because more than 50% of patients with LEMS have a malignancy, most commonly small cell carcinoma, a concomitant paraneoplastic sensory or sensorimotor neuropathy is common. Motor NCS are characterized by a low CMAP, often only a few 100 μV. After 10 to 20 seconds of exercise (isometric muscle contraction), the CMAP amplitude will increase by more than 100% because of the accumulation of calcium in the presynaptic terminal, which increases ACh release. If exercise is performed for longer than 20 seconds, this facilitation may be replaced by postexercise exhaustion in which no increase in amplitude is seen. Low RNS will produce a decrement similar to that seen in MG except that repair of the decrement following exercise is much pronounced and accompanied by a large increase in amplitude as previously described. This response lasts 20 to 30 seconds and is then once again replaced by a low CMAP, which decreases with repetitive nerve stimulation. In all patients with low CMAPs, a brief period of exercise should be given and another CMAP elicited to look for a presynaptic neuromuscular transmission defect. In severely weak patients who are unable to exercise, rapid repetitive stimulation may be applied for 1 to 2 seconds to generate an increment in CMAP amplitude. In LEMS, an increment in CMAP with exercise usually can be detected in any muscle examined. Once the increment has been demonstrated, there is no need to repeat the study in additional muscles. In mild early cases, an increment may be isolated to proximal muscles.

The hallmark of NEE in patients with LEMS is moment-to-moment amplitude variation in all muscles examined, independent of clinical weakness. Because only a few muscle fibers per motor unit may fire, the MUAPs may be short in duration, low amplitude, and polyphasic, with a myopathic appearance. With sustained voluntary contraction, MUAPs may increase in amplitude and duration, losing their myopathic appearance. This feature can help distinguish them from the firing pattern seen in myopathies. Fibrillation potentials and PSWs are not present. SFEMG shows markedly increased jitter and blocking in all muscles, unlike MG whereby jitter is increased in only the most severely affected muscles. In LEMS, both jitter and blocking decrease as firing rate increases.[46]

Botulism

The EXD findings in botulism are similar to those seen in LEMS with a few key differences. The CMAP amplitude is not as severely reduced, and the incremental response to exercise is somewhat less dramatic but should be at least 40%. The increase in CMAP amplitude persists much longer than in LEMS, often for as long as 4 minutes. In infants, it may last up to 20 minutes. In severe cases of botulism, rapid RNS may not result in facilitation because of the complete block of ACh release by the toxin. In these cases, the endplates break down because of the lack of ACh and functional denervation occurs resulting in the presence of fibrillation potentials and PSWs. Unlike LEMS, only clinically weak muscles show EMG changes. Bulbar muscles should be examined in mild cases because they are usually affected first and most severely.[43]

Myopathies

The myopathic disorders include the progressive muscular dystrophies, congenital myopathies, metabolic myopathies, mitochondrial myopathies, acquired inflammatory myopathies, and some ion channel disorders. The EDX examination is less sensitive for detecting myopathies compared with other groups of neuromuscular diseases. It is also rarely helpful in differentiating between the various myopathic disorders. The patchy distribution of abnormalities presents a challenge during EMG of a suspected myopathy. EDX abnormalities seen with myopathies are nonspecific and are also seen in some nonmyopathic disorders. NCS are usually normal in myopathies unless the underlying muscle being tested is atrophic. Sensory NCS are always normal unless there is an underlying peripheral neuropathy. The NEE may show several types of spontaneous activity, including fibrillations potentials, PSWs, CRDs, and myotonic discharges. Insertional activity may be normal, increased, or decreased depending on the type of myopathy, distribution, and stage of disease. The recruitment pattern is early, with the addition of MUAPs with a low level of effort. In mild disease, the presence of early recruitment is not as obvious. Motor units may be in various stages of demise and may show low amplitudes, increased polyphasia, and decreased duration. Decreased MUAP duration is the most sensitive indicator of a myopathic process and quantitative EMG can assist in the detection. Presentations vary on NEE. Some myopathies present with isolated abnormal spontaneous activity, whereas some severe end-stage chronic myopathies develop a neurogenic appearance when only a few motor units per muscle remain. EMG abnormalities are most likely to be found in the limb girdle muscles and paraspinals.

Progressive muscular dystrophies

With the availability of molecular genetic testing for the identification of increasing numbers of progressive muscular dystrophies, the role of EDX examination is decreasing. In all of the progressive muscular dystrophies, the needle feel on insertion and the ease of needle advancement changes as the muscle is replaced by fat and connective tissue. The muscle develops a gritty feel and physical resistance to needle movement develops over time. The EDX findings in the muscular dystrophies are similar to those found in other myopathies, with a few unique characteristics. In Duchenne muscular dystrophy (DMD) and Becker muscular dystrophy (BMD), fibrillation potentials and PSWs are widespread, although they are somewhat less prominent in BMD. Occasionally, CRDs and myotonic discharges are present but they are not prominent.[47] In addition to myopathic-appearing MUAPs, large-amplitude and increased-duration MUAPs may be seen. These MUAPs are a result of muscle fiber hypertrophy or increased fiber density motor units caused by remodeling following muscle degeneration. In facioscapulohumeral muscular dystrophy (FSHD), fibrillation potentials and PSWs may or may not be present. When they are present, they are less abundant than in DMD. Unlike DMD, large-amplitude, long-duration motor units are not seen. The earliest muscles involved are facial muscles, but NEE is often not helpful because typical facial muscle MUAPs may seem myopathic when compared with limb muscles. Other affected muscles that may be tested are the scapular stabilizers, biceps, and triceps. The tibialis anterior is the first muscle affected in the lower limbs. Similar findings can be seen in individuals with limb girdle muscular dystrophies (LGMDs) in clinically weak muscles. The main difference between FSHD and LGMD is that MUAPs amplitudes tend to be larger in the latter. The NEE findings in Emery-Dreifuss muscular dystrophy are similar those found in other progressive muscular dystrophies, with a mixed pattern of small and large MUAPs. A unique characteristic of Emery-Dreifuss is more severe involvement of biceps and triceps than more proximal upper extremity muscles.

Myotonic muscular dystrophy has unique EDX features, including the presence of myotonic discharges and response to high-rate RNS. At low-rate RNS, no CMAP decrement is present. However, at high-rate RNS, a progressive decrement is seen. Myotonic potentials are induced by both needle movement and voluntary muscle contraction. They are most notable in the distal muscles and may not be present in all of the muscles examined. Fibrillation potentials are present and may be caused by spontaneous discharges of innervated single muscle fibers or by denervation. An accompanying peripheral neuropathy has been detected in some individuals with myotonic dystrophy.

Congenital myopathies

The most common congenital myopathies are central core disease, multicore disease, nemaline myopathy, centronuclear myopathy (also called myotubular myopathy), and congenital fiber-type disproportion. In general, the congenital myopathies have nonspecific myopathic changes on EDX. However, a normal examination can be seen with congenital fiber-type disproportion. Abnormal spontaneous activity is uncommon except in centronuclear myopathy, which often has fibrillation potentials, PSWs, CRDs, and occasionally myotonic discharges (Hawkes).[48] A concomitant defect in NMJ transmission has been described in a few patients with centronuclear myopathy.[49]

Mitochondrial myopathies

Mitochondrial myopathies also have nonspecific EDX findings. In mild cases, the EDX can be normal. Despite the common complaint of activity-induced fatigue, RNS studies are normal. Some individuals with mitochondrial disease have EDX findings showing a concomitant peripheral neuropathy.[50]

Metabolic myopathies

The metabolic myopathies include disorders of glycogen metabolism, lipid metabolism, and myoadenylate deaminase deficiency (MADD). There are 5 known glycogen metabolism disorders that have EDX abnormalities: glycogen storage disease (GSD) type II (acid maltase deficiency, Pompe disease), GSD type III (debranching enzyme deficiency), GSD type IV (branching enzyme deficiency), GSD type V (myophosphorylase deficiency, McArdle disease), and type VII (phosphofructokinase deficiency, Tarui disease). Acid maltase deficiency is unique in that it produces profuse spontaneous activity, including fibrillations, PSWs, CRDs, and myotonic discharges. Spontaneous activity is most prominent in the paraspinal muscles. Findings of myotonic discharges in the paraspinal muscles of an adult with proximal limb and respiratory weakness suggest Pompe disease/acid maltase deficiency.[51] Debranching enzyme deficiency (GSD type III) can be distinguished by a concomitant peripheral neuropathy in some patients. They may also have fibrillation potentials and CRDs, although to a lesser degree than GSD type II. Myotonic discharges are not a common finding with debranching enzyme deficiency. Patients diagnosed with McArdle disease experience frequent muscle cramping and contracture. On NEE, muscle contracture is electrically silent despite obvious prolonged muscle contractions. At the onset of a contracture, the interference pattern amplitude declines as does the number of MUAPs firing. Gradually over minutes, electrical silence occurs.[52] In many patients, the NEE is normal when they are not experiencing muscle cramping. When the disease is severe enough to cause permanent weakness, myopathic-appearing MUAPs can be seen. Patients with late-onset disease are likely to have fibrillation potentials, PSWs, and CRDs.[53] An abnormal response to low-rate and high-rate RNS has been reported in some patients with McArdle disease, suggesting a concomitant defect in neuromuscular transmission. Data on the EDX findings in Tarui disease are minimal but may be similar to those found in McArdle disease in some patients.

The EDX findings in lipid metabolism disorders that result in weakness, carnitine deficiency, and carnitine palmitoyltransferase deficiency (CPT) are nonspecific and not well described. In most cases of carnitine deficiency, myopathic-appearing MUAPs are seen. In severe disease, extremely weak muscles show fibrillation potentials, PSWs, and CRDs.[54] A superimposed sensorimotor peripheral neuropathy has also been reported in patients with CPT. The EDX is normal in MADD.

Inflammatory myopathies

Although clinical features and muscle biopsy findings of polymyositis and dermatomyositis can distinguish the two disorders, their electrodiagnostic findings are identical. NEE of proximal muscles and paraspinals at multiple levels should be examined. In some cases, findings are only seen in the paraspinal muscles. Abnormal findings on NEE may be patchy in distribution necessitating multiple needle insertions within the same muscle. If no abnormalities are detected in a clinically weak muscle, then a second or even third insertion site should be evaluated. Fibrillation potentials and PSWs are common and their quantity may be reflective of the severity of disease, although no correlative studies have been done. However, serial EDX studies are not recommended to evaluate the response to treatment. The EDX can be used to help distinguish between exacerbation of the inflammatory myopathy and the progression of weakness as a result of steroid myopathy in those individuals receiving treatment with corticosteroids. CRDs are common in chronic stages of the disease, and the muscle may have a gritty feel on needle insertion because of the replacement of muscle tissue with connective tissue. MUAP morphology changes are similar to those seen in other myopathies. In chronic stages of the disease, there may be some large-amplitude MUAPs among the typical myopathic motor units that are small with polyphasia.

Inclusion body myositis (IBM) may be distinguished from polymyositis by its pattern of muscle weakness, clinic course, EDX findings, and distinctive features on muscle biopsy. EDX findings are similar to those found in polymyositis and dermatomyositis; however, fibrillation potentials and PSWs are more prominent in IBM and may be found in almost every muscle examined. CRDs, myotonic discharges, and fasciculations may also be more prominent in IBM. MUAPs vary in amplitude and duration depending on the chronicity of the illness and may seem myopathic, neuropathic, or mixed. In addition to proximal muscle involvement, distal muscles, including the forearm flexors, hand intrinsics, and tibialis anterior, are involved. The quadriceps muscles are typically involved as seen by NEE, whereas the glutei are often spared.[55]

Channelopathies

The ion channel disorders encompass both myotonic disorders and the periodic paralyses. Myotonic dystrophy involves abnormalities in the sodium channel and calcium-activated potassium channel. Myotonia congenita is a chloride channel disorder, hypokalemic periodic paralysis is a calcium channel disorder, and hyperkalemic periodic paralysis and paramyotonia congenital are sodium channel disorders.

There are 2 variants of myotonia congenita. Thomsen disease is autosomal dominant and Becker disease is autosomal recessive. In both forms, diffuse myotonic discharges are seen in most muscles and may prevent the assessment of individual MUAPs. MUAPs seem normal with Thomsen disease but may be short in duration and amplitude with long-standing Becker disease. Amplitude decrement with rapid RNS is seen in Thomsen disease, whereas a similar decrement is seen with both rapid and slow rates of RNS with Becker disease.

Clinically, paramyotonia congenita and myotonia congenita are often confused. On EDX evaluation, there are distinct differences. In paramyotonia congenita, a decrement in CMAP occurs either after cooling the muscle or immediately after several minutes of forceful exercise and the CMAP amplitude does not return to baseline for more than 1 hour. In myotonia congentia, a smaller decrement is seen following exercise and it often recovers within a few minutes after stopping exercise. On NEE, cooling the limb with ice water or exercising the limb can cause decreased recruitment that approaches an electrically silent contracture in some individuals with paramyotonia congenita. Between episodes of muscle stiffness, MUAPs are normal but may be difficult to assess because of the persistent and diffuse myotonia, particularly in the distal limb muscles. Fibrillation potentials, PSWs, and increased myotonic discharges may be observed during episodes of weakness, before the onset of complete electrical silence. Abnormal spontaneous activity is not observed during asymptomatic periods.

Attacks of hyperkalemic periodic paralysis are triggered by rest following cold exposure, exercise, immobilization, fasting, and heavy meals. After exercise, a CMAP decrement is noted. It is preceded by a CMAP increment and gradually reaches its nadir by 20 minutes following exercise. Clinical and electrical myotonia may or may not be present. Patients may only display electrical myotonia, which is usually present in all muscles on NEE, even during asymptomatic periods. At the beginning of an attack, complete electrical silence may occur. Some affected individuals eventually develop mild weakness, and myopathic-appearing MUAPs are present on NEE between attacks.

Attacks of hypokalemic periodic paralysis are triggered by rest following carbohydrate loading, strenuous exercise, and stress. During attacks, the muscle membrane becomes unexcitable. CMAP amplitudes decline severely or disappear altogether.

While the CMAP is in the process of declining, rapid (10 Hz) RNS can be used to reverse the decline in amplitude. As an attack progresses, recruitment and MUAP amplitude and duration decreases. Eventually at the nadir of the attack, electrical silence occurs. Fibrillation potentials and PSWs may be observed between the onset of the attack and electrical silence. Myotonic potentials are not seen. In most patients, the NEE is normal between attacks. A few patients with permanent weakness have myopathic-appearing MUAPs and fibrillation potentials.

SUMMARY

EMG is an important diagnostic tool for the assessment of individuals with various neuromuscular diseases. It should be an extension of thorough history and physical examination. Some prototypical EMG and NCS characteristics and findings are discussed; however, a more thorough discussion can be found in textbooks and resource sited earlier. With increases in molecular genetic diagnostics, EMG continues to play an important role in the diagnosis and management of patients with neuromuscular diseases and also provides a cost-effective diagnostic workup before ordering a battery of costly genetic tests.

REFERENCES

1. Uluc K, Isak B, Borucu D, et al. Medial plantar and dorsal sural nerve conduction studies increase the sensitivity in the detection of neuropathy in diabetic patients. Clin Neurophysiol 2008;119:880–5.
2. Kaku D, Parry G, Malamut R, et al. Uniform slowing of conduction velocities in Charcot-Marie-Tooth polyneuropathy type 1. Neurology 1993;43:2664–7.
3. Murphy SM, Laurá M, Blake J, et al. Conduction block and tonic pupils in Charcot-Marie-Tooth disease caused by a myelin protein zero p.Ile112Thr mutation. Neuromuscul Disord 2011;21:223–6.
4. Banchs I, Casasnovas C, Albertí A, et al. Diagnosis of Charcot-Marie-Tooth disease. J Biomed Biotechnol 2009;2009:985415 Epub 2009 Oct 8.
5. Gabreëls-Festen A. Dejerine-Sottas syndrome grown to maturity: overview of genetic and morphological heterogeneity and follow-up of 25 patients. J Anat 2002;200:341–56.
6. Dyck PJ, Lambert EH, Sanders K, et al. Severe hypomyelination and marked abnormality of conduction in Dejerine-Sottas hypertrophic neuropathy: myelin thickness and compound action potential of sural nerve in vitro. Mayo Clin Proc 1971;46:432–6.
7. Andersson PB, Yuen E, Parko K, et al. Electrodiagnostic features of hereditary neuropathy with liability to pressure palsies. Neurology 2000;54:40–4.
8. Dumitru D. Hereditary neuropathies. In: Dumitru D, editor. Electrodiagnostic medicine. Philadelphia: Hanley & Belfus; 2002. p. 899–936.
9. Hughes RA, Cornblath DR. Guillain-Barré syndrome. Lancet 2005;366:1653–66.
10. Albers JW, Donofrio PD, McGonagle TK. Sequential electrodiagnostic abnormalities in acute inflammatory demyelinating polyradiculoneuropathy. Muscle Nerve 1985;8:528–39.
11. Baraba R, Sruk A, Sragalj L, et al. Electrophysiological findings in early Guillain-Barré syndrome. Acta Clin Croat 2011;50:201–7.
12. Murray NM, Wade DT. The sural sensory action potential in Guillain-Barré syndrome. Muscle Nerve 1980;3:444.
13. Albers JW, Kelly JJ Jr. Acquired Inflammatory demyelinating polyneuropathies: clinical and electrodiagnostic features. Muscle Nerve 1989;12:435–51.

14. Sander HW, Latov N. Research criteria for defining patients with CIDP. Neurology 2003;60:S8–15.
15. Haq RU, Fries TJ, Pendlebury WW, et al. Chronic inflammatory demyelinating polyradiculoneuropathy: a study of proposed electrodiagnostic and histologic criteria. Arch Neurol 2000;57:1745–50.
16. Dumitru D. Acquired neuropathies. In: Dumitru D, editor. Electrodiagnostic medicine. Philadelphia: Hanley & Belfus; 2002. p. 937–1042.
17. Mauermann ML, Sorenson EJ, Dispenzieri A, et al. Uniform demyelination and more severe axonal loss distinguish POEMS syndrome from CIDP. J Neurol Neurosurg Psychiatry 2012;83(5):480–6.
18. Van Asseldonk JH, Franssen H, Van den Berg-Vos RM, et al. Multifocal motor neuropathy. Lancet Neurol 2005;4:309–19.
19. Rossor AM, Kalmar B, Greensmith L, et al. The distal hereditary motor neuropathies. J Neurol Neurosurg Psychiatry 2012;83:6–14.
20. Mitsumoto H, Wilbourn AJ. Causes and diagnosis of sensory neuropathies: a review. J Clin Neurophysiol 1994;11:553–67.
21. Caruso G, Santoro L, Perretti A, et al. Friedreich's ataxia: electrophysiologic and histologic findings in patients and relatives. Muscle Nerve 1987;10:503–15.
22. Santoro L, Perretti A, Crisci C, et al. Electrophysiological and histological follow-up study in 15 Friedreich's ataxia patients. Muscle Nerve 1990;13:536–40.
23. Verhoeven K, Timmerman V, Mauko B, et al. Recent advances in hereditary sensory and autonomic neuropathies. Curr Opin Neurol 2006;19:474–80.
24. Said G. Focal and multifocal diabetic neuropathy. In: Veves A, Malik R, editors. Diabetic neuropathy: clinical management. Totowa (NJ): Humana Press; 2007. p. 367–76.
25. Ackil AA, Shahani BT, Young RR, et al. Late response and sural conduction studies. Usefulness in patients with chronic renal failure. Arch Neurol 1981;38:482–5.
26. Dumitru D. Disorders affecting motor neurons. In: Dumitru D, editor. Electrodiagnostic medicine. Philadelphia: Hanley & Belfus; 2002. p. 581–651.
27. Dubowitz V. Muscle disorders in children. Philadelphia: WB Saunders; 1978.
28. Daube JR. Electrodiagnostic studies in amyotrophic lateral sclerosis and other motor neuron disorders. Muscle Nerve 2000;23:1488–502.
29. Hausmanowa-Petrusewicz I, Friedman A, Kowalski J, et al. Spontaneous motor unit firing in spinal muscular atrophy of childhood. Electromyogr Clin Neurophysiol 1987;27:259–64.
30. Krivickas LS. Amyotrophic lateral sclerosis and other motor neuron diseases. Phys Med Rehabil Clin N Am 2003;14:327–45.
31. Ferrante MA, Wilbourn AJ. The characteristic electrodiagnostic features of Kennedy's disease. Muscle Nerve 1997;20:323–9.
32. Siddique T, Ajroud-Driss S. Familial amyotrophic lateral sclerosis, a historical perspective. Acta Myol 2011;30:117–20.
33. Brooks BR. El Escorial World Federation of Neurology criteria for the diagnosis of amyotrophic lateral sclerosis. Subcommittee on Motor Neuron Diseases/Amyotrophic Lateral Sclerosis of the World Federation of Neurology Research Group on Neuromuscular Diseases and the El Escorial "clinical limits of amyotrophic lateral sclerosis" workshop contributors. J Neurol Sci 1994;124(Suppl):96–107.
34. de Carvalho M, Dengler R, Eisen A, et al. Electrodiagnostic criteria for diagnosis of ALS. Clin Neurophysiol 2008;119:497–503.
35. Eisen A, Kuwabara S. The split hand syndrome in amyotrophic lateral sclerosis. J Neurol Neurosurg Psychiatry 2012;83:399–403.

36. Behnia M, Kelly JJ. Role of electromyography in amyotrophic lateral sclerosis. Muscle Nerve 1991;14:1236–41.
37. Isaacs JD, Dean AF, Shaw CE, et al. Amyotrophic lateral sclerosis with sensory neuropathy: part of a multisystem disorder? J Neurol Neurosurg Psychiatry 2007;78:750–3.
38. Gawne AC, Pham BT, Halstead LS. Electrodiagnostic findings in 108 consecutive patients referred to a post-polio clinic. The value of routine electrodiagnostic studies. Ann N Y Acad Sci 1995;753:383–5.
39. Tsai HC, Hung TH, Chen CC, et al. Prevalence and risk factors for upper extremity entrapment neuropathies in polio survivors. J Rehabil Med 2009;41:26–31.
40. Trojan DA, Gendron D, Cashman NR, et al. Electrophysiology and electrodiagnosis of the post-polio motor unit. Orthopedics 1991;14:1353–61.
41. Farbu E, Gilhus NE, Barnes MP, et al. EFNS guideline on diagnosis and management of post-polio syndrome. Report of an EFNS task force. Eur J Neurol 2006;13: 795–801.
42. Rutkove SB, et al. Effects of temperature on neuromuscular electrophysiology. Muscle Nerve 2001;24:867–82.
43. Dumitru D. Neuromuscular junction disorders. In: Dumitru D, editor. Electrodiagnostic medicine. Philadelphia: Hanley & Belfus; 2002. p. 1127–228.
44. Sanders DB. AAEM minimonograph #25: single-fiber electromyography. Muscle Nerve 1996;19:1069–83.
45. Cruz-Martinez A, Ferrer MT, Diez Tejedor E, et al. Diagnostic yield of single fiber electromyography and other electrophysiological techniques in myasthenia gravis. I. Electromyography, automatic analysis of the voluntary pattern, and repetitive nerve stimulation. Electromyogr Clin Neurophysiol 1982;22:377–93.
46. O'Neill JH, Murray NM, Newsom-Davis J, et al. The Lambert-Eaton myasthenic syndrome. A review of 50 cases. Brain 1988;111:577–96.
47. Dumitru D. Hereditary myopathies. In: Dumitru D, editor. Electrodiagnostic medicine. Philadelphia: Hanley & Belfus; 2002. p. 1265–370.
48. Hawkes CH, Absolon MJ. Myotubular myopathy associated with cataract and electrical myotonia. J Neurol Neurosurg Psychiatry 1975;38:761–4.
49. Liewluck T, Shen XM, Milone M, et al. Endplate structure and parameters of neuromuscular transmission in sporadic centronuclear myopathy associated with myasthenia. Neuromuscul Disord 2011;21:387–95.
50. Kamieniecka Z. Myopathies with abnormal mitochondria. Acta Neurol Scand 1977;55:57–75.
51. Barohn RJ, McVey AL, DiMauro S. Adult acid maltase deficiency. Muscle Nerve 1993;16:672–6.
52. Dycken ML, Smith DM, Peake RL. An electromyographic diagnostic screening test in McArdle's disease: a case report. Neurology 1967;17:45–50.
53. Pourmand R, Sanders DB, Corwin HM. Late-onset McArdle's disease with unusual electromyographic findings. Ann Neurol 1983;40:347–77.
54. Vandyke DH, Griggs RC, Markesbery W, et al. Hereditary carnitine deficiency of muscle. Neurology 1975;25:154–9.
55. Dumitru D. Acquired myopathies. In: Dumitru D, editor. Electrodiagnostic medicine. Philadelphia: Hanley & Belfus; 2002. p. 1371–432.

A Practical Approach to Molecular Diagnostic Testing in Neuromuscular Diseases

W. David Arnold, MD[a],*, Kevin M. Flanigan, MD[b,c]

KEYWORDS

- Neuromuscular diseases • Molecular diagnostic testing • Genomic technologies
- Genetic disorders

KEY POINTS

- Molecular testing is an important aspect in the care of patients with neuromuscular disorders.
- Some potential benefits include diagnostic certainty, the identification of current and future therapeutics, and information to help guide accurate genetic counseling and family planning.
- Once a genetic condition is considered, it is usually imperative to establish as precise a clinical diagnosis as possible before proceeding with targeted molecular diagnostic testing.
- The future of molecular testing will likely shift away from targeted genetic analysis toward genomic technologies to allow for a nontargeted approach.

INTRODUCTION

Genetic testing plays an increasingly important role in neuromuscular medicine. Over the last 2 decades, there has been rapid progress in molecular genetics, leading to a continually increasing number of identified diagnostic entities and clinically available diagnostic tests. As genetic testing becomes more efficient from a cost and throughput standpoint, it will become an increasingly useful part of patient care. This practicality is particularly likely as treatments become available; as our understanding of hereditary neuromuscular disorders increases and potential treatment strategies are identified, genetic testing will become critical to provide personalized

[a] Division of Neuromuscular Disorders, Department of Neurology, Wexner Medical Center at the Ohio State University, The Ohio State University, 395 W. 12th Avenue, 7th Floor, Columbus, OH 43210, USA; [b] The Center for Gene Therapy, Nationwide Children's Hospital, 700 Children's Drive, Columbus, OH 43205, USA; [c] The Ohio State University, Nationwide Children's Hospital, 700 Children's Drive, Columbus, OH 43205, USA
* Corresponding author.
E-mail address: William.Arnold@osumc.edu

Phys Med Rehabil Clin N Am 23 (2012) 589–608
http://dx.doi.org/10.1016/j.pmr.2012.06.002
1047-9651/12/$ – see front matter © 2012 Elsevier Inc. All rights reserved.

care. For the clinician, this growth in genetic testing may be daunting, and the approach to obtaining a molecular diagnosis may seem challenging.

The utility of genetic testing is often questioned by physicians, patients, or insurers when specific treatments are unavailable for most of the known hereditary conditions. However, the accepted benefits of genetic testing extend beyond treatment alone. Perhaps most importantly, genetic testing can often provide a definitive diagnosis, shortening the diagnostic odyssey for a family and avoiding unnecessary and often expensive additional testing; provide information for accurate genetic counseling and family planning guidance; suggest appropriate surveillance testing; and identify current and future therapeutic interventions. Benefits beyond standard clinical care include the identification of specific mutations, potentially allowing clinical trial participation, or participation in genotype/phenotype correlation and natural history studies.

These benefits may come at a significant financial burden, and striking a balance between sufficient and excessive use of testing is not always easy or straightforward. Many patients require multiple tests to achieve a diagnosis, and testing may exceed thousands of dollars. In some cases, despite extensive testing, a specific mutation may not be identified. In such cases, the possibility of an underlying hereditary condition may not be entirely excluded because of the incomplete understanding of the hereditary causes of most neuromuscular disorders. Additional potential drawbacks of genetic testing include psychological stress and anxiety and potential stigmatization and discrimination with the confirmation of a genetic disorder. The identification of a genetic disorder in presymptomatic patients may cause unnecessary psychological stress. Additionally, genetic testing in an affected individual carries significant potential implications for family members at risk of carrier or affected status.

For these reasons, the clinician involved in the care of neuromuscular disease needs a working understanding of the principles of genetics and genetic diagnoses as well as the indications for performing and the limitations of common genetic tests. Furthermore, they must be prepared to provide genetic testing results along with (or with access to) appropriate genetic counseling.

HEREDITARY BASIS OF DISEASE

For most disorders related to single gene inheritance, disease phenotype is caused by the inheritance of a mutated copy or copies of a gene. The pattern of inheritance is determined by whether the mutated gene is on an autosome (chromosomes 1–22) or on a sex-linked chromosome (chromosome X or Y) and whether the disorder is dominant or recessive (**Fig. 1**). Autosomal disorders affect both sexes and can be transmitted by either sex. Individuals with autosomal dominant disorders usually have at least one affected parent, and subsequent generations of an affected parent have a 50% chance of being affected. A gene is considered dominant if one copy is sufficient to determine the presence of a particular trait. Autosomal recessive disorders are caused by having 2 mutated copies of a gene, one copy from each parent. Parents of an affected individual are usually asymptomatic but carry one mutated copy of a gene. Children of 2 asymptomatic carriers have a 25% chance of being affected.

X-linked disorders may occur in a dominant or recessive fashion. Females have 2 X chromosomes, one of paternal origin and the other of maternal origin. Males have one Y chromosome of paternal origin and one X chromosome of maternal origin. X-linked recessive disorders usually only affect males born to asymptomatic parents. The father is unaffected and (usually) the mother is an asymptomatic carrier. In X-linked disorders, there is no male-to-male transmission. Because of lyonization, or inactivation of one X chromosome in females, a proportion of females may be symptomatic

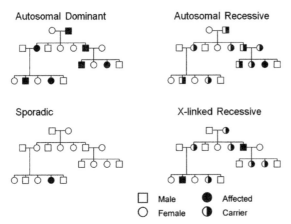

Fig. 1. Pedigree charts demonstrating autosomal dominant, autosomal recessive, X-linked recessive, and sporadic patterns on inheritance.

carriers of recessive X-linked traits and this can occur in 2% to 8% in Duchenne muscular dystrophy (DMD).[1]

Mitochondrial inheritance (not shown in see **Fig. 1**) is another important mode of inheritance. Mitochondrial DNA is transmitted from maternal origin because the mitochondria from the sperm are usually actively degraded after fertilization. The transmission occurs from a maternal lineage, and all offspring may be affected. Mitochondrial DNA mutations may subsequently be transmitted from female but not male offspring to future generations. However, it is important to note that not all mitochondrial disorders are caused by mitochondrial DNA mutations and may also be related to mutations in autosomally encoded mitochondrial proteins.

In addition to the previously discussed modes of transmission, sporadic or de novo mutations may spontaneously occur. In this instance, family history or genetic testing of parents for affected or carrier status is unrevealing. This phenomenon occurs with variable frequency and occasionally may exceed the frequency of inherited mutations in certain conditions. When family history is negative, a de novo mutation should be considered, but other possible explanations exist. Somatic mosaicism may occur in which a mutation may be in some but not all cells; if the mutation is in germline cells, it may be passed onto future generations. Other issues, including age of onset, mistaken paternity, and incomplete penetrance, can obscure a significant family history and should be taken in account when obtaining and reviewing the family history.

GENERAL APPROACH

Because of the significant costs of most molecular testing, it is imperative to establish as precise a clinical diagnosis as possible. The most important and most obvious step is the consideration that patients' symptoms may be genetic in origin. The possibility of an inherited process is not always obvious. The presence of slowly progressive or longstanding symptoms and other features listed in **Box 1** may suggest a hereditary process but such features are occasionally absent. It is not uncommon for patients to be initially unable to identify slowly progressive deficits or recognize similar symptoms in other family members, particularly if other family members have not received a confirmed diagnosis. Slowly progressive symptoms often go unnoticed until such symptoms interfere with day-to-day activities. Specific questions regarding

---
Box 1
Classical features suggestive of a hereditary disorder

Longstanding or slowly progressive deficits

Clinical signs out of proportion to the patients' described symptoms

History of similar symptoms in other family members

Early onset

Musculoskeletal abnormalities, such as pes cavus, scoliosis, contractures

---

early milestones, participation in sports, or other physically demanding activities is often necessary to reveal subtle deficits in neuromuscular function. The examination of other unaffected family members may be required to determine subtle involvement.

If a genetic cause is considered, the general approach begins with clinical localization and use of ancillary testing as necessary to determine as precise a diagnosis as possible before obtaining molecular genetic testing. Depending on the clinical phenotype, electrodiagnostic testing, laboratory testing, or tissue biopsy may be required to exclude other acquired disorders and narrow the differential diagnosis to allow for targeted molecular testing. Despite these measures, the diagnostic yield of neurogenetic testing can be low even if multiple tests are pursued. The combined yield in a retrospective study was as low as 20%.[2]

All patients who are at risk to be affected by genetic disorders should be offered genetic counseling. Inheritance patterns, risk to offspring, and potential implications for other family members should be clearly explained. With this information, families can make informed decisions to help deal with risks and potentially lessen the impact of the disease. In some cases, the information can assist in making financial, lifestyle, family planning, and career choices.

This article focuses on general patterns of hereditary neuromuscular disorders (**Table 1**) and the common hereditary conditions within each subtype. The disorders are organized by localization (nerve, muscle, motor neuron, and neuromuscular junction), and the clinical features characteristic for individual disorders are outlined. Because of the constraints of the article, not all hereditary conditions with peripheral nervous system involvement are discussed (ie, hereditary spastic paraparesis, spinocerebellar ataxia, Friedreich ataxia, porphyria, and so forth).

HEREDITARY NEUROPATHIES
Charcot-Marie-Tooth Disease

Charcot-Marie-Tooth (CMT) disease is a group of hereditary disorders with significant clinical and genetic heterogeneity characterized by variably present findings of slowly progressive distal muscle weakness and wasting, sensory loss, and reduced reflexes. The prevalence of CMT is approximately 1 in 2500. Rapid advancement in genetic understanding has brought both clarification and confusion into classification strategies because of genotypic and phenotypic variability; despite significant advances, diagnostic strategies are limited by the incomplete knowledge of mutations associated with CMT. Up to one-third of patients with clinically defined CMT will have genetically undefined disorders even if all known mutations are assessed.[3] The classification of CMT subtypes is based on electrophysiological criteria of axonal loss versus demyelination and inheritance pattern. Electrophysiology is usually stratified into demyelinating, intermediate, and axonal subtypes; diagnostic algorithms are

Table 1	
Common patterns of hereditary neuromuscular disorders	
Patterns of Hereditary Neuromuscular Disorders	**Common Features**
Myopathies	
Muscular dystrophy	Usually proximal predominant weakness
Distal myopathy	Distal muscle weakness
Congenital myopathy	Early onset with static or slowly progressive weakness
Metabolic myopathy	Slowly progressive or dynamic symptoms of weakness, ± exertional rhabdomyolysis and muscle contractures
Mitochondrial myopathies	Weakness ± other systemic features of mitochondrial cytopathy
Muscle channelopathy	Fluctuating symptoms of muscle stiffness (myotonia) or weakness (periodic paralysis)
Motor Neuron	
Proximal spinal muscular atrophy	Lower motor neuron dysfunction with proximal muscle weakness
Familial ALS	Mixed lower and upper motor neuron dysfunction
Distal spinal muscular atrophy	Distal muscle weakness
Spinobulbar muscular atrophy	Lower motor neuron dysfunction with proximal limb and bulbar weakness
Neuropathy	
Charcot-Marie-Tooth	Distal sensory loss and muscle weakness
Hereditary sensory and autonomic neuropathy	Sensory loss / Variable autonomic dysfunction / Usually less prominent weakness
Distal hereditary motor neuropathy	Distal weakness / Occasional mild sensory loss
Focal/multifocal neuropathy	Recurrent bouts of focal sensory loss and weakness
Nerve channelopathy	Generalized neuropathy with variable features of sensory loss or pain
NMJ disorders	
Congenital myasthenic syndromes	Fluctuating weakness

Abbreviations: ALS, amyotrophic lateral sclerosis; NMJ, neuromuscular junction.

available elsewhere to help guide genetic testing.[4] Demyelinating subtypes (autosomal dominant [CMT1], autosomal recessive [CMT4], and X-linked recessive [CMTX]) are characterized by electrophysiological findings of upper limb motor conduction velocities less than 38 m/s. Axonal subtypes (CMT2) are characterized by motor conduction velocities greater than 45 m/s, and intermediate subtypes are characterized by motor conduction velocities between greater than 35 m/s and greater than or equal to 45 m/s.

Nerve conduction studies are thus the starting point for the evaluation of patients with CMT and are necessary to guide rationale testing. CMT1A is the most common form of all CMT and is responsible for close to 90% of patients with demyelinating CMT with motor conduction velocities between 15 and 35 m/s.[4] It is inherited in an autosomal dominant pattern, but 10% of cases may occur related to a de novo mutation.[5] It is caused by a 1.5 Mb duplication of the *PMP22* gene on chromosome 17p11.2. In cases with intermediate upper limb motor nerve conduction velocities, CMTX (caused by mutations in the *GJB1* gene) and CMT1B (*MPZ* gene) are responsible for approximately 50% and 25% respectively.[4] Axonal forms (CMT2) make up only around 12% of CMT cases.[3] Among them, CMT2A2 (caused by mutations in the *MFN2* gene) is the most common cause at 20%.[3] Besides these specific genes, however, all other causes are exceedingly rare, making shotgun testing of all CMT genes inefficient.

Hereditary sensory and autonomic neuropathy (HSAN) is a related but distinct group of disorders associated with progressive sensory loss, variable autonomic disturbance, and less frequent/prominent loss of motor function. HSAN is significantly less common than hereditary motor and sensory neuropathy. Usually, this group of disorders is classified by clinical characteristics, inheritance pattern, and electrodiagnostic findings.[6]

Distal Hereditary Motor Neuropathies

The distal hereditary motor neuropathies (dHMN), also referred to as distal spinal muscular atrophies and sometimes classified within motor neuron disorders, are an unusual group of disorders characterized by distal weakness and muscle atrophy. Electrodiagnostic features usually show distal motor axon loss with preserved conduction velocities and normal sensory responses. dHMN is classified clinically by inheritance and associated clinical features, such as age of onset; inheritance pattern; and other distinguishing features, such as vocal cord paralysis, upper limb predominance, or upper motor neuron signs. Several genes have been identified that are associated with the clinical phenotype of dHMN. The symptoms of dHMN overlap significantly with that of CMT and are distinguished only by preserved sensation, but it is important to note that sensory loss is not invariably absent. This clinical heterogeneity is reflected in the case of mutations in *HSPB1*, which has been associated with both dHMN and CMT (CMT2F) phenotypes.

Other Hereditary Neuropathies

Focal hereditary neuropathy variants include hereditary neuropathy with predisposition to pressure palsy (HNPP) and hereditary neuralgic amyotrophy. HNPP is an autosomal dominant neuropathy associated with liability to the development of focal neuropathies at common sites of compression. It is related to a deletion in the *PMP22* gene on 17p11.2, the same gene that is duplicated in CMT1A. In a large cohort of patients with CMT, HNPP was responsible for 10% of cases.[3] It can usually be distinguished from other forms of CMT by focal clinical signs and symptoms and electrophysiological features of multifocal demyelination at common sites of entrapment.

Hereditary neuralgic amyotrophy, also called hereditary brachial plexus neuropathy, is an autosomal dominant disorder associated with bouts of severe pain and motor greater than sensory deficits in the distribution of individual nerves of the upper limb and occasional cranial nerves. About 20% of cases are related to a mutation in the *SEPT9* gene.[7,8] Patients present with clinical features that overlap significantly with that of idiopathic neuralgic amyotrophy and distinguishing between idiopathic, and hereditary cases is often difficult. In addition to the previously mentioned neuropathies, there are numerous additional rare hereditary neuropathy variants that are beyond the scope of this article.

HEREDITARY MYOPATHIES
Dystrophinopathies

The dystrophinopathies include the spectrum of X-linked recessive disorders related to a mutation in the *DMD* gene located on chromosome Xp21.2-p21.1. Two allelic variants are commonly seen. DMD, the most common muscular dystrophy, affecting 1 in 3500 boys, occurs in individuals with severe deficiency of dystrophin. Onset occurs between 3 to 5 years of age with progressive, symmetric, proximal predominant weakness. Common clinical features include dilated cardiomyopathy, scoliosis, and mild mental retardation. Treatment with corticosteroids modifies disease progression.[9-11] Becker muscular dystrophy (BMD) is a dystrophinopathy with a more variable clinical phenotype occurring 1 in 20,000 births. The onset is usually after 7 years of age, but the severity and age of onset is related to muscle dystrophin levels. Failure to walk may be variable, occurring from 16 to 80 years of age. Potential associated features include cardiomyopathy, mental retardation, muscle hypertrophy, and myalgia. Other phenotypes of dystrophinopathy include selective cardiomyopathy and manifesting female carriers. In selective cardiomyopathy (also termed X-linked dilated cardiomyopathy), patients present with dilated cardiomyopathy with minimal weakness. Female carriers may present with proximal weakness, cramps, and myalgia.

Genetic testing is the preferred method for diagnosis in the dystrophinopathies and it should be considered particularly in young boys presenting with proximal weakness before other invasive testing methods. Creatine kinase is typically markedly elevated and is a reasonable screening tool in individuals suspected to have dystrophinopathy. Demonstrating the presence of a pathogenic variant in the DMD gene provides molecular confirmation of the diagnosis. The lack of the identification of a mutation in the DMD gene lessens the chance of a dystrophinopathy, but sensitivity depends on the screening procedures used. DMD deletion/duplication testing will identify approximately two-thirds of affected males,[12,13] but clinicians should be certain that the laboratory they select uses a method that interrogates all 79 exons in the gene, such as multiplex ligation-dependent probe amplification or comparative genomic hybridization.[14-17] In cases in which a deletion or duplication is not identified and a consistent clinical phenotype is present, screening for point mutations or muscle biopsy with dystrophin quantification should be considered.

The major determinant as to whether mutations are associated with DMD or BMD is whether the mutations result in a preserved mRNA reading frame that allows translation of a protein with both N-terminal and C-terminal functionality. This rule, termed the reading frame rule, holds true in around 90% of cases of DMD and around 60% of BMD cases.[18,19] These percentages demonstrate that the phenotype cannot be predicted by genomic analysis alone and reminds the clinician that prognosis should not be based on the genetic report in isolation.[20]

Myotonic Dystrophies

Myotonic dystrophy is a highly variable, autosomal dominant disorder of skeletal muscle associated with multisystem involvement. It is the most common hereditary neuromuscular disease in adults. Two forms of myotonic dystrophy have been described: myotonic dystrophy type 1 (DM1) and myotonic dystrophy type 2 (DM2) (**Table 2**). Both disorders are characterized by clinical and electrical myotonia and progressive weakness. DM1 is characterized by myotonia and weakness that is

Table 2		
Comparison of features of myotonic dystrophy type 1 and 2		
	Myotonic Dystrophy Type 1	**Myotonic Dystrophy Type 2**
Gene mutation	DMPK	ZNF9
Weakness	Distal predominant	Proximal predominant
Myotonia	Usually prominent	Present but less severe
Pain	Unusual	Frequent

most prominent in the distal limbs, bulbar, and neck flexors. DM1 is related to an expanded and unstable CTG trinucleotide repeat localized to the 3′ untranslated region of the dystrophia myotonica protein kinase (DMPK) gene located on chromosome 19q13.3. Associated systemic features include cataracts, excessive daytime sleepiness, insulin resistance, and impaired cognitive function. Because of repeat instability, DM1 is marked by repeat expansion in subsequent generations, with anticipation in disease onset and severity. The longest repeats are associated with congenital myotonic dystrophy, the most severe form of DM1, which is present at birth. Congenital DM1 is associated with hypotonia, weakness, and difficulties with breathing, sucking, and swallowing at birth. Motor function improves significantly in early life, but motor and self-care skills are often delayed. In children with congenital DM1, learning disabilities are common. Mutational analysis is available as a polymerase chain reaction–based test for the expanded DMPK allele, but clinicians should be aware that in some congenital cases the repeat size is too large for efficient amplification of the expanded allele, resulting in false-negative tests that require the use of a different testing modality to resolve.

DM2, also known as proximal myotonic myopathy, is related to a mutation in the CCTG repeat sequence in intron 1 of the ZNF9 gene. DM2 is associated with myotonia, proximal predominant weakness, and other systemic symptoms of cardiac dysfunction, insulin insensitivity, cataracts, and testicular failure. Myotonia is not usually severe, but pain is often prominent. Unlike DM1, a congenital form of DM2 has not been reported.

Limb-Girdle Muscular Dystrophies

Limb girdle muscular dystrophy (LGMD) is a descriptive term describing a large heterogeneous group of muscle disorders associated with proximal limb weakness. The clinical presentation of several types of LGMD resembles that of the dystrophinopathies but affects male and females equally. Multiple forms of LGMD with autosomal dominant inheritance classified as type 1 (LGMD 1) and recessive inheritance classified as type 2 (LGMD 2) have been identified. In about 75% of cases, genetic testing can be used to identify the specific form.[21]

The general evaluation of possible LGMD include laboratory, electrodiagnostic, muscle biopsy, cardiac, and molecular testing. The history may provide clues to a particular form based on features of the age of onset, inheritance pattern, and other associated features. Examination, by definition, usually demonstrates proximal limb muscle weakness, but atypical features of distal limb weakness, focal weakness (ie, scapular winging), and contractures may be present and should be recognized. Creatine kinase levels may vary considerably and may be helpful in discerning between subtypes. Electrodiagnostic testing is helpful to determine the presence of a myopathic process and to exclude other conditions with proximal predominant weakness, such as spinal muscular atrophy (SMA) or congenital myasthenic syndrome, but electromyographic (EMG) findings are often nonspecific, with significant overlap between different forms of LGMD. **Table 3** outlines some clinical and laboratory features that may be associated with each autosomal dominant and recessive form of LGMD.

Muscle biopsy remains a critical aspect of the evaluation of LGMD. The muscle biopsy site should be guided using imaging and electrodiagnostic studies to obtain involved but not end-stage tissue. Biopsy tissue should be analyzed with standard histologic techniques to both confirm the presence of dystrophic features, including variation of fiber size, increased central nuclei, and endomysial fibrosis, and exclude other mimicking conditions. Most histologic changes in LGMD are nonspecific, but some histopathologic changes may suggest certain disorders. For example, significant inflammation has been described in calpainopathy and alpha2-laminin deficiency and may be a helpful diagnostic feature.[49,50] The primary value of muscle biopsy, however, lies in providing tissue for protein expression studies. Some, including dysferlinopathy (LGMD2B) and *FKRP* (LGMD2I), can generally be diagnosed by immunohistochemical analysis, whereas others, particularly calpainopathy (LGMD2A), require immunoblot analysis. Such testing may reveal patterns characteristic of a specific underlying genetic defect but should be performed in a pathology laboratory with sufficient experience in performance of testing and interpretation. Interpretation of the findings may be difficult because of the lack of availability of direct assays for all primary defects and secondary changes that may occur in certain forms of LGMD.

Direct DNA analysis for a specific gene mutation provides the most definitive method of diagnosis. Although this is often guided by protein expression studies, in some cases (generally based on clinical features), mutational analysis may be the appropriate first test; in some disorders, only DNA analysis is clinically available. (It is particularly worth noting that this is the case with the increasingly recognized LGMD2L, caused by mutations in *ANO5*, for which no diagnostic antibody has been described.) Although mutation analysis is not readily available for all LGMDs, molecular diagnostics is a rapidly evolving field, and one can expect that novel genome scale technologies will be of particular value in genetically heterogeneous categories such as the LGMDs.[51]

Facioscapulohumeral Muscular Dystrophy

Facioscapulohumeral muscular dystrophy (FSHD) is an autosomal dominant muscular dystrophy with a prevalence estimated at 1 in 20,000 but as high as 1 in 14,500 in some regions.[52] Patients usually present with slowly progressive weakness involving face, scapular stabilizers, and distal lower limb weakness, all of which are frequently asymmetric.[53,54] Phenotypic variation is significant, and patients have been described lacking facial weakness or with unusual presentations, such as isolated trunk extensor myopathy.[55,56] Life expectancy is not usually shortened, but 20% of individuals may eventually lose the ability to ambulate.[54] Creatine kinase (CK) is usually normal to only mildly elevated (3–5 times normal), and a very high CK suggests an alternate diagnosis. EMG may show myopathic changes. Muscle biopsy does not show any specific changes and is not indicated unless an alternate diagnosis is suspected. Rarely, muscle biopsy may demonstrate a mononuclear inflammatory reaction in a third of cases, partly mimicking an inflammatory process.

FSHD is related to a deletion of integral copies of the D4Z4 repeat motif located in the subtelomeric region of chromosome 4q35.[57] Normal D4Z4 alleles have 11 to 100 repeats. Alleles associated with FSHD have only 1 to 10 repeats. Most patients will have an affected parent, but a de novo mutation may occur in up to 30%.[58,59] The clinically available test will detect approximately 95% of patients with FSHD, but the clinician must be aware of exceptional cases in which results of testing may be negative and the syndrome not associated with a D4Z4 contraction.[60] A unifying model of a novel mechanism by which D4Z4 contraction (or hypomethylation, in the case of contraction-independent FSHD) results in disease has recently been proposed.[61] Under this model, these conditions provide a permissive chromatin structure that allows a transcript encoding a homeoboxlike protein DUX4 to be expressed from each D4Z4 repeat. Only the transcript from the terminal repeat uses a chromosome 4q-specific element that contains a polyadenylation signal and all other transcripts degrade without it. Overexpression of the DUX4 protein results in muscle degeneration through mechanisms as yet incompletely understood but that are likely to involve the p53 pathway.[62]

Table 3
Limb girdle muscular dystrophy genetics and clinical features

			Limb Girdle Muscular Dystrophies		
			Autosomal Dominant		
	Protein/Locus	CK[a]	Muscle Involvement	Other Features	References
LGMD1A	Myotilin	<5X	Proximal	Dysarthria, occasional contractures	Hauser et al[22] Olivé et al[23]
LGMD1B	Lamin A/C	<5X	Proximal	Cardiac conduction disease, CM, contractures	Muchir et al[24]
LGMD1C	Caveolin-3	5–10X	Distal or proximal	Rippling muscle disease, hypertrophic CM	Galbiati et al[25]
LGMD1D	DNAJB6	<5X	Distal or proximal		Speer et al[26] Sarparanta et al[27]
LGMD1E	7q		Proximal	CM, cardiac conduction disease	Greenberg et al[28]
LGMD1F	7q31.1-q32.2	<5X	Proximal>distal		Palenzuela et al[29]
LGMD1G	4q21	1–10X	Proximal	Contractures of digits	Starling et al[30]
LGMD1H	3p25.1-p23	1–10X	Proximal		Bisceglia et al[31]
			Autosomal Recessive		
	Protein	CK	Muscle Involvement	Other Features	
LGMD 2A	Calpain-3	5 to >10X	Proximal with periscapular; distal	Contractures, occasional mild mental retardation, focal atrophy	Richard et al[32]

		CK[a]	Distribution	Clinical features	References
LGMD2B	Dysferlin	>10X	Proximal; distal		Bashlr et al[33] Bejaoui et al[34]
LGMD2C	Gamma-sarcoglycan	>10X	Proximal (may mimic DMD or BMD phenotype)	Occasional cardiac involvement; respiratory	Noguchi et al[35]
LGMD2D	Alpha-sarcoglycan	>10X	Proximal with prominent periscapular and quadriceps	Rare CM	Matsumura et al[36]
LGMD2E	Beta-sarcoglycan	>10X	Proximal	Muscle hypertrophy-prominent in tongue; CM	Lim et al[37]
LGMD2F	Delta-sarcoglycan	>10X	Proximal	Dilated CM	Nigro et al[38]
LGMD2G	Telethonin	5–10X	Proximal	Dilated CM	Moreira et al[39]
LGMD2H	TRIM32	5X to >10X	Proximal	Myalgias	Saccone et al[40]
LGMD2I	FKRP	>10X	Proximal with asymmetry	CM-dilated, respiratory failure, cramps	Bushby et al[41]
LGMD2J	Titin	>10X	Proximal		Haravuori et al[42] Hackman et al[43]
LGMD2K	POMT1	>10X	Proximal	Contractures	Burcu et al[44]
LGMD2L	Anoctamin 5	5X to >10X	Proximal; distal often asymmetric	Myalgia	Bolduc et al[45]
LGMD2M	Fukutin	>10X	Proximal	Contractures, CM, response to corticosteroids	Vuillaumier-Barrot et al[46] Godfrey et al[47] Puckett et al[48]

Abbreviations: CK, creatine levels as a factor of reference values; CM, cardiomyopathy; DNAJB6, DnaJ homolog subfamily B member 6; TRIM, tripartite motif-containing protein 32; FKRP, fukutin-related protein; POMT1, protein O-mannosyl-transferase 1.

[a] CK levels may vary considerably with each form of LGMD depending on disease duration, exertion, and phenotypic severity.

Oculopharyngeal Muscular Dystrophy

Oculopharyngeal muscular dystrophy (OPMD) is an autosomal dominantly inherited muscular dystrophy with late onset (usually after 45 years of age) ptosis, dysphagia, and usually less prominent limb involvement. OPMD is related to a trinucleotide repeat in the first exon of the *PABPN1* gene on chromosome 14q11.2 that encodes polyadenylated-binding protein nuclear 1. The clinical diagnosis is based on findings of ptosis as defined by palpebral fissure separation of less than 8 mm at rest and dysphagia defined by a swallowing time of greater than 7 seconds to swallow 80 mL of water, both in the setting of an autosomal dominant family history.[63] CK is usually normal to mildly elevated. Electrodiagnostic studies may demonstrate myopathic changes. Muscle biopsy is not usually indicated but may demonstrate findings of intra-nuclear inclusions of tubular filaments and rimmed vacuoles.[64] Molecular diagnosis of OPMD is confirmed with the presence of 12 to 17 GCG trinucleotide repeats in the first exon of the *PABPN1* gene. Less commonly, autosomal recessive OPMD may occur if there is homozygous presence of 11 GCG trinucleotide repeats.

Emery-Dreifuss Muscular Dystrophies

Emery-Dreifuss muscular dystrophy (EDMD) is a group of hereditary myopathies that may be transmitted in an autosomal dominant, autosomal recessive, and X-linked recessive pattern. Three genes are associated with the clinical phenotype of EDMD. *EMD*, which encodes emerin, and Four and a half LIM domains protein 1 (*FHL1*), which encodes *FHL1*, are both associated with X-inked EDMD. *LMNA*, which encodes lamins A and C, is a cause of autosomal dominant and autosomal recessive forms of EDMD.

The clinical diagnosis is supported by findings of progressive muscle weakness and atrophy, early contractures, and cardiac disease associated with conduction defects. CK is normal at birth until 1 year of age but subsequently may range 2 to 20 times the upper limit of normal.[65] Muscle biopsy demonstrates dystrophic features. Immunode-tection of emerin is absent in 95% of patients with X-linked EDMD.[66] Immunodetection of FHL1 is available in patients with XL-EDMD.[67] Immunodetection of lamins A/C is not reliable. Molecular genetic testing is clinically available for all 3 genes associated with EDMD. If family history is apparent, testing for *EMD* and *FHL1* should be pursued in patients with X-linked EDMD and *LMNA* in patients with autosomal dominant or reces-sive EDMD. In males without a family history, immunodetection studies are helpful to guide molecular genetic testing. In females without a family history, manifesting carrier states are very rare and testing for autosomal dominant EDMD with *LMNA* testing is appropriate.

Other Myopathies

In addition to the muscular dystrophies there are several other hereditary myopathies with distinguishing features. Although most myopathic processes cause proximal prom-inent weakness, the distal myopathies, as the name implies, cause distal predominant weakness. A genetic diagnostic evaluation is available for several subtypes. Congenital myopathies are a group of early onset myopathies lacking dystrophic features on muscle biopsy and are usually characterized by a more static course. Muscle channelopathies are caused by hereditary defects in sarcolemmal ion channels. The disorders within this spectrum may demonstrate features of myotonia (hyperexcitability), paralysis (inexcit-ability), or both. Metabolic myopathies include mitochondrial cytopathies, fat oxidation defects, and glycogen storage diseases. Metabolic myopathies include disorders with isolated muscle pathologic conditions as well as combined muscle and other systemic involvement. Clinical features may include dynamic myopathic features worsened with increased metabolic demand and slowly progressive weakness with nonfluctuating signs and symptoms. Mitochondrial disorders occur as result of mutations of nuclear or mitochondrial DNA. Mitochondrial myopathy may occur in isolation, but multisystem disease is frequent because of the ubiquitous distribution of mitochondria. Mitochondrial disorders are often categorized into clinical syndromes, such as Kearns-Sayre syndrome, mitochondrial encephalopathy with lactic acidosis and strokelike episodes, chronic progressive external ophthalmoplegia, and myoclonic epilepsy with ragged-red fibers, but many patients will not fit into any particular phenotypic classification.

MOTOR NEURON DISORDERS
SMA

SMA is a neurodegenerative disorder associated with the loss of motor neurons in the anterior horn of the spinal cord and lower brainstem, resulting in progressive muscle weakness and atrophy. SMA is a heterogeneous disorder with multiple autosomal dominant, autosomal recessive, and X-linked forms but the most common form, responsible for 95% of cases, is an autosomal recessive disorder related to mutations in the survival of motor neuron gene (SMN1). It occurs in 1 in 6000 to 10, 000 infants and is the most common genetic cause of death in infants.[68]

The diagnosis of SMN-related SMA can be confirmed using molecular genetic testing with targeted mutation analysis by detection of homozygous deletions of the exons 7 and 8 of the SMN1 gene. Point mutations may occur. As a consequence, if a single deletion is identified in the setting of a clinical phenotype typical of SMA, sequencing of SMN1 should be considered. In humans, a second gene, SMN2, exists that is identical to SMN1 except for a single nucleotide substitution in exon 7. SMN2 copy number modulates disease severity in that increased copies of SMN2 result in less severity.[69,70] SMA is classified clinically into 4 groups (SMA1–SMA4) based on onset and maximum function achieved.

Recently, genes responsible for a variety of distal motor neuron syndromes have been identified, with both dominant and recessive patterns of inheritance. These syndromes have been characterized as distal SMA or dHMN and clinical features are reviewed elsewhere.[71] Clinical genetic testing is available for many of these.

X-linked Spinobulbar Muscular Atrophy

X-linked spinobulbar muscular atrophy (SBMA), also known as Kennedy disease, is a disorder of progressive degeneration of lower motor neurons associated with proximal limb and bulbar predominant weakness and atrophy associated with fasciculations. SBMA occurs because of mutations in the androgen receptor gene; because of an associated mild androgen insensitivity, gynecomastia, testicular atrophy, and reduced fertility are common. Molecular testing for an expanded CAG trinucleotide repeat is available clinically. Full penetrance is associated with 38 repeats or greater, and 34 repeats or less is considered normal. A result of 35 to 37 repeats is of uncertain clinical significance and should be interpreted in conjunction with clinical features and family history.[72]

Familial Amyotrophic Lateral Sclerosis

Amyotrophic lateral sclerosis (ALS) is a disorder of upper and lower motor neuron degeneration. The diagnosis is confirmed using clinical and electrodiagnostic criteria.[73,74] Familial and sporadic cases of ALS have similar clinical and electrodiagnostic features. More than 15 genes are associated with familial ALS (**Table 4**). Mutations in SOD1, C9ORF72, TARDBP, FUS, ANG, SETX, and ATXN2 have also been

Table 4
Familial ALS loci

Familial ALS		Locus	Gene
Autosomal Dominant	ALS1	21q22	SOD1
	ALS3	18q21	
	ALS4	9q34	SETX
	ALS6		FUS
	ALS7	20p13	
	ALS8	20q13.33	VAPB
	ALS9		ANG
	ALS10	1p36.22	TARDBP
	ALS11	6q21	FIG4
	ALS12		OPTN
	ALS13		ATXN2
	ALS14		VCP
	ALS-FTD	9p21	C9ORF72
Autosomal Recessive	ALS2	2q33	ALS2
	ALS5	15q15-q22	SPG11
X-linked dominant	ALS15	Xp11.21	UBQLN2

associated with sporadic cases, and mutations in *SOD1* and *C9ORF72* have been reported in up to 3% and 21% of sporadic cases, respectively.[75–81] Nevertheless, genetic testing is most likely to be informative in patients with an affected first or second degree relative, which occurs in approximately 5% to 10% of cases of ALS, or in cases with a juvenile onset of disease. Mutations in *C9ORF72*, *SOD1*, *FUS*, and *TARDBP* are the 4 most common causes associated with familial ALS.[76,82] The most common of these, close to 50% in some cohorts, are mutations in *C9ORF72*, whereas approximately 20% of familial cases are caused by *SOD1* mutations.[76]

CONGENITAL MYASTHENIC SYNDROMES

Congenital myasthenic syndromes (CMS) or hereditary forms of neuromuscular junction transmission failure have now been associated with mutations in genes encoding a variety of proteins essential for function at the neuromuscular synapse. As reviewed in detail elsewhere, these include choline acetyltransferase, acetylcholinesterase, β2-laminin, acetylcholine receptor, rapsyn, plectin, Nav1.4, muscle specific protein kinase, agrin, Dok-7, and glutamine–fructose-6-phosphate transaminase 1.[83] The associated disorders may present in a variety of ways. Although autoimmune myasthenia gravis is responsible for most patients with neuromuscular junction disorders, some forms of CMS may closely mimic the presentation of autoimmune myasthenia gravis with the lack of responsiveness to immunomodulatory treatment frequently being the only distinguishing feature. Genetic confirmation of CMS may help avoid unnecessary or potentially harmful immunomodulatory treatments. In general, mutational analysis is guided by clinical and sometimes morphologic features. For example, mutations in *DOK7* are often associated with a proximal and axial myopathy suggestive of LGMD, and mutations in *GFPT* are typically associated with tubular aggregates on muscle biopsy.[83]

The treatment of CMS is usually supportive. Symptomatic treatments using agents to increase neuromuscular junction transmission usually provide at least a partial benefit. Acetylcholinesterase inhibitors; 3,4 diaminopyridine, a potassium channel antagonist; certain serotonin reuptake inhibitors; ephedrine; and other medications may be helpful in select cases. The response to a particular agent is usually gene specific, with some agents being ineffective or even harmful in certain forms of CMS.

SUMMARY

DNA analysis is the gold standard of diagnostic certainty in hereditary conditions. A specific diagnosis allows for accurate genetic counseling and medical management. Genetic testing has made a precise diagnosis possible in many forms of hereditary neuromuscular disorders, but availability of reliable testing remains incomplete. Molecular diagnostic tests are constantly being updated, making online testing databases increasingly necessary. For current testing availability it is recommended that the reader refer to an online database, such as www.genetests.org.[84]

During an era of developing therapeutic interventions for hereditary disorders, genetic testing will be critical to identify potential subjects for therapeutic trials and eventually treatment. The current challenges faced include the heavy economic burden of expensive testing and incomplete understanding of testing limitations. Currently, molecular diagnostic testing relies on recognizing characteristic clinical phenotypes and assessing genes known to commonly be associated with such phenotypic expression. In some disorders, such as SMA or DMD, this task is simplified; when the diagnosis is considered, other ancillary testing, such as muscle biopsy or electrodiagnosis, is unnecessary. In such cases, genetic testing is the most economically sound approach to diagnosis. In other disorders, such as LGMD or CMT, pursuing a specific diagnosis can be a much more daunting task; often, despite extensive testing, a specific diagnosis is elusive. The future of molecular testing will likely shift away from targeted genetic analysis toward genomic technologies, such as whole genome or exome sequencing, that will become increasingly rapid and cost-efficient and allow for a nontargeted approach.[85] With these advances will come future difficulties of managing incidental identification of disorders, particularly those that are presymptomatic and untreatable.

REFERENCES

1. Soltanzadeh P, Friez MJ, Dunn D, et al. Clinical and genetic characterization of manifesting carriers of DMD mutations. Neuromuscul Disord 2010;20(8):499–504.
2. Edlefsen KL, Tait JF, Wener MH, et al. Utilization and diagnostic yield of neurogenetic testing at a tertiary care facility. Clin Chem 2007;53(6):1016–22.
3. Saporta AS, Sottile SL, Miller LJ, et al. Charcot-Marie-Tooth disease subtypes and genetic testing strategies. Ann Neurol 2011;69(1):22–33.
4. Miller LJ, Saporta AS, Sottile SL, et al. Strategy for genetic testing in Charcot-Marie-disease. Acta Myologica 2011;30(2):109–16.
5. Nelis E, Van Broeckhoven C, De Jonghe P, et al. Estimation of the mutation frequencies in Charcot-Marie-Tooth disease type 1 and hereditary neuropathy with liability to pressure palsies: a European collaborative study. Eur J Hum Genet 1996;4(1):25–33.
6. Dyck PJ, Thomas PK, editors. Peripheral neuropathy. 4th edition. Philadelphia: W.B. Saunders; 2005.
7. Kuhlenbaumer G, Hannibal MC, Nelis E, et al. Mutations in SEPT9 cause hereditary neuralgic amyotrophy. Nat Genet 2005;37(10):1044–6.
8. Hannibal MC, Ruzzo EK, Miller LR, et al. SEPT9 gene sequencing analysis reveals recurrent mutations in hereditary neuralgic amyotrophy. Neurology 2009;72(20): 1755–9.

9. Mendell JR, Moxley RT, Griggs RC, et al. Randomized, double-blind six-month trial of prednisone in Duchenne's muscular dystrophy. N Engl J Med 1592;320(24): 1592–7.

10. Manzur AY, Kuntzer T, Pike M, et al. Glucocorticoid corticosteroids for Duchenne muscular dystrophy. Cochrane Database Syst Rev 2004;(2):CD003725; PMID: 15106215. Cochrane Database Syst Rev 2008;1.

11. Bushby K, Muntoni F, Urtizberea A, et al. Report on the 124th ENMC International Workshop. Treatment of Duchenne muscular dystrophy; defining the gold standards of management in the use of corticosteroids. 2-4 April 2004, Naarden, The Netherlands. Neuromuscul Disord 2004;14(8–9):526–34.

12. Dent KM, Dunn DM, von Niederhausern AC, et al. Improved molecular diagnosis of dystrophinopathies in an unselected clinical cohort. Am J Med Genet A 2005; 134(3):295–8.

13. Prior TW, Bridgeman SJ. Experience and strategy for the molecular testing of Duchenne muscular dystrophy. J Mol Diagn 2005;7(3):317–26.

14. Lalic T, Vossen RH, Coffa J, et al. Deletion and duplication screening in the DMD gene using MLPA. Eur J Hum Genet 2005;13(11):1231–4.

15. Hegde MR, Chin EL, Mulle JG, et al. Microarray-based mutation detection in the dystrophin gene. Hum Mutat 2008;29(9):1091–9.

16. Saillour Y, Cossée M, Leturcq F, et al. Detection of exonic copy-number changes using a highly efficient oligonucleotide-based comparative genomic hybridization-array method. Hum Mutat 2008;29(9):1083–90.

17. Gaudio DD, Yang Y, Boggs BA, et al. Molecular diagnosis of Duchenne/Becker muscular dystrophy: enhanced detection of dystrophin gene rearrangements by oligonucleotide array-comparative genomic hybridization. Hum Mutat 2008; 29(9):1100–7.

18. Monaco AP, Bertelson CJ, Liechti-Gallati S, et al. An explanation for the pheno-typic differences between patients bearing partial deletions of the DMD locus. Genomics 1988;2(1):90–5.

19. Flanigan KM, Dunn DM, von Niederhausern A, et al. Mutational spectrum of DMD mutations in dystrophinopathy patients: application of modern diagnostic tech-niques to a large cohort. Hum Mutat 2009;30(12):1657–66.

20. Flanigan KM, Dunn DM, von Niederhausern A, et al. Nonsense mutation-associated Becker muscular dystrophy: interplay between exon definition and splicing regulatory elements within the DMD gene. Hum Mutat 2011;32(3): 299–308.

21. Bushby K. Diagnosis and management of the limb girdle muscular dystrophies. Pract Neurol 2009;9(6):314–23.

22. Hauser MA, Horrigan SK, Salmikangas P, et al. Myotilin is mutated in limb girdle muscular dystrophy 1A. Hum Mol Genet 2000;9(14):2141–7.

23. Olivé M, Goldfarb LG, Shatunov A, et al. Myotilinopathy: refining the clinical and myopathological phenotype. Brain 2005;128(10):2315–26.

24. Muchir A, Bonne G, van der Kooi AJ, et al. Identification of mutations in the gene encoding lamins A/C in autosomal dominant limb girdle muscular dystrophy with atrioventricular conduction disturbances (LGMD1B). Hum Mol Genet 2000;9(9): 1453–9.

25. Galbiati F, Razani B, Lisanti MP. Caveolae and caveolin-3 in muscular dystrophy. Trends Mol Med 2001;7(10):435–41.

26. Speer MC, Vance JM, Grubber JM, et al. Identification of a new autosomal dominant limb-girdle muscular dystrophy locus on chromosome 7. Am J Hum Genet 1999;64(2):556–62.

27. Sarparanta J, Jonson PH, Golzio C, et al. Mutations affecting the cytoplasmic functions of the co-chaperone DNAJB6 cause limb-girdle muscular dystrophy. Nat Genet 2012;44(4):450–5.
28. Greenberg SA, Salajegheh M, Judge DP, et al. Etiology of limb girdle muscular dystrophy 1D/1E determined by laser capture microdissection proteomics. Ann Neurol 2012;71(1):141–5.
29. Palenzuela L, Andreu AL, Gàmez J, et al. A novel autosomal dominant limb-girdle muscular dystrophy (LGMD 1F) maps to 7q32.1-32.2. Neurology 2003;61(3): 404–6.
30. Starling A, Kok F, Passos-Bueno MR, et al. A new form of autosomal dominant limb-girdle muscular dystrophy (LGMD1G) with progressive fingers and toes flexion limitation maps to chromosome 4p21. Eur J Hum Genet 2004;12(12): 1033–40.
31. Bisceglia L, Zoccolella S, Torraco A, et al. A new locus on 3p23-p25 for an autosomal-dominant limb-girdle muscular dystrophy, LGMD1H. Eur J Hum Genet 2010;18(6):636–41.
32. Richard I, Broux O, Allamand V, et al. Mutations in the proteolytic enzyme calpain 3 cause limb-girdle muscular dystrophy type 2A. Cell 1995;81(1):27–40.
33. Bashlr R, Strachan T, Keers S, et al. A gene for autosomal recessive limb-girdle muscular dystrophy maps to chromosome 2p. Hum Mol Genet 1994;3(3):455–7.
34. Bejaoui K, Hirabayashi K, Hentati F, et al. Linkage of Miyoshi myopathy (distal autosomal recessive muscular dystrophy) locus to chromosome 2p12-14. Neurology 1995;45(4):768–72.
35. Noguchi S, McNally EM, Ben Othmane K, et al. Mutations in the dystrophin-associated protein gamma-sarcoglycan in chromosome 13 muscular dystrophy. Science 1995;270(5237):819–22.
36. Matsumura K, Tome FM, Collin H, et al. Deficiency of the 50K dystrophin-associated glycoprotein in severe childhood autosomal recessive muscular dystrophy. Nature 1992;359(6393):320–2.
37. Lim LE, Duclos F, Broux O, et al. [beta]-sarcoglycan: characterization and role in limb-girdle muscular dystrophy linked to 4q12. Nat Genet 1995;11(3):257–65.
38. Nigro V, de Sá Moreira E, Piluso G, et al. Autosomal recessive limb girdle muscular dystrophy, LGMD2F, is caused by a mutation in the [delta]-sarcoglycan gene. Nat Genet 1996;14(2):195–8.
39. Moreira ES, Wiltshire TJ, Faulkner G, et al. Limb-girdle muscular dystrophy type 2G is caused by mutations in the gene encoding the sarcomeric protein telethonin. Nat Genet 2000;24(2):163–6.
40. Saccone V, Palmieri M, Passamano L, et al. Mutations that impair interaction properties of TRIM32 associated with limb-girdle muscular dystrophy 2H. Hum Mutat 2008;29(2):240–7.
41. Bushby K, Anderson LV, Pollitt C, et al. Abnormal merosin in adults. A new form of late onset muscular dystrophy not linked to chromosome 6q2. Brain 1998;121(Pt 4): 581–8.
42. Haravuori H, Vihola A, Straub V, et al. Secondary calpain3 deficiency in 2q-linked muscular dystrophy: titin is the candidate gene. Neurology 2001;56(7): 869–77.
43. Hackman P, Vihola A, Haravuori H, et al. Tibial muscular dystrophy is a titinopathy caused by mutations in TTN, the gene encoding the giant skeletal-muscle protein titin. Am J Hum Genet 2002;71(3):492–500.
44. Burcu BB, Gökhan GU, Pervin PD, et al. An autosomal recessive limb girdle muscular dystrophy (LGMD2) with mild mental retardation is allelic to Walker-Warburg

syndrome (WWS) caused by a mutation in the POMT1 gene. Neuromuscul Disord 2005;15(4):271–5.

45. Bolduc V, Marlow G, Boycott KM, et al. Recessive mutations in the putative calcium-activated chloride channel anoctamin 5 cause proximal LGMD2L and distal MMD3 muscular dystrophies. CORD Conference Proceedings. Am J Hum Genet 2010; 86(2):213–21.

46. Vuillaumier-Barrot S, Quijano-Roy S, Bouchet-Seraphin C, et al. Four Caucasian patients with mutations in the fukutin gene and variable clinical phenotype. Neuromuscul Disord 2009;19(3):182–8.

47. Godfrey C, Escolar D, Brockington M, et al. Fukutin gene mutations in steroid-responsive limb girdle muscular dystrophy. Ann Neurol 2006;60(5):603–10.

48. Puckett RL, Moore SA, Winder TL, et al. Further evidence of Fukutin mutations as a cause of childhood onset limb-girdle muscular dystrophy without mental retardation. CORD conference proceedings. Neuromuscul Disord 2009;19(5):352–6.

49. Gallardo E, Rojas–García R, de Luna N, et al. Inflammation in dysferlin myopathy: immunohistochemical characterization of 13 patients. Neurology 2001;57(11): 2136–8.

50. Pegoraro E, Cianno BD, Hoffman EP, et al. Congenital muscular dystrophy with primary laminin α2 (merosin) deficiency presenting as inflammatory myopathy. Ann Neurol 1996;40(5):782–91.

51. Piluso G, Dionisi M, Del Vecchio Blanco F, et al. Motor chip: a comparative genomic hybridization microarray for copy-number mutations in 245 neuromuscular disorders. Clin Chem 2011;57(11):1584–96.

52. Flanigan KM, Coffeen CM, Sexton L, et al. Genetic characterization of a large, historically significant Utah kindred with facioscapulohumeral dystrophy. Neuromuscul Disord 2001;11(6–7):525–9.

53. Kilmer DD, Abresch RT, McCrory MA, et al. Profiles of neuromuscular diseases. facioscapulohumeral muscular dystrophy. Am J Phys Med Rehabil 1995; 74(Suppl 5):S131–9.

54. Lunt PW, Harper PS. Genetic counselling in facioscapulohumeral muscular dystrophy. J Med Genet 1991;28(10):655–64.

55. Felice KJ, North WA, Moore SA, et al. FSH dystrophy 4q35 deletion in patients presenting with facial-sparing scapular myopathy. Neurology 1927;54(10):1927–31.

56. Jordan B, Eger K, Koesling S, et al. Camptocormia phenotype of FSHD: a clinical and MRI study on six patients. J Neurol 2011;258(5):866–73.

57. Sposito R, Pasquali L, Galluzzi F, et al. Facioscapulohumeral muscular dystrophy type 1A in northwestern Tuscany: a molecular genetics-based epidemiological and genotype-phenotype study. Genet Test 2005;9(1):30–6.

58. Bakker E, Van der Wielen MJ, Voorhoeve E, et al. Diagnostic, predictive, and prenatal testing for facioscapulohumeral muscular dystrophy: diagnostic approach for sporadic and familial cases. J Med Genet 1996;33(1):29–35.

59. Zatz M, Marie SK, Passos-Bueno MR, et al. High proportion of new mutations and possible anticipation in Brazilian facioscapulohumeral muscular dystrophy families. Am J Hum Genet 1995;56(1):99–105.

60. de Greef JC, Lemmers RJ, Camaño P, et al. Clinical features of facioscapulohumeral muscular dystrophy 2. Neurology 2010;75(17):1548–54.

61. Lemmers RJ, van der Vliet PJ, Klooster R, et al. A unifying genetic model for facioscapulohumeral muscular dystrophy. Science 2010;329(5999):1650–3.

62. Wallace LM, Liu J, Domire JS, et al. RNA interference inhibits DUX4-induced muscle toxicity in vivo: implications for a targeted FSHD therapy. Mol Ther 2012. [Epub ahead of print]. http://dx.doi.org/10.1038/mt.2012.68.

63. Brais B, Xie YG, Sanson M, et al. The oculopharyngeal muscular dystrophy locus maps to the region of the cardiac alpha and beta myosin heavy chain genes on chromosome 14q11.2-q13. Hum Mol Genet 1995;4(3):429–34.
64. Tome FM, Fardeau M. Nuclear inclusions in oculopharyngeal dystrophy. Acta Neuropathol 1980;49(1):85–7.
65. Bialer MG, Bruns DE, Kelly TE. Muscle enzymes and isoenzymes in Emery-Dreifuss muscular dystrophy. Clin Chem 1990;36(3):427–30.
66. Yates JR, Wehnert M. The Emery-Dreifuss muscular dystrophy mutation database. Neuromuscul Disord 1999;9(3):199.
67. Gueneau L, Bertrand AT, Jais JP, et al. Mutations of the FHL1 gene cause Emery-Dreifuss muscular dystrophy. Am J Hum Genet 2009;85(3):338–53.
68. Kolb SJ, Kissel JT. Spinal muscular atrophy: a timely review. Arch Neurol 2011; 68(8):979–84.
69. Mailman MD, Heinz JW, Papp AC, et al. Molecular analysis of spinal muscular atrophy and modification of the phenotype by SMN2. Genet Med 2002;4(1):20–6.
70. Elsheikh B, Prior T, Zhang X, et al. An analysis of disease severity based on SMN2 copy number in adults with spinal muscular atrophy. Muscle Nerve 2009;40(4): 652–6.
71. Rossor AM, Kalmar B, Greensmith L, et al. The distal hereditary motor neuropathies. J Neurol Neurosurg Psychiatry 2012;83(1):6–14.
72. Kuhlenbaumer G, Kress W, Ringelstein EB, et al. Thirty-seven CAG repeats in the androgen receptor gene in two healthy individuals. J Neurol 2001;248(1): 23–6.
73. Brooks BR, Miller RG, Swash M, et al, World Federation of Neurology Research Group on Motor Neuron D. El Escorial revisited: revised criteria for the diagnosis of amyotrophic lateral sclerosis. Amyotroph Lateral Scler Other Motor Neuron Disord 2000;1(5):293–9.
74. de Carvalho M, Dengler R, Eisen A, et al. Electrodiagnostic criteria for diagnosis of ALS. Clin Neurophysiol 2008;119(3):497–503.
75. Andersen PM, Nilsson P, Keränen ML, et al. Phenotypic heterogeneity in motor neuron disease patients with CuZn-superoxide dismutase mutations in Scandinavia. Brain 1997;120(10):1723–37.
76. Renton AE, Majounie E, Waite A, et al. A hexanucleotide repeat expansion in C9ORF72 is the cause of chromosome 9p21-linked ALS-FTD. Neuron 2011; 72(2):257–68.
77. Kabashi E, Valdmanis PN, Dion P, et al. TARDBP mutations in individuals with sporadic and familial amyotrophic lateral sclerosis. Nat Genet 2008;40(5):572–4.
78. Lai SL, Abramzon Y, Schymick JC, et al. FUS mutations in sporadic amyotrophic lateral sclerosis. Neurobiol Aging 2011;32(3):550.e1–4 [Epub 2010 Feb 6].
79. Greenway MJ, Andersen PM, Russ C, et al. ANG mutations segregate with familial and 'sporadic' amyotrophic lateral sclerosis. Nat Genet 2006;38(4):411–3.
80. Xiong HL, Wang JY, Sun YM, et al. Association between novel TARDBP mutations and Chinese patients with amyotrophic lateral sclerosis. BMC Med Genet 2010; 11(1):8.
81. Zhao ZH, Chen WZ, Wu ZY, et al. A novel mutation in the senataxin gene identified in a Chinese patient with sporadic amyotrophic lateral sclerosis. Amyotroph Lateral Scler 2009;10(2):118–22.
82. DeJesus-Hernandez M, Mackenzie Ian R, Boeve BF, et al. Expanded GGGGCC hexanucleotide repeat in noncoding region of C9ORF72 causes chromosome 9p-linked FTD and ALS. Neuron 2011;72(2):245–56.

83. Engel AG. Current status of the congenital myasthenic syndromes. Neuromuscul Disord 2012;22(2):99–111.
84. Genetests–Geneclinics home page. Seattle (WA): University of Washington. Available at: http://www.ncbi.nlm.nih.gov/projects/GeneTests/static/about/aboutindex.shtml. Accessed March 22, 2012.
85. Lupski JR, Reid JG, Gonzaga-Jauregui C, et al. Whole-genome sequencing in a patient with Charcot–Marie–Tooth neuropathy. N Engl J Med 2010;362(13):1181–91.

Muscle Biopsy Evaluation in Neuromuscular Disorders

Nanette C. Joyce, DO[a],*, Björn Oskarsson, MD[b],
Lee-Way Jin, MD, PhD[c]

KEYWORDS

- Muscle biopsy • Neuromuscular disease • Neurogenic atrophy • Myopathic
- Histopathology

KEY POINTS

- Muscle biopsy has an integral role in the diagnostic workup of patients presenting with quantifiable acute or chronic-progressive weakness.
- Electrodiagnostic testing, magnetic resonance or ultrasound imaging can aid in selection of an appropriate muscle for biopsy, and care should be taken to avoid biopsying muscle damaged by electromyography or trauma.
- There are 2 major categories of histopathologic abnormalities observed in muscle disease: neurogenic atrophy and myopathic changes. These structural changes often occur in tandem in myopathies.
- Immunohistochemical staining, biochemical testing, and electron microscopy can add to the diagnostic yield of routine muscle histology staining when indicated; however, the tissue samples must be handled and processed appropriately for each specialty technique to ensure optimal results.
- The best results are obtained from a muscle biopsy when there is good communication between the ordering clinician and the interpreting pathologist, the procedure is well thought out, and tissue retrieval, processing, and shipping are planned in advance to avoid common pitfalls.

INTRODUCTION

Muscle biopsy is an important tool for the evaluation and diagnosis of patients presenting to clinic with acute or progressive weakness who are suspected of having

Dr Joyce is supported by a grant from the Association of Academic Physiatrists and National Institutes of Health.
[a] Department of Physical Medicine and Rehabilitation, University of California Davis School of Medicine, 4860 Y Street, Suite 3850, Sacramento, CA 95817, USA; [b] Department of Neurology, University of California Davis School of Medicine, 4860 Y Street, Suite 3700, Sacramento, CA 95817, USA; [c] Department of Pathology and Laboratory Medicine, University of California Davis School of Medicine, 4400 V Street, Sacramento, CA 95817, USA
* Corresponding author.
E-mail address: Nanette.joyce@ucdmc.ucdavis.edu

Phys Med Rehabil Clin N Am 23 (2012) 609–631
http://dx.doi.org/10.1016/j.pmr.2012.06.006
1047-9651/12/$ – see front matter © 2012 Elsevier Inc. All rights reserved.

an underlying neuromuscular disorder. Alongside the clinical examination, electro-diagnostic, laboratory, and molecular genetic testing, muscle biopsy has a critical role, providing diagnostic evidence that either establishes the cause of disease or focuses the differential diagnosis. For example, in the setting of rapidly progressive muscle weakness, a muscle biopsy is the most expeditious diagnostic study to allow the clinician to distinguish between a necrotizing, metabolic, or inflammatory myopathy and facilitate rapid, appropriate therapeutic management. Or, as in the case of a young boy who presents with progressive proximal weakness and hyperckemia, and whose genetic tests do not confirm a dystrophinopathy, immunohistochemical staining of the muscle biopsy specimen can often identify the pathologic protein defect and pave the way for genetic confirmation of the disease.

The muscle biopsy itself is a straightforward procedure with little risk. However, to get the full benefit of the procedure several experts need to be involved, including a surgeon, processing laboratory and pathologist, which requires planning. Different from biopsies of other organs for which simple preservation in formalin is the routine procedure, a successful muscle biopsy requires optimal cryoprocessing of the fresh specimen to preserve viable macromolecules for enzyme histochemistry and metabolic assays. Therefore, the ordering physician must orchestrate the collection, packaging, and processing of tissues to ensure the desired testing can be performed, and to avoid the need for a repeat procedure because of limited, inappropriate, or poor sample quality. To this end, it is important that the ordering clinician is familiar with the procedure, knows the common pitfalls, and understands what each member of the team requires to provide an optimal outcome. Although it is not within the scope of this article to provide the depth of knowledge required of a neuropathologist to read and interpret a muscle biopsy, it is our hope that it provides the basic information needed to plan a biopsy procedure, instruct a team, get tissues successfully to the laboratory, and interpret the report once it is in hand.

INDICATIONS FOR MUSCLE BIOPSY AND MUSCLE SELECTION

We choose to do a muscle biopsy in the setting of quantifiable weakness and when we are certain that a diagnosis will not likely be reached in a less expensive, less invasive manner. For example, we order serum molecular genetic testing to rule out a dystrophinopathy before considering a muscle biopsy when presented with a male child who has progressive weakness, hyperckemia, calf hypertrophy, and who uses a Gower maneuver to stand. The same is true for the patient with classic signs and symptoms of myotonic muscular dystrophy type I, where the clinical examination is predictive of the diagnosis. However, in most cases, when the differential diagnosis is more extensive, we order a muscle biopsy in the early stage of care to home in on a diagnosis.

When choosing the site for biopsy, the most important step is to locate a muscle that is affected by the disease. Although this sounds simple, it is not always straightforward and can be challenging. If the disease process is chronic, progressive, and seems diffuse and symmetric, choosing the site for biopsy is typically easy and Medical Research Council (MRC) strength grading or electrodiagnostic testing can be used. Choosing a muscle with MRC grade 4/5 strength is often sufficient and provides tissue that reveals the disease and not just end-stage morphology. A muscle with MRC grade 3/5 strength is often too severely affected, with extensive nonspecific end-stage changes that may preclude identification of the muscle disease because of the lack of muscle fibers (**Fig. 1**). However in acute-onset weakness, when there is little concern that end-stage disease is present, a muscle that is severely to moderately affected should be chosen.[1]

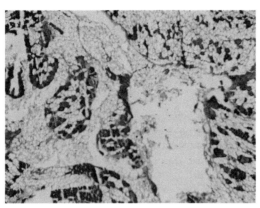

Fig. 1. End-stage muscle precluding histologic assessment of cause on trichrome.

Electromyographic (EMG) testing can aid in identifying affected muscle; however, care should be taken to ensure that the biopsy is not performed on tissue with needle trauma from the examination, because this can also confound interpretation. Limiting the EMG study to a single side of the body allows the biopsy to be performed on a corresponding muscle on the opposite side. However, if the pathologic process seems patchy or multifocal, it is often better to use magnetic resonance imaging or ultrasonography to identify an involved muscle.[2–4] When using EMG to locate affected muscle, if the disease is asymmetric, it is possible to inadvertently sample normal tissue. If you suspect an asymmetric process, imaging should be completed before the biopsy to confirm muscle involvement (**Fig. 2**).

Muscles traditionally chosen for biopsy include the deltoid, biceps, and quadriceps. These muscles all have sufficient norms established for fiber type percentages and muscle fiber size for comparison.[5,6] However, in a study by Lai and colleagues,[7] the diagnostic usefulness of a biopsy taken from the deltoid proved superior to that of the biceps. The investigators surmised this was likely the case because of the proximal location of the deltoid muscle in the setting of myopathic diseases, which often have a proximal to distal

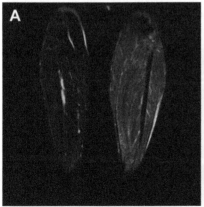
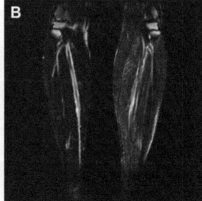

Fig. 2. (*A*, *B*) Magnetic resonance imaging of the lower limbs in the case of a toxic myopathy. The T2 images show asymmetric involvement affecting only the left lower limb. Had a muscle biopsy been taken from the right gastrocnemius, the pathologic tissue would have been missed.

gradient of muscle involvement. The gastrocnemius and tibialis anterior muscles are appropriate choices in diseases with distal limb signs and symptoms. The peroneus brevis muscle, located close to the superficial peroneal nerve, is a favored biopsy site when nerve biopsy is also indicated, as in the case of a suspected vasculitis.[8]

The examining pathologist needs to be provided with information identifying the location of the biopsy site. Muscles vary in their normal ratio of type I to type II fibers, making this information necessary.[6] In addition, the pathologist should have access to the patient's medical history, including age, sex, physical condition, disease onset and progression, signs and symptoms, serum creatine kinase and other biochemical laboratory values, electrodiagnostic test results, medication and family history.[9] Clear communication between the caring physician and the pathologist regarding clinicopathologic correlation is of vital importance for an accurate diagnosis or a list of differentials that points the way for the next step of care.

OPEN MUSCLE BIOPSY PROCEDURE

A muscle biopsy is a small procedure that is best performed in a procedure room, but can be performed in a regular examination room if good lighting and a reasonable area for sterile equipment are ensured. Performing the procedure under general anesthesia is rarely indicated because of the risks and cost, but for young children and patients unable to remain still during the procedure, general anesthesia is often preferred. The essential equipment includes a self-retractor, scalpel, scissors, mosquito forceps, and pick-up forceps.

After identifying the biopsy site, the distal limb should be inspected. Pulses should be palpated and the limb assessed for signs of poor circulation. The skin overlying the muscle should be examined and the muscle palpated. If no concerning local or distal signs are seen in the limb, then the site should be prepared. First, the area should be cleaned with a surgical skin cleanser (eg, betadine or chlorhexidine). A sterile draping should then be placed around the surgical area. To achieve anesthesia in the skin and subcutaneous tissue, a local anesthetic should be injected, avoiding puncture and infiltration of the underlying muscle tissue (**Fig. 3**). We routinely use 5 to 20 mL of 1% lidocaine. Lidocaine with epinephrine 1:100,000 effectively reduces bleeding. The epinephrine normally precludes the need for cautery or ligature. The anesthetic should be injected along the whole incision line to provide adequate anesthesia, which sets in within 2 minutes. The use of a buffered anesthetic removes much of the pain

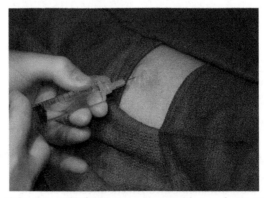

Fig. 3. Infiltration of the skin and subcutaneous tissue with anesthetic. Care should be taken to avoid needle perforation or infiltration of the muscle.

associated with this otherwise most painful part of the biopsy. The skin can then be incised with a scalpel (**Fig. 4**). Skin is thicker in young adults compared with older adults, and proximal limbs have thicker covering than distal limbs. The subcutaneous adipose tissue, between the skin and muscle, is of varying thickness. When the subcutaneous tissue is deep, the length of the skin incision needs to be longer to allow reasonable exposure of the muscle. The subcutaneous tissue is best separated by blunt dissection and retracted (**Fig. 5**). Beneath the subcutaneous tissue, the muscle is covered by a layer of fascia (**Fig. 6**). Most human muscles do not have thick fascial layers, but the quadriceps muscle, a popular site for biopsy, has a thick fascia. If the muscle has a thick fascial covering, it needs to be incised using scissors or a blade to expose the muscle. When the muscle has been exposed, a group of fibers should be separated out bluntly from the belly of the muscle, avoiding the tendinous regions where muscle fibers normally are smaller, with increased connective tissue (**Fig. 7**). It is helpful to surround the separated muscle fibers with a suture before cutting the ends of the fibers (**Fig. 8**).

The amount of muscle tissue excised depends on planned testing and the nature of the underlying disease. If a multifocal or patchy disease process is suspected, multiple specimens may be needed to increase the likelihood of obtaining pathologic tissue. In general, a sample measuring 1 cm in length and 0.5 cm in diameter (about the size of 2 pencil erasers) excised in parallel to the length of the muscle fiber is adequate. Although many laboratories prefer working with clamped tissue, in which the sample is fixed in an isometric muscle clamp or stitched at both ends to a tongue blade or cork to keep it from retracting, we do not use a muscle clamp technique and have not had technical difficulties interfering with the quality of our biopsies. Check with your laboratory to determine if they prefer all or part of the specimen clamped.

If tissue needs to be sent for specialized testing, a larger sample may be required and the laboratory providing the processing should be contacted for specifications (**Table 1**). Once removed, the specimen should be inspected (**Fig. 9**) and then packaged as described in the section on shipping and handling.

Bleeding at the surgical site should be stopped by irrigation with epinephrine and applied pressure. If bleeding continues, then cautery or ligation should be performed. Before beginning closure, it is necessary that hemostasis is achieved. If fascia was sectioned, it should be sutured (**Fig. 10**) to prevent muscle herniation, which otherwise can be a chronic nuisance for the patient. After closing the fascia, the subcutaneous tissue should be sutured and the skin closed. We use 4:0 or 3:0 resorbable suture material to close the fascia, subcutaneous tissue, and the skin (**Figs. 11** and **12**). After skin closure,

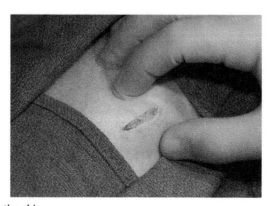

Fig. 4. Incision of the skin.

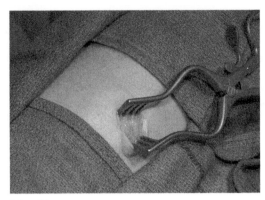

Fig. 5. Retraction of the skin.

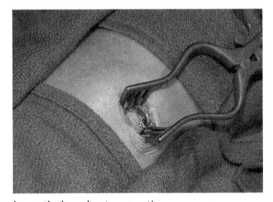

Fig. 6. Fascial layer beneath the subcutaneous tissue.

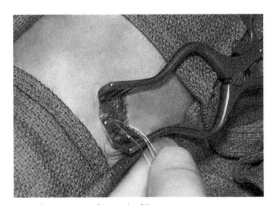

Fig. 7. Blunt dissection of a group of muscle fibers.

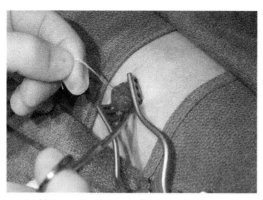

Fig. 8. Separating muscle fibers with suture before cutting the ends of the fiber.

the biopsy site should be bandaged. We normally use Steri-Strips (3M USA, St. Paul, MN, USA), nonstick gauze, and occlusive dressing (**Fig. 13**). If the site can be wrapped with an elastic wrap, a light pressure bandage can be applied and left on for a few hours.

The patient should be instructed in observing the surgical site for signs of infection or bleeding, but no follow-up visits after the muscle biopsy are normally necessary.

NEEDLE BIOPSY

Needle biopsy instead of an open procedure can be performed and is the preferred method at some institutions. The methods are similar, but the incision need only be 5 to 10 mm versus at least 30 mm for an open biopsy. Sharp dissection is performed down

Table 1
The amount of tissue that is optimal for the required technique and immediate handling instructions for the biopsied tissue

Assessment Technique	Use	Ideal Amount of Tissue	Immediate Processing Requirements
Frozen section	Muscle fiber morphology and enzyme histochemistry Most diagnostic information with light microscopy	1 cm^3	Wrap in lightly moist gauze and ship to processing laboratory
Paraffin embedding	Inflammation and morphology of inflammatory cells	0.5 cm x 1 cm	Wrap in lightly moist gauze and ship to processing laboratory
EM	Ultrastructural analysis Visualization of endomysial capillaries, inclusions, mitochondria, myofilaments, collagen, and so forth	1–2-mm-thick section	4% glutaraldehyde
Biochemical testing	Assessing storage and mitochondrial diseases	50–550 mg of tissue, but depends on anticipated testing	Rapid freezing in liquid nitrogen at site of biopsy. Ship frozen on dry ice overnight

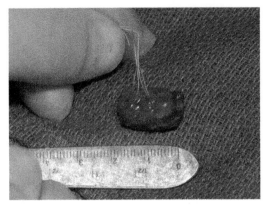

Fig. 9. Inspecting the muscle specimen to ensure quality and adequate quantity of muscle excised.

to the fascia. A 5-mm Bergström or similar needle is then inserted and a specimen withdrawn. The specimens obtained are smaller (~100 mg), and therefore are not well suited for routine histochemistry. Strategies to improve tissue yield have more recently been developed. Tarnopolsky and colleagues[10] developed a suction-modified Bergström technique that provides larger tissue samples adequate for histology and that maintains safety.

Once removed, it is advisable to inspect the tissue under a dissecting microscope to ensure that adequate muscle tissue has been obtained. Depending on the clinical question at hand a ~100-mg specimen may be more than adequate for immunohistochemistry or biochemical analysis. Limitations of needle biopsy include the inability to directly inspect the tissue before excision, increased possibility of missing pathologic tissue, particularly in a multifocal disease process (such as inflammatory myopathies), and bleeding can occur without the source being visible. Most bleeding occurrences can be stopped by applying pressure on the biopsy site, but on occasion a conversion to an open procedure is necessary to ligate a bleeding vessel. Proponents of the needle biopsy technique find it simpler than open biopsy.[11]

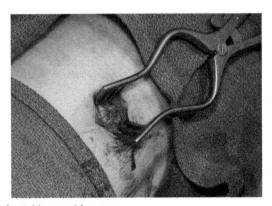

Fig. 10. Close the fascial layer with suture.

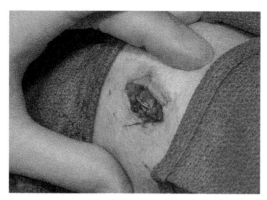

Fig. 11. Closing the subcutaneous layers before suturing the skin.

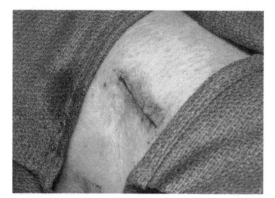

Fig. 12. Closure of the skin.

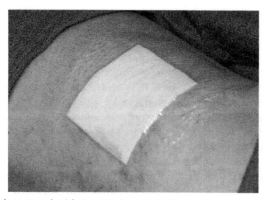

Fig. 13. Covering the wound with Steri-Strips, nonstick gauze, and occlusive dressing.

SHIPPING AND HANDLING

The specimen should quickly be packaged for shipment to the pathology laboratory. If biochemical testing is required, a smaller separate specimen (50–500 mg depending on planned tests) should be wrapped in foil and placed directly into liquid nitrogen while in the procedure room (snap-freezing). This step should be planned in advance so that liquid nitrogen is available in the procedure room. This strategy enables biochemical testing, when delay before freezing results in rapid deterioration of the quality of the specimen. The tissue for biochemical testing should be kept frozen by storing it in a −70°C freezer until it is shipped, on dry ice, to the reference laboratory via overnight express delivery.

If there is a delay of more than a few hours before processing the remaining tissue, a second small piece of muscle (50 mg of tissue no thicker than 2 mm) can be separated for fixation in 4% glutaraldehyde for electron microscopy (EM). Although EM is not a standard test, it is best to process tissue for EM so that testing can be completed if indicated after histologic evaluation. This process is not as time sensitive as that for biochemical testing and is simple to perform.

The main portion of the muscle specimen should be placed in lightly moist (not soaked) gauze, closed in an airtight container, and then placed on wet ice to keep the tissue cold while it is transported to the laboratory. If the specimen is soaked in saline or wrapped in gauze that is too damp, liquid is absorbed into the tissue and ice crystals form during freezing. This situation causes artifact, which makes pathologic interpretation of the sample difficult if not impossible. If the destination of the tissue is to a distant laboratory, the specimen for frozen and paraffin-embedded sections should be shipped cold but not frozen. The tissue is best transported over long distances using a cooler with dry ice or water ice. Please refer to your laboratory for local regulations, handling, and shipping instructions.

REFERENCE LABORATORIES

There are many academic and a few commercial laboratories that can provide good-quality, basic muscle histology processing. For more extensive testing, services may need to be provided by a specialized laboratory. Although there is no specific directory for locating these specialized laboratories, major academic centers with neuromuscular medicine programs either have laboratories capable of performing these tests or may be willing to provide references.

INTERPRETING MUSCLE BIOPSY RESULTS

Detailed interpretation of muscle histology is outside the scope of this article, but we would like to convey a basic understanding of the common techniques and stains used when assessing muscle biopsy specimens. Routine histochemistry, which is typically performed on frozen tissue, commonly includes the stains listed in **Table 2**. Frozen sections provide the most diagnostic information by light microscopy. The various stains allow the assessment of muscle fiber morphology, and identification of many pathologic and often diagnostic signs, such as those of inflammation, obvious mitochondrial abnormalities, and both glycogen and lipid storage abnormalities. Specialized immunohistochemical studies directed at disease-associated targets can also be performed on frozen tissue. These studies use antibodies against muscle-associated proteins such as dystrophin, emerin, sarcoglycan, major histocompatibility complex 1, and so forth to localize and often quantify these proteins (**Table 3**).[11]

Paraffin-embedded sections are typically stained with hematoxylin and eosin (H&E) and are the most informative when assessing inflammation and identifying the

Table 2
Routine stains used for muscle biopsy analysis

Class of Stain	Stain	Use
Morphology	H&E	General morphology including fiber size, split fibers, location of nucleii, regenerating and degenerating fibers, connective tissue, inflammatory cells, inclusions and storage material
	Modified Gömöri trichrome	Mitochondrial abnormalities, inclusion bodies, nemalin rods, and connective tissue
	Verhoeff van Gieson	Connective tissue and elastin in vessels
Fiber type enzymes	Adenosine triphosphatase pH 9.4: pale type I/dark type II pH 4.6: subtyping type II pH 4.3: pale type II/dark type I	Performed at different pHs to visualize different fiber types. Shows fiber type grouping and fiber type predominance
Oxidative enzymes	Nicotinamide adenine dehydrogenase	Intracellular structures and myofibrillar organization
	Succinate dehydrogenase	Mitochondrial disease
	Cytochrome oxidase	Mitochondrial disease
Hydrolytic Enzymes	Esterase	Denervated fibers, lysosomes, macrophages
	Acid phosphatase	Lysosomes, macrophages, vacuoles
	Alkaline phosphatase	Increased perimysial staining in inflammatory myopathies
Storage material	Periodic acid-Schiff (PAS)	Glycogen, presence of ring fibers
	Oil red O or Sudan black	Lipids

morphology of invading inflammatory cells. They are also useful for assessing vasculitis and degree of endomysial fibrosis. EM, as previously stated, is not routinely performed on each specimen. However, it provides ultrastructural analysis of specific abnormalities and clear visualization of inclusions (such as in inclusion body myosities), organelles

Table 3
Available immunohistochemical antibodies for muscle biopsy analysis

Protein	Disease
Dystrophin	Duchenne and Becker muscular dystrophy
Myotillin	Limb-girdle 1A
Caveolin-3	Limb-girdle 1C
Desmin	Limb-girdle 1E
Dysferlin	Limb-girdle 2B
Sarcoglycan	Limb-girdle 2C - F
Emerin	Emery-Dreifuss muscular dystrophy
α2-Laminin	Merosin-deficient congenital muscular dystrophy
B-Dystroglycan	Congenital muscular dystrophy
Collagen VI	Ullrich congenital muscular dystrophy
Major histocompatibility complex class I	Inflammatory myopathies

Data from Meola G, Bugiardini E, Cardani R. Muscle biopsy. J Neurol 2012;259(4):601–10.

(such as mitochondria), myofibrils, sarcolemma, basement membrane, and abnormal depositions (such as collagen or amyloid) that are not possible by light microscopy and sometimes add to the diagnostic information. If tissue is not prepared immediately after the biopsy for EM, stored frozen tissue prepared later for EM may provide important, albeit limited, histopathologic information.[12] In addition, light microscopic examination of 1-μm-thick resin sections, prepared for ultrathin sectioning used in EM imaging, can sometimes yield valuable information.

Normal Muscle Structure and Appearance

Normal human muscle is composed of many individual muscle fibers bundled together by layers of connective tissue that are arranged in a nesting-doll–like fashion. The innermost structure, the single muscle fiber, is covered by a thin layer of primarily reticular fibers called the endomysium. The endomysium is inconspicuous, and muscle fibers appear to be in direct contact with each other. The finest capillaries, nerve twigs, and lymphatic capillaries are found within the endomysium. Groups of muscle fibers are bound together by the thicker perimysium, forming structures called fascicles. Capillaries, nerve fibers, and lymphatic vessels also track in the perimysium.

Bundles of fascicles are encased within the dense irregular connective tissue of the epimysium. These connective tissue layers provide mechanical protection for the muscle fibers and increase the tensile strength of the muscle. The layers are continuous with the tendon, which provides attachment to bone.

Individual muscle fibers are syncytia, formed by embryonic fusion of many myoblasts or later, myosatellite cells. Each muscle fiber contains many nuclei, peripherally positioned immediately adjacent to the sarcolemmal membrane (**Fig. 14**). In healthy muscle, only 3% to 5% of fibers contain nuclei that are located internally, within the cell, but many disease processes lead to internal nuclei. Each nucleus provides a segment of the cell with needed translated protein products.[13]

In cross-section, individual myofibers appear polygonal except in the infant, in whom round fibers are normal.[14] Cells vary in diameter based on age, gender, and the specific muscle being evaluated. In the infant, the average muscle fiber diameter is 16 μm, which increases to the adult size (40–60 μm) by 12 to 15 years.[15]

Neural input, as a function of the motor unit, determines the metabolic signature of the muscle fiber. The motor unit, by definition, consists of a single α-motor neuron and all of the corresponding muscle fibers it innervates. Muscle fibers belonging to a single

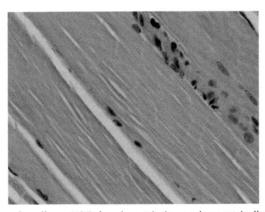

Fig. 14. Skeletal muscle cells on H&E showing striation and eccentrically located nuclei.

motor unit have the same metabolic type and are interspersed between fibers from other motor units, creating a patchwork pattern of varying fiber types visible with adenosine triphosphatase (ATPase) stains.[16] There are 2 major muscle fiber types: type I fibers, which are considered slow twitch, use oxidative metabolism, and have higher amounts of lipids and mitochondria within the sarcoplasm; and type II or fast twitch fibers, which predominantly use glycogen for energy production. However, there are multiple subtypes of type II fibers that are identified by varying cell characteristics, the most common being the capacity to use the oxidative metabolic pathway for ATP production.[6,16] Type II fibers are generally larger in diameter then type I fibers, and are larger in men than women.[15] ATPase stains, commonly performed under 3 different pH values, are used to identify fiber type: (1) pH 9.4 ATPase stains type I fibers light and type II fibers dark, (2) pH 4.3 ATPase stains type I fibers dark and type II fibers light, and (3) pH 4.6 ATPase stains type I fibers dark, type IIA fibers light, and type IIB fibers an intermediate shade.[9] The percentage of type IIB fibers increases with age, deconditioning, and obesity.[15]

The sarcoplasm contains myoglobin, glycogen, mitochondria, lysosomes and lipid vacuoles and is approximately 40% of the cell volume. The contractile unit of a muscle fiber is the myofibril. It comprises a long chain of sarcomeres that orient in parallel with the long axis of the fiber, and is constructed from proteins including actin, myosin, and titin.

Patterns of Neuromuscular Disease

There are 2 major characteristic myopathologic patterns of neuromuscular disease: (1) neurogenic, resulting from diseases of the innervating neuron; and (2) myopathic, caused by intrinsic diseases of the muscle fiber that can be inherited or acquired, including the muscular dystrophies, congenital, inflammatory, metabolic, and toxic myopathies. However, it is not uncommon to have pathohistologic findings of both neurogenic and myopathic processes in a single biopsy. Aggressive and chronic myopathies often lead to denervation of the muscle fiber and therefore neurogenic findings superimposed on a myopathic pattern on biopsy.[14]

Neurogenic atrophy

Diseases of the α-motor neuron cause muscle weakness and hypotonic muscle atrophy. The earliest structural change in neurogenic atrophy seen on muscle biopsy is the loss of the polygonal shape of the muscle fiber.[14] A pattern of scattered, atrophic muscle fibers involving both type I and II fibers is another early finding. The atrophic fibers become small and angulated. If reinnervation occurs, then fiber-type grouping is evident with ATPase staining and the normal patchwork pattern is no longer evident. Instead, groups of similar fiber types lie adjacent to one another (**Fig. 15**). This phenomenon occurs after denervation followed by reinnervation, when a single remaining nearby motor neuron sprouts and reinnervates multiple atrophied muscle fibers, altering the fiber type to reflect the metabolic signature of the reinnervating motor neuron.[17]

Other structures commonly associated with neurogenic atrophy are; (1) nuclear bags, which appear as clumps of nuclei encircled by the remaining sarcolemmal membrane; and (2) target or targetoid fibers, which are best observed with nicotinamide adenine dinucleotide-tetrazolium (NADH-TR) staining. Target fibers are characterized by the presence of 3 zones, each with varying stain intensity, within the cell. The pale central zone results from reduced oxidative enzymatic activity, disorganized myofibrils, and a paucity of mitochondria. The central zone is encircled by a darkly stained zone, which is enriched with mitochondria and has increased enzymatic

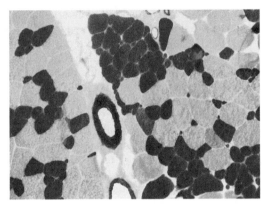

Fig. 15. ATPase stain revealing fiber type grouping.

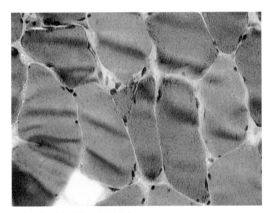

Fig. 16. Split fiber stained with Gömöri trichrome.

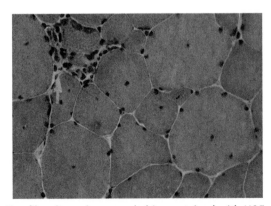

Fig. 17. Degenerating fiber (*arrow*) on muscle biopsy stained with H&E.

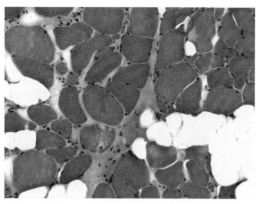

Fig. 18. Increased endomysial (*arrow*) and perimysial fibrosis in muscle stained with H&E.

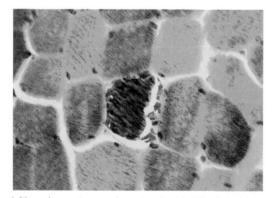

Fig. 19. Ragged red fiber shown in muscle stained with Gömöri trichrome.

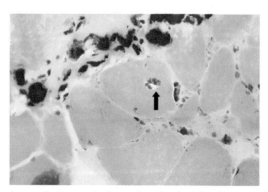

Fig. 20. Red rimmed vacuole in muscle (*arrow*) stained with Gömöri trichrome. The biopsy was taken from a patient eventually diagnosed with inclusion body myositis.

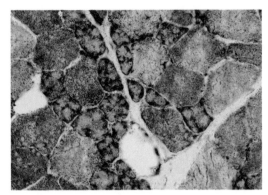

Fig. 21. Lobulated fibers (*arrow*) stained with succinate dehydrogenase stain. These fibers are observed in many myopathies, including limb-girdle 2A.

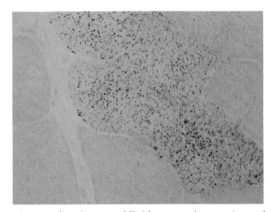

Fig. 22. Oil red O stain revealing increased lipid storage in type I muscle fibers.

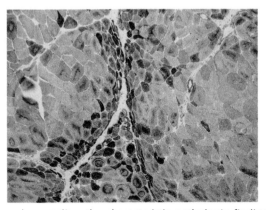

Fig. 23. Skeletal muscle revealing the characteristic pathologic finding of perifascicular atrophy in a patient diagnosed with dermatomyositis. The muscle is stained with NADH.

Table 4
Histopathologic features found in select muscular dystrophies

Category of Disease	Disease	Technique	Histologic Finding
Muscular dystrophy	Duchenne	H&E, Gömöri trichrome	Myopathic pattern with breaks in the sarcolemma
			Necrosis myophagocytosis
		Immunohistochemistry for dystrophin	Reduced or absent dystrophin seen around the sarcolemmal membrane
		Western blotting	Reduction in molecular size and quantity of dystrophin
	Limb-girdle	H&E, Gömöri trichrome	Myopathic pattern
			Calpainopathy (type 2A) commonly has lobulated fibers (see **Fig. 22**)
		Blue with H&E Red staining with Gömöri trichrome Intense blue staining with NADH-TR	Ring fibers
			Calpainopathy with eosinophilic infiltrate
		Immunohistochemistry for dystrophin-associated glycoproteins	Reduced or absent proteins
	Fascioscapulohumeral	H&E, Gömöri trichrome	Myopathic pattern
			May have mononuclear cell infiltrate
	Oculopharyngeal	H&E, Gömöri trichrome	Myopathic pattern
			Rimmed vacuoles in angulated fibers
		ATPase	Type I angulate fibers
	Congenital	H&E, Gömöri trichrome	Myopathic pattern
			Significantly increased endomysial fibrosis
		Immunohistochemistry	Reduced collagen VI (Ullrich)
	Myotonic	H&E, Gömöri trichrome	Significantly increased number of internal nuclei (~15% of fibers)
			Pyknotic nuclear clumps
		ATPase	Type I atrophy
		Blue with H&E Red staining with Gömöri trichrome Intense blue staining with NADH-TR	Ring fiber (wrapping of the diseased fiber around itself)

activity. The third zone stains normally, and is at the periphery of the myofiber. Target fibers are found most commonly in type I muscle fibers.[18]

Targetoid fibers are similarly found in the setting of neurogenic atrophy. They resemble target fibers but have only 2 discrete regions within the cell. The clinical significance of target and targetoid fibers is essentially the same, reflecting neurogenic atrophy.[19]

Myopathic changes

Myopathic changes observed on biopsy often include both a common underlying pattern of muscle disease with superimposed disease-specific structural alterations. The changes, particularly if early in the disease, may cause focal myofiber damage as in mitochondrial disorders, segmental damage as may occur in the dystrophies, or multifocal damage as occurs in the inflammatory myopathies.[20,21] Common myopathic features include fiber size variation with both atrophied and hypertrophied muscle fibers. The atrophied fibers are often rounded, as opposed to the sharply angulated atrophic fibers observed in neurogenic atrophy. The hypertrophied fibers, as they enlarge, may eventually divide into 2 fibers and are referred to as split fibers (**Fig. 16**).

Degenerating and regenerating fibers are scattered throughout myopathic muscle (**Fig. 17**). Degeneration usually begins in a segmental fashion, affecting a portion of a fiber. This finding is best appreciated on longitudinal sections. Small regenerating fibers can easily be identified by enlarged nuclei, and a bluish stain of the interior of the fiber with H&E staining. The bluish stain is caused by the increased concentration of RNA within the cell.

Old damage can be identified by the increase of internalized nuclei, which are common in many myopathies. An extreme example of this phenomenon is observed

Table 5
Common histopathologic findings in select congenital myopathies

Category of Disease	Disease	Technique	Histologic Finding
Congenital myopathies	Centronuclear/ myotubular	H&E, Gömöri trichrome	Myopathic pattern
			Increased number of central nuclei (~70% and greater)
			Perinuclear region with decreased myofilaments and increased glycogen, mitochondria, and lysosomes
		ATPase	Type I fiber predominant involvement
	Nemaline rod	H&E, Gömöri trichrome	Myopathic pattern
		Red staining with Gömöri trichrome	Perinuclear or subsarcolemmal threadlike inclusions
		ATPase	Inclusions found predominantly in type I fibers
		EM	Inclusions with filamentous pattern similar to the z-band
	Central core disease	H&E: frozen and paraffin sections Also seen with NADH-TR	Myopathic pattern with dark staining material in interior of cell
		ATPase	Above finding almost exclusively found in type I fibers

in centronuclear myopathy, in which 20% to 100% of fibers show this abnormality.[22,23] Internal nuclei may also be significantly increased in myotonic muscular dystrophy and have been previously reported to affect approximately 15% of fibers. In myotonic muscular dystrophy type I, type I fibers show a predominance of internal nuclei as opposed to myotonic muscular dystrophy type II, in which internal nuclei are more commonly seen in type II fibers.[24] A characteristic feature of these diseases is the phenomenon of a train of nuclei, closely packed, and lined up along the center of a muscle fiber. Endomysial and perimysial thickening occurs with chronic progression of most myopathic diseases (**Fig. 18**).

Disease-specific changes

Although most diseases of muscle have some or all of the above findings, a few appear normal on muscle biopsy, with only minimal hints of disease. This situation may be because the disease is patchy and the tissue sampled during biopsy missed pathologic muscle. Or, the disease does not typically cause structural abnormalities. Examples of muscle diseases that often have normal muscle structure on routine histochemical staining, although diseased, are several of the metabolic myopathies,

Table 6
Common histopathologic findings in select glycogen storage metabolic myopathies

Category of Disease	Disease	Technique	Histologic Finding
Metabolic myopathy: glycogen metabolism	Acid maltase deficiency: Pompe disease	H&E, Gömöri trichrome Periodic acid-Schiff + diastase sensitive	Myopathic pattern Glycogen accumulation in the lysosomes Vacuolization of the sarcoplasm
		Acid phosphatase EM	Present in vacuoles Membrane-bound glycogen granules and free glycogen
	Myophosphorylase deficiency: McArdle disease	H&E, Gömöri trichrome	Glycogen free beneath the sarcolemmal membrane or in vacuoles
		Myophosphorylase testing EM	Absence of phosphorylase Increased glycogen
	Phosphofructokinase deficiency	Periodic acid-Schiff Diastase resistant	Increased glycogen
		Phosphofructokinase testing	Absence of phosphofructokinase May have polysaccharide inclusions
	Debrancher enzyme	Periodic acid-Schiff Diastase sensitive Blue with H&E Red staining with Gömöri trichrome Intense blue staining with NADH-TR	Subsarcolemmal course glycogen vacuoles Ring fibers
			Increase of glycogen in Schwann cells

including carnitine palmitoyl transferase deficiency and myoadenylate deaminase deficiency, in which the tissue sections may appear normal unless sampled shortly after an episode of rhabdomyolysis.[25]

Others myopathies have histologic abnormalities considered strongly indicative for a certain disease, such as ragged red fibers, which are common in mitochondrial disease (**Fig. 19**); central cores, found in central core disease; and rimmed vacuoles, found in inclusion body myositis (**Fig. 20**).[26–28] However, each of these histopathologic findings may be seen in other myopathies, adding to the complexity of reading a muscle biopsy and reaching a conclusion. For example, ragged red fibers have been reported in inclusion body myositis and are also a common finding with normal aging.[26] If standard staining techniques do not offer definitive diagnostic information, immunohistochemical staining and biochemical testing may provide evidence of a specific disease process (**Figs. 21–23**).

Tables 4–9 list a select group of neuromuscular diseases with some of their common histopathologic findings. These tables are meant to help facilitate understanding of a muscle biopsy report, and they also show one of the potential shortcomings of muscle biopsy, that most if not all abnormalities are found in more than just 1 disease. However, the pattern of findings in a muscle biopsy should be considered in the context of the clinical history and examination and can then be powerful and provide an accurate diagnosis.

On occasion, the pathologist is only able to conclude that the specimen provides findings consistent with an unspecified myopathy. This is perhaps the least helpful result from the perspective of the clinician who is searching for diagnostic answers. In this situation, a large differential remains. As previously reviewed, this result may occur for a variety of reasons; such as the excised tissue may not have been taken

Table 7
Common histopathologic findings in select lipid storage and mitochondrial myopathies

Category of Disease	Disease	Technique	Histologic Finding
Metabolic myopathy: lipid metabolism	Carnitine deficiency	Oil red O	Markedly increased lipid droplets
		ATPase	More marked in type I fibers (see **Fig. 23**)
	Carnitine palmitoyl transferase deficiency	H&E, Gömöri trichrome	Often normal unless previous episodes of myoglobinuria, then may have necrotic fibers and regenerating fibers
		Oil red O	Lipid normal or mildly elevated
	Myoadenylate deaminase deficiency	H&E, Gömöri trichrome	Structurally normal
		Myoadenylate deaminase testing	Absence of myoadenylate deaminase
Metabolic myopathy: mitochondrial	Mitochondrial	Gömöri trichrome	Ragged red fibers Numerous myofibrillar mitochondria
		EM	Intramitochondrial paracrystalline inclusions Dense bodies Increased glycogen
		Oil red O	Increased lipid

Table 8
Common histopathologic findings in select inflammatory myopathies

Category of Disease	Disease	Technique	Histologic Finding
Inflammatory myopathy	Dermatomyositis	H&E, Gömöri trichrome	Regenerating/degenerating Necrotic fibers Microinfarcts Macrophages and lymphocytes in the perivascular and perimysial region
		NADH-TR	Perifascicular atrophy (see **Fig. 23**)
		Major histocompatibility complex 1	Complement components membrane attack complex around small blood vessels
	Inclusion body myositis	H&E, Gömöri trichrome	Inflammatory infiltrate in the endomysium Eosinophilic cytoplasmic inclusions Ragged red fibers Autophagic/rimmed vacuoles
		Cytochrome oxidase	Cytochrome oxidase- negative fibers
		EM	Intranuclear filamentous inclusions
	Polymyositis	H&E frozen, Gömöri trichrome	Myopathic pattern with lymphocytes and macrophages invading nonnecrotic fibers
		H&E paraffin sections	Myeloid dendritic cells and plasma cells in the endomysium
	Autoimmune necrotizing myositis	H&E, Gömöri trichrome	Scattered necrotic fibers Edema
		EM	Pipestem capillaries

Table 9
Common histopathologic findings in select toxic myopathies

Category of Disease	Disease	Technique	Histologic Finding
Toxic myopathies	Amiodarone	Gömöri trichrome	Scattered fibers with autophagic vacuoles Neurogenic atrophy
		EM	Myofibrillar disorganization
		Nerve biopsy	Myeloid inclusions
	Statin	H&E frozen and paraffin, Gömöri trichrome	Muscle fiber necrosis with phagocytosis Regenerating fibers
		Oil red O	Lipid-filled vacuoles
	Steroid	ATPase	Atrophy of type II fibers
		Oil red O	Lipid in type I fiber
		EM	Rare mitochondrial abnormalities

from a disease-fulminant region, or the disease process is in its infancy and the findings are not yet specific for a single disease process. Under these circumstances, although infrequent, it is not unreasonable to repeat a muscle biopsy, particularly in the setting of progressive weakness.

SUMMARY

Muscle biopsy is a valuable diagnostic tool when the clinician is faced with the challenge of assessing a patient with weakness caused by an underlying neuromuscular disease. The data gained from a biopsy can add to the clinical examination, electrodiagnostic, and laboratory findings, and provide essential information that may lead to diagnosis and initiation of appropriate treatment. Although the procedure is straightforward, the clinician needs to plan ahead, identify a team, determine if specialized tests are necessary, determine how much tissue is needed for processing, and then supervise the collection and delivery of the tissues to prevent artifact and ensure high-quality results. Maintaining good communication and strong working relationships with surgeons, processing and reference laboratories, and the neuropathologist ensures the highest-quality results and provides the most information from a muscle biopsy.

REFERENCES

1. Dubowitz V, Sewry C. The procedure of muscle biopsy. In: Muscle biopsy: a practical approach. 3rd edition. Saunders Elsevier; 2007. p. 3–20.
2. Mercuri E, Pichiecchio A, Allsop J, et al. Muscle MRI in inherited neuromuscular disorders: past, present, and future. J Magn Reson Imaging 2007;25(2):433–40.
3. Mercuri E, Jungbluth H, Muntoni F. Muscle imaging in clinical practice: diagnostic value of muscle magnetic resonance imaging in inherited neuromuscular disorders. Curr Opin Neurol 2005;18(5):526–37.
4. Zaidman CM, Holland MR, Anderson CC, et al. Calibrated quantitative ultrasound imaging of skeletal muscle using backscatter analysis. Muscle Nerve 2008;38(1):893–8.
5. Staron RS, Hagerman FC, Hikida RS, et al. Fiber type composition of the vastus lateralis muscle of young men and women. J Histochem Cytochem 2000;48(5):623–9.
6. Schiaffino S, Reggiani C. Fiber types in mammalian skeletal muscles. Physiol Rev 2011;91(4):1447–531.
7. Lai CH, Melli G, Chang YJ, et al. Open muscle biopsy in suspected myopathy: diagnostic yield and clinical utility. Eur J Neurol 2010;17(1):136–42.
8. Collins MP, Mendell JR, Periquet MI, et al. Superficial peroneal nerve/peroneus brevis muscle biopsy in vasculitic neuropathy. Neurology 2000;55(5):636–43.
9. Hiton-Jones D, Squier M, Taylor D, et al. Metabolic myopathies. In: Major problems in neurology. Philadelphia: WB Saunders; 1995. p. 30–54.
10. Tarnopolsky MA, Pearce E, Smith K, et al. Suction-modified Bergström muscle biopsy technique: experience with 13,500 procedures. Muscle Nerve 2011;43(5):717–25.
11. Meola G, Bugiardini E, Cardani R. Muscle biopsy. J Neurol 2012;259(4):601–10.
12. Giagnacovo M, Cardani R, Meola G, et al. Routinely frozen biopsies of human skeletal muscle are suitable for morphological and immunocytochemical analyses at transmission electron microscopy. Eur J Histochem 2010;54(3):e31.
13. Exeter D, Connell DA. Skeletal muscle: functional anatomy and pathophysiology. Semin Musculoskelet Radiol 2010;14(2):97–105.

14. De Girolani U, Nachmanoff D, Specht L. Disease of skeletal muscle. In: Garcia J, editor. Neuropathology: the diagnostic approach. St Louis (MO): Mosby; 1997. p. 717–64.
15. Bossen E. Muscle biopsy. In: Wortmann R, editor. Disease of skeletal muscle. Philadelphia: Lippincott Williams & Wilkins; 2000. p. 333–48.
16. Scott W, Stevens J, Binder-Macleod SA. Human skeletal muscle fiber type classifications. Phys Ther 2001;81(11):1810–6.
17. Sorarù G, D'Ascenzo C, Nicolao P, et al. Muscle histopathology in upper motor neuron-dominant amyotrophic lateral sclerosis. Amyotroph Lateral Scler 2008; 9(5):287–93.
18. Schmitt HP, Volk B. The relationship between target, targetoid, and targetoid/core fibers in severe neurogenic muscular atrophy. J Neurol 1975;210(3):167–81.
19. Buxton PH. Pathology of muscle. Br J Anaesth 1980;52(2):139–51.
20. Dalakas MC. Muscle biopsy findings in inflammatory myopathies. Rheum Dis Clin North Am 2002;28(4):779–98.
21. Scola RH, Pereira ER, Lorenzoni PJ, et al. Toxic myopathies: muscle biopsy features. Arq Neuropsiquiatr 2007;65(1):82–6.
22. Peyronnard JM, Charron L, Ninkovic S. Type I fiber atrophy and internal nuclei. A form of centronuclear myopathy? Arch Neurol 1982;39(8):520–4.
23. Jeannet PY, Bassez G, Eymard B, et al. Clinical and histologic findings in autosomal centronuclear myopathy. Neurology 2004;62(9):1484–90.
24. Pisani V, Panico MB, Terracciano C, et al. Preferential central nucleation of type 2 myofibers is an invariable feature of myotonic dystrophy type 2. Muscle Nerve 2008;38(5):1405–11.
25. William N. Fishbein myoadenylate deaminase deficiency: inherited and acquired forms. Biochem Med 1985;33(2):158–69.
26. Rifai Z, Welle S, Kamp C, et al. Ragged red fibers in normal aging and inflammatory myopathy. Ann Neurol 1995;37(1):24–9.
27. Jungbluth H, Sewry CA, Muntoni F. Core myopathies. Semin Pediatr Neurol 2011; 18(4):239–49.
28. Huizing M, Krasnewich DM. Hereditary inclusion body myopathy: a decade of progress. Biochim Biophys Acta 2009;1792(9):881–7.

Physical Therapy Evaluation and Management in Neuromuscular Diseases

Linda B. Johnson, BS, PT[a],*, Julaine M. Florence, PT, DPT[b],
R. Ted Abresch, MS[c]

KEYWORDS

- Physical therapy • Neuromuscular diseases • Outcome measures • Exercise

KEY POINTS

- Physical therapists (PTs) have extensive specialized training in musculoskeletal evaluation and assessment, which enables them to provide skilled interventions and prophylactic care maximizing function in neuromuscular disorders (NMDs).
- PTs must use their clinical judgment to differentiate between musculoskeletal symptoms that respond to conventional therapy interventions and those symptoms related to NMDs that do not.
- Evidence for the effectiveness of physical therapy treatments in the NMD population is lacking and future research into the efficacy and benefits of PT treatment interventions in NMDs is recommended.
- The development of reliable and valid outcome measures that are responsive to changes in the disease course and treatment interventions is needed to improve the evaluation and management of NMDs.

NMDs are a group of myopathic or neuropathic diseases that directly or indirectly affect the functioning of muscle. Myopathic diseases primarily result in muscular degeneration rather than affecting the nerves themselves. Neuropathic diseases include motor neuron diseases that involve motor neurons in the brain, spinal cord, and periphery, leading to impaired muscle function. Many mechanisms account for the pathology in NMDs, including hereditable genetic deficits (eg, dystrophinopathies, metabolic

[a] Physical Therapy Department, University of California Davis, Suite 1100, 4860 Y Street, Sacramento, CA 95817, USA; [b] Neuromuscular Division, Department of Neurology, Washington University School of Medicine, Box 8111, 660 South Euclid, St Louis, MO 63110, USA; [c] Department of Physical Medicine & Rehabilitation, Rehabilitation Research and Training Center, University of California Davis, MED:PM&R, TB191, One Shields Avenue, Davis, CA 95616, USA
* Corresponding author.
E-mail address: linda.johnson@ucdmc.ucdavis.edu

Phys Med Rehabil Clin N Am 23 (2012) 633–651
http://dx.doi.org/10.1016/j.pmr.2012.06.005
1047-9651/12/$ – see front matter © 2012 Elsevier Inc. All rights reserved.

myopathies, and spinal muscular atrophies), environmental-genome interactions (eg, acute idiopathic demyelinating polyradiculoneuropathy), and environmental causes (eg, tick paralysis and polio). The primary symptoms associated with most neuromuscular diseases include muscular weakness and fatigue but may also include rigidity, loss of muscular control, spasms, and muscle-associated pain. The disability associated with NMDs depends on the specific disease, its pathogenesis, the extent of clinical involvement, and the rate of progression.

PTs have extensive specialized training in musculoskeletal evaluation and assessment, giving them the tools to address and treat the significant needs of this population. Their knowledge of the pathophysiology and progression of disabling symptoms enables them to provide skilled hands-on interventions and prophylactic care. They provide services for NMD patients in a multitude of settings and across all ages. PTs are participating at the forefront of NMD research, developing outcome measures, assessing treatment interventions, and documenting the natural history progression of NMDs. Many of the standard practices of PTs, however, are only validated within a healthy population. This article reviews the role of PTs in assessing and treating patients with NMDs and discusses the available evaluation techniques and interventions with an effort to differentiate between treatments specific to this population and the more conventional practice of PTs. The status of current outcome measures available in research and their applicability to the clinic are also presented. Discussion regarding exercise and pain management related to NMDs is not addressed but can be found in the articles Abresch et al and Carter et al elsewhere in this issue.

THE ROLE OF THE PHYSICAL THERAPIST IN NEUROMUSCULAR DISEASES
In the NMD Clinic

In the clinic, a seasoned NMD PT has the expertise to perform many roles, from evaluator to educator and from equipment specialist to patient/family advocate. These services can provide crucial timely intervention and improve patient flow in an NMD clinic: addressing immediate concerns, facilitating communication between a patient's community therapist or durable medical equipment (DME) provider and clinic staff, and providing specialized advice to direct outpatient services to maximize the therapy benefit for the client. Clinic therapists should be able to rapidly assess disease-specific symptoms or complaints and determine if immediate intervention will improve the issue. Their assessments should be focused, enabling them to determine the stage and rate of disease progression and to anticipate the development of future disease-related disability and initiate preventative or palliative measures. Clinic therapists then have a primary responsibility to communicate patient status changes to PTs who are responsible for patients in alternate settings.

Recognizing that each clinic functions differently, having varied resources, the services a clinic PT provides ultimately depends on the needs of the multidisciplinary team, who define the clinic roles according to staffing and expertise. Regional differences in delivery of care exist and reimbursement may drive the availability of a clinic therapist. Therapy reimbursement is typically based on productivity and billable time. The multidisciplinary clinic often does not have a mechanism for billing for services in this manner and then PT services may only be available if time is contracted to a clinic. Although insurance requirements, Medicare, and the increasing need for preauthorization may hinder staffing clinics with a therapist, standard of care recommends the participation of a PT in an NMD clinic.[1,2] When a clinic therapist is not available or if the symptoms require ongoing intervention, a referral to outpatient therapy should be generated.

A clinic PT may use a multitude of assessments to document improvement or decline. When pharmaceutical intervention is initiated and ongoing for disease management, quantitative measures can be especially informative to a physician and provide evidence of treatment efficacy. Timed motor performance measures can be used to document objective functional changes in a patient's mobility and may help a clinician identify rates of disease progression.[3,4] Functional measures that document levels of functional mobility are helpful in making exercise or equipment recommendations. Outcome measures are discussed later.

The clinic is an excellent place to begin patient education regarding disease management. Designing a good home exercise program, to begin early after diagnosis, benefits patients and may encourage better long-term compliance. The structure of a clinic provides the opportunity to introduce only a few exercises and avoid overwhelming patients. Instruction in range-of-motion (ROM) exercises is important before the onset of joint contracture and follow-up at each subsequent visit can be used to correct techniques and add additional stretches as the disease progresses. In conjunction with stretching, patients may need education in proper positioning. Habitual poor postures, such as sacral sitting, thoracic flexion, leaning on a single wheelchair arm rest, sitting with unsupported feet, and prolonged immobilization, increase the risk of joint contractures in patients with NMD. Assessment of a patient's wheelchair and other mobility assistive devices provides the opportunity to identify a poorly fitting wheelchair and quickly rectify the problem. When a patient complains of weakness and fatigue that interfere with activities of daily living, energy conservation techniques should be discussed. In addition, education regarding pulmonary hygiene with instruction in breathing exercises, airway clearance, and assisted cough techniques is easily done in clinic.

Therapists should assess functional mobility and recommend appropriate home equipment. A detailed history of the home environment, including existing DME and architectural details as well as the ability of the caregiver to provide transfer support, must be documented. With the progressive nature of many NMDs, equipment recommendations must be based on both present and future needs of a patient. A tub transfer bench may work now but if transfers will no longer be functional within the year, investing in a full bath transfer system is a better long-term solution. Power mobility recommendations must be made with a 5-year functional outcome in mind because reimbursement for power equipment is usually limited to 1 device every 5 years. Sometimes, a home health referral to evaluate a home for equipment and safety is appropriate.

In the Outpatient Clinic

Outpatient therapists traditionally treat symptoms, such as weakness, pain, or impaired mobility, related to a primary NMD. A referral for outpatient therapy should reference the specific symptom or disability requiring treatment intervention in addition to the NMD diagnosis. The therapist performs a thorough evaluation using strength testing, mobility assessment, musculoskeletal function, and alignment to confirm the diagnosis and determine a course of treatment. Finding and referring to a PT with experience in NMD is key to establishing appropriate goals and treatment plans. In this population, shoulder pain may not simply be due to the more common diagnosis of rotator cuff impingement but may involve the inability to stabilize proximal joints and/or prolonged muscle and nerve stretch due to weakened proximal muscles combined with limb dependence as well as overuse syndrome. Familiarity with NMD known patterns of weakness and gait deviations assists with treatment planning. A clinic NMD therapist should be available to consult with the treating therapist to ensure safe and effective treatment.

PTs establish a specific problem list with a corresponding treatment plan and set objective goals to be met within a specified time frame. Modalities are selected for their effectiveness on specific pathology, such as pain or muscle spasms. Exercise prescription, including body posture, stabilization, exercise repetitions, and duration, are established. Close monitoring for response to exercise, including levels of fatigue, changes in weakness, and reporting of pain, is necessary. Movement analysis of gait and transfers is followed with training in gait strategies and energy-efficient techniques. Trial with various ambulatory or transfer assistive devices is used to maximize mobility.

A unique but important role is performed by outpatient pediatric PTs. These therapists have expertise in normal and abnormal developmental movement patterns. Experienced therapists are able to recognize early signs and symptoms suggestive of an NMD, such as lack of developmental progression despite intervention in a floppy infant, and initiate referral to an NMD specialist for early diagnostic work-up and intervention. A pediatric therapist also provides developmental therapy to a young NMD infant or child, maximizing function and assisting progression through developmental stages.

In the Home

Home-based PT is reserved for homebound patients who cannot access a therapy facility for medical reasons. The home setting is unique in that the therapist may address a patient's mobility limitations in the daily living space and recommend changes to the environment for optimal safety and mobility. Assessments may be performed to determine the most appropriate DME for a patient's home. Problem solving and improvising with available home items is possible and can be valuable for easing the challenges of care giving. Providing treatment in the home affords greater privacy and, for the very ill, maximizes the energy available for treatment. Many home therapists, however, have little experience with NMD clients and may need to consult with a clinic NMD therapist.

Home therapists perform evaluation and assessment of a patient's condition and set a treatment plan and goals that can be achieved in the home. Therapeutic exercises may be restricted due to limited availability of equipment but can include ROM exercises, resistance or isometric exercises, dynamic stabilization, gait training, or transfer training. Portable modalities may be available but are usually limited in scope. Home is a good place for caregiver training with focus on positioning and transfers. Educating caregivers in proper body mechanics and safety as well as community resources is invaluable. Once patients may safely leave the home to access outpatient therapy services, care should be transferred to an outside provider if they have continued functional therapy goals. In the United States, insurance companies do not usually cover physical therapy for maintenance or prophylactic services, so therapy must be discontinued when a patient does not have further functional goals.

In the School

The pediatric population spends a significant amount of time in the school environment. School-based therapy is often available and focuses primarily on educational goals, which are reflected in the treatment plan. Mobility, positioning, and staff training are frequent interventions to ensure accessibility and adaptability for pediatric NMD patients. Good communication between the NMD clinic therapist and the school therapist is important for implementing changes in DME or reporting changes in functional status that may have an impact on a patient's performance in school.

Mobility is assessed as it relates to the classroom or school facility. Gait devices must be determined appropriate and safe for the classroom. Standers or gait trainers may be appropriate and allow a nonambulatory child to be upright for classroom activities or enable independent mobility for a marginally ambulatory child. Some children may be able to safely ambulate in the classroom but not beyond due to uneven terrain or risk of falls in a crowded hallway. A wheelchair may need to be provided before the complete loss of ambulation so a child can traverse the campus or participate in field trips. Power wheelchairs with recline, tilt, or standing functions must be accommodated into the classroom for nonambulatory children.

The most important role of the school therapist is to ensure that a child is able to participate in all educational tasks. Successful ergonomics in the classroom include a student's posture and positioning at the desk, upper extremity support and position when writing, and type of writing utensils and/or communication device. The therapist may provide additional trunk support, modify seating, try alternate positioners, modify writing utensils, or apply wrist splints to decrease pain. For the more involved child with spinal muscular atrophy (SMA) or congenital muscular dystrophy, extensive adaptations may be necessary and involve the full educational team. PTs participate in developing an individual education plan for each child that guarantees students receive everything necessary to accommodate their disability in the classroom.

Finally, the school PT instructs the school staff in the safest methods to assist a child who has transfer needs for toileting and recommends appropriate transfer and or toileting equipment. Thorough training of the school staff in transfers ensures the safety for both child and staff caregiver.

In the Workplace

The Americans with Disability Act requires that employees with qualifying disabilities be reasonably accommodated in the workplace.[5] An NMD clinic therapist may help determine when an adult needs special accommodation in a place of employment. These recommendations may include modification of the workstation, mobility device specific for the occupation, and bathroom equipment and workplace accessibility.

In Research

PTs have played a role in clinical research for NMD since the mid-1970s, participating in the design, standardization, implementation, and documentation of reliability of clinical outcome measures and assessments. They have and continue to serve as clinical evaluators for therapeutic trials, performing the physical and functional assessments that serve as outcome measures and endpoints. PTs also have the opportunity to be clinical evaluators in natural history studies, helping to document the phenotype in several genotype/phenotype studies in NMD.

OUTCOME MEASURES IN NEUROMUSCULAR DISEASES

Although promising and novel therapeutic agents have recently emerged for muscular dystrophies and other neuromuscular diseases, significant barriers to the development of adequate clinical trials in these diseases remain.[6] Crucial deficiencies include lack of a detailed understanding of the characteristics and natural history of specific neuromuscular diseases, lack of objective clinical outcome measures that are sufficiently sensitive to changes in disease course, and lack of data that directly link changes in clinical outcome measures to patient-perceived well-being.[7-9]

To understand whether a specific therapeutic intervention is effective in NMDs requires explicit identification of the context of the population being studied (diagnosis, demographics, and so forth), assessing the health status before an intervention is performed with an appropriate clinical endpoint, delivering the prescribed intervention, and measuring health status after the prescribed intervention has been delivered.[10] All 3 dimensions (context, intervention, and outcome measures) must be addressed. Until recently, the diagnosis, pathophysiology, and genetics of many of the NMDs were not understood. For example, in many studies, the dystrophinopathies were aggregated together based on similar progressive muscle wasting, without understanding the different pathophysiologies of the individual diseases. The intervention, whether a pharmaceutical treatment, exercise regimen, social support, or other intervention, needs to be clearly defined and documented with regard to dose, frequency, and timing. Studies need to be performed to show that the outcome measure chosen for a clinical trial is reliable, valid, and responsive to change with the number of subjects chosen for the trial and the length of the trial.

For trials in NMDs, which are rare diseases, the burden of determining a reliable and responsive outcome measure is much greater than in cancer and cardiovascular disease, where a much larger number of patients can be used to power the study. Because most NMDs are rare diseases, the outcome measures need to demonstrate that a therapeutic intervention will make a clinical meaningful difference over the short time period (6–12 months) typically assessed in a clinical trial with limited numbers of subjects. The correct choice of outcome measures in clinical trials is critical to generate meaningful data that enable a therapy to move toward regulatory approval.

The 6-minute walk test (6MWT) has been chosen as the primary clinical endpoint for several recent clinical trials of ambulant subjects with Duchenne muscular dystrophy (DMD), Becker muscular dystrophy, SMA, Pompe disease, mucopolysaccharidosis, facioscapulohumeral muscular dystrophy (FSHD), fibromyalgia, glycogen storage disease, and polio.[11] The 6MWT has been shown valid, reliable, and responsive to change in several different disease populations and has already received regulatory approval by the US Food and Drug Administration and the European Medicines Agency. Some of the advantages of the 6MWT are that it is easy to understand, easy to perform, valid, reliable, and responsive to change. The 6MWT uses an interval scale (distance) that permits the use of parametric statistical analysis (use of mean, SD, correlation, regression, and analysis of variance). A change of approximately 30 meters in the 6-minute walk distance (6MWD) has been accepted as a clinically meaningful difference.

Although the 6MWT has received regulatory approval, it is not the ideal outcome measurement for all clinical trials in NMDs. The 6MWT is only applicable in ambulant subjects, which limits its usefulness in a wide range of potential studies, and it does not necessarily change linearly with disease progression. In a PTC Therapeutics trial of Ataluren for boys with DMD, the subject population was limited to boys greater than 4 years of age who could ambulate at least 75 meters.[12] Even with this limitation, the 6MWT outcome measure was not ideal for this 12-month trial of 174 subjects. Several boys lost their ability to ambulate during the trial and the change in 6MWD was not linear. Because loss of muscle function in DMD occurs against the background of normal childhood growth and development, younger children with DMD can show an increase in distance walked during 6MWT over 1 year despite progressive muscular impairment.[13] The analysis of the percent-predicted 6MWD data (using an age and height–based equation fitted to normative data), however, may reduce the variability of the 6MWD and account for normal growth and development. Henricson and colleagues[14] have shown that increases in 6MWD are proportional to normal growth up to approximately age 7 in boys with DMD, which is consistent with the commonly held concept of the honeymoon period in DMD during which functional gains, that result from growth and development, outpace disease progression such that percent-predicted 6MWD is stable at approximately 80% of healthy controls. Past age 7, boys with DMD experience substantial declines in percent-predicted 6MWD.

Because NMDs are diverse and have a large range of symptoms, choosing an optimal outcome measure for clinical trials has been challenging. It is now recognized that it is unlikely that one outcome measure can be used for all studies of NMDs. Instead, the outcome measure should be selected according to the population included in the trial, functional status of the patients at recruitment, duration of the study, and possible effect of the treatment. In some diseases, such as spinal muscular atrophy (SMA) or myotonic dystrophy, patients may be relatively stable over time, whereas other NMDs are relentlessly progressive (amyotrophic lateral sclerosis [ALS] and DMD). Therefore, the outcome measures used to assess changes in a patient with SMA are significantly different from those used in a patient with ALS.

Outcome measures that have been used to assess interventions in NMDs have (1) assessed functional capacity using timed function test or quantitative measures of strength with interval or ratio outcome measures, (2) assessed function or activity using ordinal scales that are typically evaluated by PTs, (3) assessed cognitive and psychological function using ordinal neuropsychological scales, and (4) assessed health status by measuring health status with person-reported quality-of -life scales.

Outcome measures that have been used to assess functional capacity using timed motor performance tests in individuals with NMDs include the measures listed in **Table 1**. The advantages of these outcome measures are that they are interval and ratio scales and are able to be analyzed using parametric statistics. The difficulties in using these measures are that, in themselves, they provide little information regarding clinical meaningfulness. It is not inherently known what a 5-second difference in time to run or walk 10 meters means to a patient. If these data are combined with natural history data in DMD, as done by McDonald and colleagues,[3] the data can be used to predict the likelihood that a boy with DMD would lose his ability to ambulate 1 year later. The timed motor performance and strength data can also be correlated with personal reported outcomes of health status of individuals to determine the clinical meaningfulness of changes of these outcomes. Another way to better understand the meaning of these outcomes is to develop a percent-predicted value similar to the Centers for Disease Control and Prevention growth charts or spirometry values for pulmonary function.

Table 1
Commonly used functional capacity measures

Timed Motor Performance Measures	Ordinal Measures of Function
Time to stand from floor	Medical Research Council manual muscle test
Time to stand from chair	ALS Functional Rating Scale
10-Meter walk time test	Barthel index
Time to climb 4 stairs	Brooke upper limb scale
Time to descend 4 stairs	Vignos lower limb scale
Timed up and go	Gross motor function measure
Timed get up and go	Egen Klassifikation scale
9-Hole peg test	Motor function measure
2-Minute walk test	Hammersmith functional motor scale
6-Minute walk test	Children's Hospital of Philadelphia Infant Test of Neuromuscular Disorders

Functions of NMD subjects have typically been evaluated by trained PTs using ordinal scales of measurement (see **Table 1**; **Table 2**). Although these scales have been validated, they are ordinal scales that require the use of nonparametric statistics (medians, modes, and percentiles) for analyses. These items are based on classical test theory that recruits items arbitrarily, without weighting. These scales describe the order, but not the relative size or degree of difference, between the items measured.[15,16] Therefore, summing these scores can lead to misinterpretation of the data. No information is provided regarding the minimally clinical important difference for these measures.

Research has shown that a combination of outcomes measures may better document motor function than a single measure.[17] In addition to measures of physical function, PTs have used a host of scales to assess the cognitive function, neuropsychological function, and health-related quality of life of individuals with NMDs (see **Table 2**). Although most of these measures use ordinal scales, most have been related to normal control values and provide clinical significance.

To overcome some of the limitations of ordinal scales, new techniques using Rasch model and item response theory have been used to transform ordinal scores, which are scale dependent and of limited accuracy, into linearly weighted interval measures that are scale independent.[18] This methodology has already been applied to the ACTIVLIM,[19] the National Institutes of Health (NIH) Neuro-QOL[20] quality-of-life scale, and the North Star Ambulatory Assessment of DMD.[21] These activities significantly improve the usefulness of these outcome measures, allow the examination of confounding factors, improve the sensitivity of these scales, test for unidimensionality, and potentially permit the development of a scale that can reliably and responsively assess results from individuals who experience a much broader range of impairments. The responsiveness of these scales over time needs to be examined as personal reported outcomes of health status are collected to determine the clinically meaningful important differences.

Table 2
Cognitive function, neuropsychological, and quality-of-life measures

Cognitive and Neuropsychological Measures	Quality-of-Life Measures
California Verbal Learning Test	Individualized Neuromuscular Quality of Life
Category fluency test and color word test	PedsQL
Delis-Kaplan executive function system	NIH Neuro-Qol
Design fluency test	Euroqol (EQ-5D)
Five-factor inventory	Perceived Quality of Life Scale
Hooper visual organization test	Quality of Well-Being Scale
Letter and category fluency test	SF-36v2 Health Survey
Proverb test Raven standard progressive matrices	Schedule for the Evaluation of Individual Quality of Life
Rey-Osterrieth complex figure test Rosenberg self-esteem scale 20	Questionnaire for Adults Health-Related Quality of Life
Self-efficacy scale, sorting test	
Stroop color and word test	
Trail making test	
Twenty questions test	
Wechsler Adult Intelligence Scale–revised	
Word context test	

The lack of validated outcome measures has been identified as a major barrier that has held back therapeutic development in NMDs and limited the translation of promising research results into clinical trials and treatments. Therefore, the development of specific and sensitive tools for assessing the effects of treatments in patients with NMDs is starting to receive a significant amount of attention.[22] The TREAT-NMD Neuromuscular Network is working to harmonize the use of the most appropriate outcome measures for different diseases at different stages of their progression and is collating information about existing outcome measures into a single and freely available online resource.[23] As outcome measures gain clinical significance, PTs will start using them in clinics to document response to therapeutic interventions and disease progression.

PHYSICAL THERAPY EVALUATION IN NEUROMUSCULAR DISEASES

PTs have access to many evaluation methods of performing a focused examination of a patient's symptom. Patients are referred with a treatment diagnosis, such as weakness, pain, gait impairment, or frequent falling, that may be related to their NMDs. Therapists must determine the source of these symptoms through skilled evaluation of the musculoskeletal and nervous system. Identifying specific pathology directs treatment intervention and improves treatment outcome. Objective measures are performed for documentation of baseline status. Functional mobility and safety are assessed. Throughout the evaluation, therapists must use their clinical judgment to determine an effective therapy intervention for NMD patients.

Strength Testing

Because weakness is a primary symptom of NMDs, manual muscle testing (MMT) is performed at initial evaluation. Therapists have extensive training and practice in performing MMT. They monitor patients closely to detect compensations and muscle substitutions, both common occurrences in NMD patients. For accurate and reproducible MMT, therapists must use standardized positions and stabilize proximal joints during testing. More important than strength to therapists is the quality of the contraction, the timing of recruitment, the active arc of motion and the ability to sustain a contraction. These help determine if weakness, motor control, pain, or fatigue is limiting strength.

Because MMT has its own limitations due to subjectivity, many therapists are using quantitative muscle testing (QMT) to evaluate strength. A fixed QMT system has been shown more reliable than MMT as an outcome measure.[24] QMT provides an ordinal numeric value when measuring strength, which allows therapists to document progress. A protocol should be followed to ensure reproducibility at each visit. A make test is most often used in the NMD population, which consists of patients performing their maximum voluntary isometric contraction against a stationary handheld device. Handheld QMT is not appropriate if patients are able to overcome the ability of the therapist to maintain a myometer in a stationary position. Limitations to QMT include the inability to position properly, maintain stabilization, and prevent substitution of compensatory muscles.

Contractures

Measurement of ROM is necessary for biomechanical analysis of movement and for documentation of progress. The measurements are performed using a goniometer and standard testing positions. Again, in the NMD population, formal positions may not be possible. Active and passive ROM should be tested. Lack of full active ROM is most often due to weakness but all other causes must be investigated. Therapists note the end feel of movement. Locating limitations in the joint capsule, muscle, or tendon dictates the therapy intervention. Comparison of the agonist and antagonist length and elasticity is performed. Specific joints are known to be at risk in the different NMDs and should be evaluated carefully. Pain (discussed later) is also a limiting factor in ROM and should be documented and addressed in treatment plan and patient goals.

Functional Mobility

Although it may not be the primary reason for referral to therapy, functional mobility should be assessed in each patient. Often, presenting symptoms are the result of improper biomechanics of patient mobility. Functional mobility and gait may be quantified with functional outcome measures, such as timed motor performances or disease-specific functional scales. In addition, therapists assess the amount of assistance needed to perform a given function. Functional mobility should include bed mobility, transfers, gait, floor recovery, and wheelchair mobility, if appropriate. Therapists observe initiation of movement, weight shifts, postural alignment, timing, and effort required to complete the movement. A patient's balance, base of support, and use of assistive devices are noted. The amount of effort it takes for a patient to accomplish a task and the energy expenditure should be documented. Realistic mobility goals should be set based on the evaluation and known progression of the disease.

Pain

Pain is a frequent complaint in NMDs, with as many as 82% of patients with certain diagnoses complaining about pain.[25] There are differences in pain patterns found between diagnoses, although location of pain is similar in many conditions with the lower extremities and back as primary sites of pain.[25,26] Pain has been documented in pediatric NMD patients as young as 11 years old. Pain correlates with lower functional scores, mobility limitations, and use of mobility assistive devices.[25,27]

Physical therapy offers an option for treatment of pain in NMD patients when the evaluation identifies a musculoskeletal diagnosis correlating with the pain. A thorough pain history focuses the examination of the patient. Characteristics of the pain, duration, and progression since onset help determine which modalities might be effective. Location, intensity, description of pain symptoms, and pain triggers may direct treatment toward manual intervention. Examination of the soft tissue looks for muscle imbalance, trigger points, overstretched joints, and muscle spasms. Therapists work through a cascade of techniques, with each finding directing the next technique. A treatment plan is developed, addressing the possible sources of pain, including weakness, poor skeletal alignment, and myofascial or soft tissue pain.

DME Evaluations

DME is expensive and highly technical. Physical therapy or occupational therapy evaluations are required by Medicare to document the medical and functional needs of a patient to ensure appropriate equipment is issued for each patient. Therapists keep abreast with the changing technologies in DME. They assess the strength, ROM, sensation, skin integrity, and respiratory status to determine the power mobility device that meets the needs of a patient. They are familiar with what is reimbursable and what may be an extra purchase for a patient. Where available, loan closets may be a source for equipment recommended by the therapist. Therapists also assess and recommend ambulatory assistive devices, transfer assists, bathroom equipment, and hospital beds.

PHYSICAL THERAPY INTERVENTIONS FOR NMD PATIENTS

PTs must complete an assessment or evaluation to determine the pathology or symptoms to receive intervention. Each treatment intervention should be focused with a specific outcome in mind. Several techniques may be needed to address a single pathology or a single technique may address multiple symptoms. Unfortunately, little research exists to validate therapy treatment interventions in NMDs and treatments are based on expert opinion. The following is a summary of treatment interventions commonly used in NMDs.

Stretching Exercises

Evidence of contractures is present in various NMDs, especially those with excessive fibrosis and fatty infiltration into the muscle, such as dystrophic myopathies.[28] In healthy subjects, contractures may constitute shortening of the skin, subcutaneous tissue, muscle, ligament, joint capsule or intra-articular surface.[29] All clauses must be considered when treating contractures in NMDs. In addition, there are dependent contractures caused by passive positioning or the inability to actively move the extremity through full ROM due to weakness. Shortening of the hip and knee flexor muscles in prolonged sitting, and tight long finger flexors from hand weakness and habitual positioning for use of wheelchair controls or computer games are examples of this. There are functional contractures that develop to compensate for a biomechanical disadvantage in the presence of weakness. Plantar flexion contractures occur due to repetitive forceful contractions of the triceps surae, acting as ancillary extensors of the knee as the quadriceps are failing, thereby changing the gait pattern in DMD. This is an example of the proposal by Gaudreault et al that "the passive moments produced by joint contractures can benefit the gait of patients with muscle weakness."[30] Restriction in ROM of ankle dorsiflexion helps to prevent spontaneous falls by limiting a sinking into ankle and knee flexion.

Stretching is recommended whenever a patient is at risk for or has evidence of contractures. The response to stretch has been well researched in healthy populations but due to the muscle pathology of NMDs, standard treatment techniques may not apply. In a healthy population, a warm-up of the involved muscle is recommended. This may entail heat application, simple exercise, or contraction of the antagonist. None of these has been studied or used in the NMD population. Static stretching, which is commonly used for treatment in NMDs, involves taking the muscle to its maximal length across the affect joint while keeping the joint in proper alignment and stabilizing the joints that are not being moved. When end feel of movement has been reached, the position is held for at least 10 seconds and then repeated. Daily stretching is recommended.

Research is lacking in the NMD population regarding the frequency and duration of static stretch. In healthy subjects, stretching performed 1 to 2 times per day, 3 to 7 days per week, demonstrated that ROM increased with the frequency of stretching and improvement was retained up to 4 weeks after stopping the exercises.[31] Research shows that short 5-minute static stretching causes change in the muscle-tendon unit.[32] Longer sustained stretch of 60 minutes in the presence of spasticity in a stroke patient has demonstrated an increase in ROM and a change in muscle tendon property.[33] Further research is needed in the NMD population to determine the optimal frequency and duration of ROM exercises.

Resting splints for ankles and wrists are often prescribed to allow neutral resting positions and are used during the sleeping hours with the intent of limiting the progression of contracture. There is no evidence to direct the timing of the initiation of splinting or the most effective wear time, but early intervention has become standard of care. Research has shown a decrease in tendoachilles contracture with the use of a night splint compared with intermittent stretching in DMD.[34] No increase in dorsiflexion ROM was found while wearing night splints in Charcot-Marie-Tooth disease (CMT).[35] Serial casting in DMD was also found to increase ROM with no loss of function during casting.[36] Serial casting can be used in the presence of a contracture, but it was found to have no sustained benefit in a trial with subjects with CMT.[37] Upright weight bearing is an alternate method of stretching for the lower extremities. A standing frame or standing wheelchair may be appropriate when a patient is losing ambulatory status. Surgical tendon lengthening is available to improve joint motion and alignment and may be done for comfort and positioning; however, it should be approached with caution in ambulatory children who may rely on some end resistance of dorsiflexion beyond neutral to prevent falls and sinking into flexion. In DMD, Achilles tendon lengthening increased ROM but did not improve function and in some cases decreased function; subjects relapsed by 24 months.[38]

Pain

Pathology of pain in NMDs is not well documented. During an evaluation, the therapist determines if there is a musculoskeletal or soft tissue pathology that is appropriate for therapy intervention. Conventional PT has many well-studied modalities for pain, which include ultrasound, transcutaneous nerve stimulation (TENS), cold, heat, and massage. There have been few studies assessing these treatment modalities for pain in the NMD population. Jensen and colleagues[39] found that although multiple pain treatments were used in their study sample, none was effective for all participants.

In a normal population, ultrasound is used for its thermal effect to increase tissue temperature at a depth of 3 cm or greater.[40] Thermal ultrasound is indicated for soft tissue shortening, inflammation, and tissue healing. Heat in the form of hot packs may be applied superficially to decrease muscle spasms or to prepare a muscle for stretching. Cold is applied to decrease inflammation or increase pain threshold. Ice cup massage is most effective over trigger points or smaller areas of pain, such as tendonitis.

TENS has the broadest application because it is thought to alter the pain pathway. Working theories on the mechanism of action include selective activation of large diameter fibers and presynaptic and postsynaptic inhibition. High-frequency TENS at 80 pulses per second, delivered over 20 minutes, has been shown superior to lower-frequency TENS at increasing the pressure pain threshold.[41] TENS is easily applied to sites of musculoskeletal pain in NMD patients. No research, however, has measured the effect of TENS in this population.

In the presence of weakness, joint pain is often associated with improper alignment or overstretching of the joint capsule. The goal of therapy is to restore proper alignment to the joint. Each NMD has a different pattern of weakness and this must be considered before choosing the appropriate treatment. When muscle weakness precludes self-stabilization, external splinting devices may be applied to approximate normal muscle length. For instance, when abdominal muscles become too weak to stabilize the back, an abdominal binder may be applied. When there is shoulder subluxation, external shoulder splints may decrease pain.

A careful evaluation of DME is needed to ensure that their assistive devices are not source of pain. For cosmetic reasons, ambulatory patients often prefer to use a single point cane when they first require an assistive device. The stress of carrying a cane or the asymmetry of use, however, may cause upper extremity pain. Changing to a 4-wheeled walker avoids lifting and provides equal bilateral support. Walker height is sometimes lowered for clients with upper extremity weakness so they can lean onto fully extended arms; however, this forward lean may aggravate back pain. In this case, if a patient changes to a rollator walker, with forearm supports, back strain may be reduced. For the wheelchair user, shoulder pain is associated with poorly fitting armrests and positioned armrests that do not keep the humerus aligned in the gleno-humeral joint. Back and hip pain correlate to improperly fitted leg rests, causing inappropriate knee to hip height. An appropriate wheelchair cushion is essential for skin integrity and pain control. Static positioning without pressure relief decreases blood flow and produces pain in a patient who uses a wheelchair full time. Bed positioning in dependent patients is extremely important because they cannot reposition themselves for pressure relief. Anatomic alignment, using external supports, such as pillows, to support the arm in side lying, should be taught to every family. Provision of pressure-relieving cushions and mattresses, electric beds, and rotating beds need to be considered for severely affected patients.

Strengthening/Aerobic Exercises

Strength exercises are controversial in progressive NMDs because the benefit of and response to exercise may be remarkably different depending on disease pathogenesis. NMDs present with a primary weakness from muscle pathology and secondary disuse or deconditioning weakness. The consensus in the literature is that a gentle strengthening program consisting of submaximal effort is safe and appropriate to avoid disuse atrophy, especially in the slowly progressive diseases.[42,43] The goal of exercise is to maintain existing strength or to slow progression of weakness, not to strengthen the weakened muscles. The type and intensity of exercise depends on diagnosis and severity of disease. In a quickly progressing diseases, exercise is more controversial. A full discussion of exercise in the NMD population can be found in the article by Abresch et al elsewhere in this issue.

Progression of weakness and patterns of weakness are disease specific. In DMD, there is a rapid progression of weakness in childhood, with trunk musculature and proximal muscles weakening first. In limb-girdle muscular dystrophy, the scapular/humeral and pelvic areas are involved, and in FSHD, the scapulothoracic muscles weaken. ALS often causes asymmetric weakness and usually has adult-onset with rapid progression. The consulting therapist should be familiar with each disease entity and know these patterns of progression and when intervention is optimal. Observation of functional movement as well as strength tests confirm the level of weakness and phase of disease progression in a patient. The NMD specialist should provide input and assistance in the development of an exercise program.

When indicated, exercises should begin with a limited number of repetitions with little or no resistance. Higher-resistance exercises have been shown no more effective than moderate exercises and may cause deleterious effects on skeletal muscle.[44] A PT reassesses tolerance and increase frequency, duration, or resistance as appropriate. A maximum of 30 to 45 minutes, divided throughout the day, limits fatigue. Patients can be taught to self-monitor their level of exertion using the Borg scale of perceived exertion.[45] Care should be taken to avoid damaging already weakened muscles with overstretching or overuse. Inevitably, some clients already are working at a maximal level while performing their normal activities of daily living and should not add work to these muscles by exercising. Other patients may benefit from more challenging exercises but should be monitored closely.

Fatigue has been reported to play a large role in NMDs, especially FSHD, myotonic dystrophy, and hereditary motor and sensory neuropathy.[46] In a review of the literature, Abresch and colleagues[42] described the lack of adequate evidence regarding exercise in NMDs but concluded that there is the potential for aerobic training to improve the cardiopulmonary condition of individuals with an NMD. Aerobic exercises, such as walking, swimming, and biking, provide overall fitness with less stress to the musculoskeletal system. For children, exercise may be incorporated into their daily play routines. If a patient experiences pain, excessive fatigue, an increase in fasciculations, or muscle spasms within 24 hours of exercising, the exercise should be curtailed and re-evaluated. Periodic evaluations should be performed to adjust the exercise program to reflect the progression of the disease.

Aquatic therapy is an excellent mode of exercise for this population. Water buoyancy supports the weakened muscles but allows maximal functional movement. Full assisted ROM is possible in all planes of movement with proper instruction. Pool exercises maximize a patient's aerobic capacity while treating all the muscle groups. This is efficient for patients with limited energy resources. A case study for a child with SMA III demonstrated that 45-minute aquatic exercises 2 times per week for 3 months increased walking velocity, stride length, and single-limb stance time in gait.[47] The limitations of pool therapy include poor accessibility and lack of reimbursement for aquatic programs.

Early-onset NMDs in infancy provides a challenge to PTs because care can range from palliative to recreational exercise. Despite poor prognosis, if appropriate, an infant with SMA I should be referred for a therapy consultation to educate parents in positioning, handling, and sensory stimulation. Knowing how to handle and engage their child enriches the parent-child bonding experience. SMA I children develop little antigravity strength and are challenged to move through the normal stages of sensorimotor development that affect cognitive development. They cannot experience body exploration, midline orientation, toy manipulation, or cause and effect. Developmental exercise should be focused on gravity-eliminated positions. Midline toy play can be performed in side lying. Prone positioning can be performed on an incline with additional supports to minimize gravitational forces. When an infant is positioned in a reclined seat, support behind the upper arm assists in bringing the arms to midline into a child's field of vision. Creative parents and therapists often invent devices that support the upper extremities so children can move their arms with gravity eliminated. These children may be taught to activate switch toys with the long-term goal of using a communication device. Children with SMA II develop upright sitting and antigravity extremity strength but their progressive weakness leads to significant contractures and scoliosis if not supported. They need intensive stretching, splinting, and positioning programs. Active monitoring for DME needs should be ongoing.

Impaired Gait and Balance

Gait impairments become evident with the onset of weakness and fatigue in NMDs. Frequent falls are reported, which often increases the fear of falling and causes reduced activity. Therapy interventions must address strength, compensatory strategies, and secondary comorbidities to maximize safe functional ambulation.

Gait impairments are directly related to the patterns of weakness and presence of contractures. Proximal weakness causes instability of the trunk with resulting lordosis. Hip abductor weakness causes either a bilateral Trendelenburg hip dipping gait or a waddling gait with a lateral side sway over the supporting leg. Use of the triceps surae to assist knee extension leads to toe walking or the less-evident external rotation of hip and pronated feet. Hip flexor and extensor weakness decreases stride length. Knee extensor weakness reduces the knee flexion moment in midstance.[48] Dorsiflexion weakness or plantar flexion contractures impede toe clearance in the swing phase of gait.

Improving gait patterns in NMD patients may include endurance training, assistive device education, and orthotic recommendations. There is some evidence that weakness and fatigue of lesser involved muscles may impair gait. In CMT, hip flexors fatigue in the presence of a steppage gait pattern, decrease hip flexor velocity, and reduce walking duration.[49] In SMA, there are often changes in the hip rotator action entering stance phase accompanied by changes in ankle plantar flexor activity related directly to the external flexion moment acting on the knee.[50] These studies have proposed that strengthening of isolated or compensatory muscles may improve function and decrease fatigue in gait. Therapists must assess the gait of individual patients and form a treatment plan as it relates to stage of disease.

Energy expenditure in gait increases in the NMD population.[51,52] Aerobic exercises may be used to improve the cardiopulmonary status of mildly affected dystrophinopathy patients or NMD patients who are early in the course of their disease.[42] Aquatic therapy or stationary bicycles provide general conditioning with minimal demand on muscles. Therapists use their professional judgment to decide if a patient's gait will likely benefit from aerobic training, choose the best mode of exercise for the level of disease, and monitor patients closely for tolerance of the exercise.

As weakness develops, use of an assistive device or orthotic can improve the gait pattern, energy efficiency, and safety. The wrong device, however, can impede gait by altering the optimal gait pattern of a patient. A history of falls requires assessment of balance, gait, sensation, proprioception, and home environment. An assistive device to improve balance may be as simple as a single point cane or as sturdy as a 4-wheeled walker. In other situations, stabilizing the upper extremities by using an assistive device works its way down the chain, stabilizing the trunk and improving lower extremity function. Not all patients benefit from assistive devices, however. Use of ambulatory devices for boys with DMD prevents their adaptive gait patterns and interferes with functional gait.

Orthotic recommendations may be made by the therapist, orthotist, or physician. Orthotic considerations include desired function, weight, and tolerance for the device. An ankle foot orthosis (AFO) may assist dorsiflexion and/or prevent plantar flexion and control the knee by limiting forward tibial progression. Traditional double upright orthotics have great flexibility to assist or limit both dorsiflexion and plantar flexion but are heavy and limited to a single pair of footwear. Polypropylene AFOs are custom made and can correct foot deformities while adding ankle control. Dorsiflexion assist, plantar flexion stop, or full ankle articulation is possible. Patients must have enough strength to control an articulating joint; otherwise, a solid AFO is the most appropriate. Off-the-shelf lightweight orthotics, such as a carbon fiber AFO, prevent foot drop and add less weight so as not to fatigue patients. These do not control foot/ankle deformities, however. A new dynamic form of a floor reaction AFO allows the energy-storing component to assist weak musculature while the yielding motion allows for forward progression necessary for efficient gait. Patients must have good sensation and tolerate the pressure of any type of orthoses. Gait training should accompany the prescription of a new orthosis to educate patients in its optimal use.

Breathing Exercises

PTs may be tasked with evaluating and treating the progressive respiratory impairment in NMD patients. These patients suffer from weakness of the diaphragm and accessory muscles with resulting restrictive lung disease and ineffective cough. Spinal deformities reduce chest wall compliance and further limit lung volume.[53] Patients with bulbar symptoms have increased secretions and inability to close the glottis, which is necessary for effective coughing. If a weak cough is diagnosed in NMDs, it allows for timely provision of airway clearance techniques, including air stacking, manually assisted cough, and mechanically assisted cough.[54]

Breathing exercises involve teaching patients to maximize their lung expansion. Diaphragmatic breathing exercises, air stacking, or deep sigh breathing can be performed independently by patients. Lung expansion therapy or air stacking uses a bag value mask or mechanically assisted hyperinsufflation to increase lung volumes to maximum insufflation capacity beyond forced inspiratory vital capacity. Kang and Bach[55] determined that maximum insufflation therapy is important in increasing peak cough flow for NMD patients with vital capacity less than 1500 mL. Intermittent positive-pressure breathing-assisted hyperinsufflation has been shown to improve peak cough flow in pediatric NMDs.[56] Maximum expansion should be followed by manual assisted cough techniques. Use of a positive expiratory pressure device also assists secretion mobilization. When using the simple positive expiratory pressure device, patients inhale freely then exhale against gentle resistance, which increases back pressure, preventing atelectasis, while airflow mobilizes secretions. Chest physical therapy was the traditional method of airway clearance and may still be taught to this population. It involves positioning a patient in multiple positions and clapping over the chest wall to loosen secretions followed by vibrations and coughing to clear secretions. Many positions are head down in Trendelenburg, side lying, or prone and are often poorly tolerated in the NMD population.

Cough-assist techniques should be taught to all patients before cough becomes ineffective. A peak cough flow below 160 L/min has been the cutoff for establishing cough assistance in NMDs; however, in recent publications, a maximum assisted peak cough flow of less than 300 L/min was used to initiate mechanical cough assistance.[55,57] Manual cough assistance is done by applying pressure to the abdomen or to the lateral rib cage while a patient produces an active cough. These techniques may be performed in several positions and in many lifestyle environments and do not require equipment. The mechanical cough assist (insufflation/exsufflation) is an example of an airway clearance device, which delivers a preset volume of air to fill lungs (insufflation) and then reverses the cycle to withdraw air quickly (exsufflation) pulling with it the retained secretions. Use of any pulmonary equipment must be monitored by a physician, respiratory therapist, or trained therapist.

SUMMARY

NMDs as a group of myopathic or neuropathic diseases primarily present with weakness, fatigue, and loss of function. PTs have the knowledge and clinical expertise to provide comprehensive evaluation, assessment, and treatment for these clients. PTs play a crucial role on the NMD team, providing services across the spectrum of clinical health care settings. The NMD therapy specialist is a valuable resource, communicating therapy needs and reporting changes in functional status to community therapists, who directly treat this population. This is especially important because conventional therapy interventions may not apply to the NMD population. Research providing evidence for the effectiveness of PT treatments in the NMD population is lacking. Future studies are needed to evaluate the efficacy of current therapeutic strategies and determine best-of-care practices for PT interventions in NMDs.

REFERENCES

1. Bushby K, DMD Care Considerations Working Group. Diagnosis and management of duchenne muscular dystrophy—part 1. Diagnosis, pharmacological and psychological management. Lancet Neurol 2010;9:77–93.

2. Bushby K, DMD Care Considerations Working Group. Diagnosis and management of duchenne muscular dystrophy—part 2. Implementation of multidisciplinary care. Lancet Neurol 2010;9(2):177–89.
3. McDonald CM, Abresch RT, Carter GT, et al. Profiles of neuromuscular diseases. Duchenne muscular dystrophy. Am J Phys Med Rehabil 1995;74(Suppl 5): S70–92.
4. Bushby K, Connor E. Clinical outcome measures for trials in Duchenne muscular dystrophy: report from International Working Group meetings. Clin Investig (Lond) 2011;1(9):1217–35.
5. Available at: www.ada.gov. Accessed June 26, 2012.
6. Cossu G, Sampaolesi M. New therapies for Duchenne muscular dystrophy: challenges, prospects and clinical trials. Trends Mol Med 2007;13(12):520–6.
7. NIH Workshop on Translational Research in Muscular Dystrophy. Silver Spring (MD): June 25–27, 2007.
8. Muscular Dystrophy Association. Clinical research coalition meeting, Tucson (AZ), 2004.
9. NIH Department of Health and Human Services. Action plan for the muscular dystrophies. Plan developed by the Muscular Dystrophy Coordinating Committee Scientific Working Group, August 16-17, 2005. Bethesda (MD): Muscular Dystrophy Coordinating Committee; 2005.
10. Long A, Jefferson J. The significance of outcomes within European health sector reforms: towards the development of an outcomes culture. Int J Publ Admin 1999; 22(3):385–424.
11. Available at: clinicaltrials.gov. Accessed June 28, 2012.
12. Safety and Efficacy Study of PTC124 in Duchenne Muscular Dystrophy. Available at: ClinicalTrials.gov. Accessed June 28, 2012. Identifier: NCT00592553.
13. McDonald CM, Henricson EK, Han JJ, et al. The 6-minute walk test in Duchenne/ Becker muscular dystrophy: longitudinal observations. Muscle Nerve 2010;42(6): 966–74.
14. Henricson E, Abresch R, Han JJ, et al. Percent-predicted 6-minute walk distance in duchenne muscular dystrophy to account for maturational influences. PLoS Curr 2012;3:RRN1297.
15. Merbitz C, Morris J, Grip JC. Ordinal scales and foundations of misinference. Arch Phys Med Rehabil 1989;70:308–12.
16. Wright BD, Linacre JM. Observations are always ordinal; measurements, however, must be interval. Arch Phys Med Rehabil 1989;70:857–60.
17. Mazzone E, Martinelli D, Berardinelli A, et al. North Star Ambulatory Assessment, 6-minute walk test and timed items in ambulant boys with Duchenne muscular dystrophy. Neuromuscul Disord 2010;20(11):712–6.
18. Bond TG, Fox CM. Applying the Rasch model: fundamental measurement for the human sciences. New York: Lawrence Erlbaum Associates; 2001.
19. Vandervelde L, Van den Bergh PY, Goemans N, et al. ACTIVLIM: a Rasch-built measure of activity limitations in children and adults with neuromuscular disorders. Neuromuscul Disord 2007;17:459–69.
20. Lai JS, Nowinski C, Victorson D, et al. Quality-of-life measures in children with neurological conditions: pediatric Neuro-QOL. Neurorehabil Neural Repair 2012;26(1):36–47.
21. Mayhew A, Cano S, Scott E, et al. North star clinical network for paediatric neuromuscular disease. Moving towards meaningful measurement: Rasch analysis of the North Star Ambulatory Assessment in Duchenne muscular dystrophy. Dev Med Child Neurol 2011;53(6):535–42.

22. Mercuri E, Mayhew A, Muntoni F, et al. Towards harmonisation of outcome measures for DMD and SMA within TREAT-NMD; report of three expert workshops. Neuromuscul Disord 2008;18:894–903.
23. Available at: www.researchrom.com. Accessed June 28, 2012.
24. Escolar DM, Henricson EK, Mayhew J, et al. Clinical evaluator reliability for quantitative and manual muscle testing measures of strength in children. Muscle Nerve 2001;24(6):787–93.
25. Jensen MP, Hoffman AJ, Stoelb BL, et al. Chronic pain in persons with myotonic dystrophy and facioscapulohumeral dystrophy. Arch Phys Med Rehabil 2008; 89(2):320–8.
26. Engel JM, Kartin D, Carter GT, et al. Pain in youths with neuromuscular disease. Am J Hosp Palliat Care 2009;26(5):405–12.
27. Chiò A, Canosa A, Gallo S, et al. Pain in amyotrophic lateral sclerosis: a population-based controlled study. Eur J Neurol 2012;19(4):551–5.
28. McDonald CM. Limb contractures in progressive neuromuscular disease and the role of stretching, orthotics, and surgery. Phys Med Rehabil Clin N Am 1998;9(1): 187–211 Review.
29. Calliet R. Soft tissue pain and disability. 2nd edition. Philadelphia: FA Davis Company; 1998. p. 29.
30. Gaudreault N, Gravel D, Nadeau S, et al. A method to evaluate contractures effects during the gait of children with Duchenne dystrophy. Clin Orthop Relat Res 2007;456:51–7.
31. Cipriani DJ, Terry ME, Haines MA, et al. Effect of stretch frequency and sex on rate of gain and rate of loss in muscle flexibility during a hamstring stretching program: a randomized single-blind longitudinal study. J Strength Cond Res 2011. [Epub ahead of print].
32. Nakamura M, Ikezoe T, Takeno Y, et al. Acute and prolonged effect of static stretching on the passive stiffness of the human gastrocnemius muscle tendon unit in vivo. J Orthop Res 2011;29(11):1759–63.
33. Gao F, Ren Y, Roth EJ, et al. Effects of repeated ankle stretching on calf muscle-tendon and ankle biomechanical properties in stroke survivors. Clin Biomech (Bristol, Avon) 2011;26(5):516–22.
34. Hyde SA, Fłłytrup I, Glent S, et al. A randomized comparative study of two methods for controlling Tendo Achilles contracture in Duchenne muscular dystrophy. Neuromuscul Disord 2000;10(4–5):257–63.
35. Refshauge KM, Raymond J, Nicholson G, et al. Night splinting does not increase ankle range of motion in people with Charcot-Marie-Tooth disease: a randomised, cross-over trial. Aust J Physiother 2006;52(3):193–9.
36. Rose KJ, Burns J, Wheeler DM, et al. Interventions for increasing ankle range of motion in patients with neuromuscular disease. Cochrane Database Syst Rev 2010;(2):CD006973. Review.
37. Glanzman AM, Flickinger JM, Dholakia KH, et al. Serial casting for the management of ankle contracture in Duchenne muscular dystrophy. Pediatr Phys Ther 2011;23(3):275–9.
38. Rose KJ, Raymond J, Refshauge K, et al. Serial night casting increases ankle dorsiflexion range in children and young adults with Charcot-Marie-Tooth disease: a randomised trial. J Physiother 2010;56(2):113–9.
39. Jensen MP, Abresch RT, Carter GT, et al. Chronic pain in persons with neuromuscular disease. Arch Phys Med Rehabil 2005;86(6):1155–63.
40. Hayes BT, Merrick MA, Sandrey MA, et al. Three-mhz ultrasound heats deeper into the tissues than originally theorized. J Athl Train 2004;39(3):230–4.

41. Chen CC, Johnson MI. An investigation into the hypoalgesic effects of high- and low-frequency transcutaneous electrical nerve stimulation (TENS) on experimentally-induced blunt pressure pain in healthy human participants. J Pain 2010;11(1):53–61.

42. Abresch RT, Han JJ, Carter GT. Rehabilitation management of neuromuscular disease: the role of exercise training. J Clin Neuromuscul Dis 2009;11(1):7–21.

43. Aitkens SG, McCrory MA, Kilmer DD, et al. Moderate resistance exercise program: its effect in slowly progressive neuromuscular disease. Arch Phys Med Rehabil 1993;74(7):711–5.

44. Kilmer DD, McCrory MA, Wright NC, et al. The effect of a high resistance exercise program in slowly progressive neuromuscular disease. Arch Phys Med Rehabil 1994;75(5):560–3.

45. Borg GA. Psychophysical bases of perceived exertion. Med Sci Sports Exerc 1982;14(5):377–81.

46. Kalkman JS, Schillings ML, van der Werf SP, et al. Experienced fatigue in facio-scapulohumeral dystrophy, myotonic dystrophy, and HMSN-I. J Neurol Neurosurg Psychiatry 2005;76(10):1406–9.

47. Salem Y, Gropack SJ. Aquatic therapy for a child with type III spinal muscular atrophy: a case report. Phys Occup Ther Pediatr 2010;30(4):313–24.

48. Doglio L, Pavan E, Pernigotti I, et al. Early signs of gait deviation in Duchenne muscular dystrophy. Eur J Phys Rehabil Med 2011;47(4):587–94.

49. Ramdharry GM, Day BL, Reilly MM, et al. Hip flexor fatigue limits walking in Charcot-Marie-Tooth disease. Muscle Nerve 2009;40(1):103–11.

50. Matjacić Z, Olensek A, Krajnik J, et al. Compensatory mechanisms during walking in response to muscle weakness in spinal muscular atrophy, type III. Gait Posture 2008;27(4):661–8.

51. McCrory MA, Kim HR, Wright NC, et al. Energy expenditure, physical activity, and body composition of ambulatory adults with hereditary neuromuscular disease. Am J Clin Nutr 1998;67:1162–9.

52. Menotti F, Felici F, Damiani A, et al. Charcot-Marie-Tooth 1A patients with low level of impairment have a higher energy cost of walking than healthy individuals. Neuromuscul Disord 2011;21(1):52–7.

53. Unterborn JN, Hill NS. Options for mechanical ventilation in neuromuscular diseases. Clin Chest Med 1994;5(4):765–81.

54. Geiseler J, Karg O. Management of secretion in patients with neuromuscular diseases. Pneumologie 2008;62(Suppl 1):S43–8 [in German].

55. Kang SW, Bach JR. Maximum insufflation capacity: vital capacity and cough flows in neuromuscular disease. Am J Phys Med Rehabil 2000;79(3):222–7.

56. Dohna-Schwake C, Ragette R, Teschler H, et al. IPPB-assisted coughing in neuromuscular disorders. Pediatr Pulmonol 2006;41(6):551–7.

57. Ishikawa Y, Miura T, Ishikawa Y, et al. Duchenne muscular dystrophy: survival by cardio-respiratory interventions. Neuromuscul Disord 2011;21(1):47–51.

Exercise in Neuromuscular Diseases

R. Ted Abresch, MS*, Gregory T. Carter, MD, MS, Jay J. Han, MD, Craig M. McDonald, MD

KEYWORDS

- Neuromuscular disease • Exercise therapy • Randomized controlled trials
- Muscular dystrophies

KEY POINTS

- An accurate diagnosis of a specific neuromuscular disease (NMD) is essential to better understand the potential benefits and contraindications that may result from a potential exercise therapy program.
- There is inadequate evidence from randomized controlled trials with sufficient sample size to document the optimal prescriptions regarding the type, intensity, duration, frequency, and mode of delivery of exercise programs for individuals with NMDs.
- In general, there is a potential for moderate-intensity aerobic training and physical activity to improve the cardiopulmonary condition of individuals with NMD, but the level and type of training depends on the diagnosis, stage, and severity of the disease.
- Moderate aerobic exercise may reverse some of the effects of deconditioning and provide positive health benefits in terms of reduced adiposity, improved cardiorespiratory status, improved sense of well-being, and increased bone mass for individuals with NMDs.
- Low-intensity resistance exercise may be beneficial for individuals with NMDs who have antigravity strength or better.
- High-resistance exercise has not been shown to offer any advantage over a moderate-resistance training program in NMDs, and should be avoided because it may cause over-work injury.

Tremendous advances have occurred in the past decade in our understanding of the molecular genetic basis and pathophysiology of neuromuscular diseases (NMDs). These advances have led to the development of a host of promising pharmaceutical therapies for NMDs, including antisense oligonucleotide (AON) exon-skipping

Funding: This work was supported by Grant #H133B0900001 from the National Institute of Disability and Rehabilitation Research. The authors take full responsibility for the contents of this article, which do not represent the views of the National Institute of Disability and Rehabilitation Research or the United States Government.
Conflict of Interest: The authors have nothing to disclose.
Department of Rehabilitation Medicine, University of California, Davis, 4860 Y Street Suite, 3850, Sacramento, CA 95817, USA
* Corresponding author. 4860 Y Street, Suite 3850, Sacramento, CA 95817.
E-mail address: rtabresch@ucdavis.edu

therapies, gene-therapy strategies, stem-cell therapies, and a host of small-molecule therapies (eg, compounds that induce read-through of premature stop-codon mutations, promotion of muscle growth via myostatin inhibition, utrophin upregulation, and steroid analogues with improved side-effect profiles).[1] While it is recognized that these therapeutic approaches will not be curative, there is significant hope that new therapies on the horizon will significantly alter disease progression, improve function, and improve quality of life. As these therapies have various biochemical targets, clinicians may need to give combinations of drugs to minimize secondary medical comorbidity, prevent or limit physical deformity, and allow the patient to integrate into society.

In addition to pharmaceutical interventions, comprehensive rehabilitation program modalities such as resistance training, aerobic exercise training, range-of-motion activities, and bracing, may prolong ambulation, increase strength, and reduce the progression of many NMDs.[2,3] These interventions may be made at various points in the natural evolution of the disease to increase strength, reduce pain, prevent or reduce the development of contractures, and maintain function for as long as possible.[3,4] Unfortunately there is not enough evidence-based information available to make an informed assessment of the potential risks and benefits of exercise for individuals with NMDs. We do not know what types of exercise programs are most appropriate for people with NMDs, nor are there randomized clinical trials, in most instances, to justify the proper intensity, duration, and frequency of those exercise regimens that should be ideally included in a prescription for an individual with an NMD.

GENERAL BENEFITS OF EXERCISE

As everyone knows, there are many potential benefits to increased physical activity and strength-training exercise in healthy subjects. Physical activity and exercise lowers mortality and prevents morbidity by reducing the development of chronic diseases, by reduction of disease-related complications and by restoration of function.[5] Increased physical activity has been shown to reduce blood pressure, help prevent obesity, and reduce the risk of osteoporosis, heart disease, arthritis, and type 2 diabetes. Exercise also decreases anxiety, depression, and pain. It enhances a feeling of well-being, promotes sleep, and increases vitality with age. Comprehensive guidelines have been developed to combat physical inactivity,[6] which is the fourth leading independent risk factor for death caused by noncommunicable diseases.

Strength Training (Progressive Resistive Exercise)

Strength training (progressive resistive exercise) increases lean body mass, muscle protein mass, contractile force, and power, and improves physical function.[7–9] Lifting of weights during concentric (muscle shortens during contraction) or eccentric (muscle lengthens during contraction) exercise produces microinjuries to the sarcolemma and initiates transcriptional and splice mechanisms, protein turnover, and signaling pathways from hormone and cytokine receptors.[10] This process involves several proteins that shuttle between sarcomeric and nonsarcomeric localizations and convey signals to the nucleus. Satellite cells, mononuclear cells, and myogenic progenitor cells that typically exist in a state of quiescence under the basal lamina are activated and fuse to the existing fiber, leading to proliferation of nuclei in the muscle, which provides the machinery for additional contractile proteins. Resistance exercise increases the DNA content in the myofibrils, which in turn increases the number of muscle proteins, especially actin and myosin.[11]

Aerobic Exercise

Aerobic endurance training induces physiologic adaptations that differ from strength training. Aerobic training that involves the use of large muscle groups reciprocally for sufficient intensity and duration (30 minutes at 50%–85% of oxidative capacity [Vo_{2max}]) induces adaptations in the heart, peripheral circulation, and skeletal muscle systems. Greater oxygen delivery is achieved by training-induced increases in cardiac output (due to increased stroke volume), capillary density, and vascular conduction. Improved use of oxygen by trained skeletal muscle is accomplished by mitochondrial biogenesis and increased mitochondrial oxidative enzyme activity, which lead to an increased capacity to generate energy through oxidative phosphorylation in trained muscles. In healthy individuals, these adaptations play a major role in improving Vo_{2max} and endurance, and reducing fatigue, as shown by the ability to perform submaximal work with less effort for longer duration. Endurance-trained individuals produce a lower concentration of blood lactate and lower heart rates than untrained individuals at the same level of submaximal exercise. Cessation of endurance training and resistance training leads to a reversal of benefits and to partial or marked reductions in the training-induced cardiopulmonary, vascular, and skeletal muscle benefits (deconditioning).

POTENTIAL BENEFITS OF THERAPEUTIC EXERCISE FOR PERSONS WITH NMDs

Therapeutic exercise and rehabilitation management techniques have been shown to correct impairment and improve musculoskeletal function in a variety of disease states.[12] The effects of therapeutic rehabilitation interventions vary depending on the specific disease, prognosis, impairment, and objective. The interventions may include the performance of general physical activities such as household ambulation and activities of daily living, performing 60 minutes of physical activity per day, yoga or, alternatively, highly selected activities focused on specific muscles or parts of the body. The potential benefits derived from therapeutic exercise would certainly be beneficial to individuals with NMDs, whose primary symptoms are weakness, fatigue, and muscle atrophy. It has been shown that many individuals with NMDs fall frequently as a result of weakness and sensory impairment associated with their disease, and that these impairments may be modified through therapeutic exercise.[13] Exercise can be used to proactively prevent the development of painful musculoskeletal syndromes associated with the loss of mobility and disuse weakness, which further contributes to pain generation.

THE DELETERIOUS EFFECTS OF SEDENTARY STATUS, DECONDITIONING, AND DISUSE WEAKNESS IN NMDs

Appropriate therapeutic exercise should be an important modality in preventing the deleterious effects associated with inactivity and deconditioning observed in subjects with NMDs. Sedentary lifestyle leads to weight gain, additional loss of muscle mass, diminished walking endurance, increased fatigue, and musculoskeletal pain. As a result, individuals with NMDs have significantly higher risk factors for metabolic syndrome and chronic disease resulting from obesity and a sedentary lifestyle. Aitkens and colleagues[14] reported that ambulatory individuals with NMDs were more obese, spent less time in total activity (144 min/d vs 214 min/d), and exercised (11 min/d vs 45 min/d) significantly less than able-bodied individuals who were group-matched for age and body mass index. Fifty-five percent of the NMD group satisfied the criteria for metabolic syndrome, versus 0% in the control group.[14] Even NMD subjects with normal weight and body mass indices also have problems with increased body fat. A recent study revealed that subjects with facioscapulohumeral muscular dystrophy (FSHD) had 14% less lean muscle tissue in their trunk, but 76% more fat in the trunk than an age-, weight-, and height-matched control group. In addition, the FSHD subjects significantly lost muscle mass and had a concomitant increase in fat mass as they aged, which was not seen in the control population.[15] Individuals with NMDs have also been shown to have problems with joint deformity, tight muscles, altered gait, balance, flexibility, and sleep, all of which have been shown to have beneficial responses to therapeutic exercise.[3] Although diminished aerobic capacity is rarely the limiting factor in performing daily work tasks,[16] involvement of the cardiac and pulmonary musculature in NMDs may reduce cardiopulmonary fitness, compounding the effects of deconditioning.

THEORETICAL RISKS OF OVERWORK WEAKNESS IN MYOPATHIES AND OTHER NMDs

If there are so many benefits to physical activity, why have doctors not prescribed exercise for patients with NMDs? Unlike able-bodied patients, clinicians have been concerned that exercise might cause overwork weakness in patients with NMDs.[17] More than 50 years ago Bennett and Knowlton[18] raised the concern that exercise in postpolio patients may produce muscle injury if the exercise regimen equals or exceeds the maximum strength of the muscle. In 1971, Johnson and Braddom[19] warned that exercise may cause overwork weakness in individuals with all NMDs, regardless of the severity of the disease and the pathogenesis. The risk of overwork weakness is likely to be greater in individuals with muscular dystrophies, and dystrophinopathies such as Duchenne muscular dystrophy in particular, whereby sarcolemmal muscle membranes are susceptible to injury from mechanical loads and stresses. As is true in most effective pharmaceutical therapies, exercise training has potential dose-dependent risks in subjects with NMDs, and these are significantly greater than those seen in the able-bodied population. Rhabdomyolysis, myoglobinuria, and significant pain have been reported after physical activity in NMDs.[20–23] Because the exercise treatment may induce overwork weakness and other adverse events, exercise studies in subjects with NMDs must be performed using just as stringent safety and efficacy measures as are used in randomized, controlled clinical drug trials.

STUDIES DOCUMENTING BENEFITS OF EXERCISE IN NMDs

Despite the concern about overwork weakness, many investigators have reported beneficial effects of exercise in NMDs. Aitkens and colleagues[24] examined the effect of a moderate-resistance, home-based strengthening exercise program on 27 people with a mixed group of NMDs. During the first week of a 12-week exercise program the patients were instructed to strengthen their knee extensors by performing 3 sets of 4 repetitions at 30% of their maximum strength (30% of a 1-repetition maximum). The subjects gradually increased their exercise regimen, and by week 12 they were performing 3 sets of 8 repetitions at 40% of their maximal strength. In a follow-up study these investigators examined whether they could achieve greater effects with a high-resistance exercise program.[25] The NMD group demonstrated significant gains in several knee-extension isokinetic strength measures but loss of elbow-flexion eccentric peak torque and work per degree. In addition, several of the subjects complained about persistent weakness after the exercise bout. Therefore the investigators determined that a high-resistance training program seems to offer no advantage over a moderate-resistance training program in this population, and may potentially cause overwork injury.[25] Furthermore, subjects who had less than 15% normal strength were unable to achieve any strength gains from strengthening exercises. Similar results were observed by Milner-Brown and Miller.[26]

CHALLENGES IN STUDY DESIGN FOR EXERCISE CLINICAL TRIALS

Despite these encouraging studies, systematic reviews have determined that there is insufficient evidence to determine whether exercise is beneficial or detrimental for individuals with peripheral neuropathies, amyotrophic lateral sclerosis (ALS), and muscle diseases.[27,28] A major reason for the lack of good controlled studies is the rarity of NMDs. To obviate this difficulty researchers have frequently grouped subjects with dystrophinopathies alongside persons with various other neuromuscular disorders, even though the severity, rate of progression, and disease type markedly affects the exercise response. Combining individuals with various types of NMDs together creates several problems; there is no reason to believe that diseases affecting the anterior horn cells, peripheral nerves, and/or muscles would respond similarly to exercise training. Therefore, studies need to be developed in which there are adequate numbers of subjects with the same diagnosis and phenotypic characteristics, in order for informed decisions to be made. In past reports, very few studies had enough information regarding the results of exercise on a sufficient sample size with one genetically and phenotypically homogeneous group for adequate conclusions to be drawn. There has been little uniformity regarding the type of exercise interventions (aerobic, strengthening, or combinations of exercise regimens), duration of exercise, intensity of exercise therapy, initial state of physical activity and fitness, and types of outcome measures. Another major weakness in the literature is the lack of clearly identified primary and secondary outcome measures. Outcome measures that have been reported include strength, endurance, fatigue, cardiopulmonary function, functional ability, activities of daily living, anxiety, depression, well-being, and pain, among others. The systematic reviews that have been published on the effect of exercise on individuals with different types of NMD highlight the inadequacy of most of the studies in the literature.[27–30]

EXERCISE STUDIES IN SPECIFIC NMDs

To understand the effect of various types of exercise regimens, one needs to understand the underlying pathophysiology of each disease with regard to the type of exercise administered, the dose (intensity, rate, and duration of exercise), degree of weakness, and progression of the disease, along with typical demographic factors (age, gender, race, and so forth). The following sections briefly review the major exercise studies done on the hereditary muscular dystrophies, hereditary myopathies (metabolic mitochondrial myopathies), acquired inflammatory myopathies, and neuropathies of the motor neuron (eg, ALS) and peripheral nerve (eg, Charcot-Marie-Tooth [CMT] disease, postpolio syndrome [PPS]).

HEREDITARY MUSCULAR DYSTROPHIES

The hereditary muscular dystrophies are a pathogenetically heterogeneous group of hereditary muscle diseases, which present with muscle weakness. Exercise studies have been performed in individuals with dystrophinopathies (Duchenne and Becker muscular dystrophy), limb-girdle muscular dystrophy (LGMD), facioscapulohumeral dystrophy (FSHD), and myotonic muscular dystrophies. Typically the muscular dystrophies are accompanied by progressive muscle fiber damage, inflammation, necrosis, and regeneration, as noted by histopathologic evaluation. Most dystrophies are associated with defects in sarcolemmal and extracellular matrix proteins, which bind the contractile elements across the sarcolemma to the extracellular matrix (especially to laminin-2 [merosin] of basal lamina). These proteins appear to be essential in maintaining the cytoskeletal framework of the muscle fiber during muscle contraction.[31] Thus, it is conceivable that intensive muscle contractions, particularly when including an eccentric component, may damage myopathic muscle to a greater extent than in able-bodied subjects. This aspect is of particular concern in those diseases known to involve structural proteins of the muscle cell, such as Duchenne muscular dystrophy, Becker muscular dystrophy, and many of the limb-girdle syndromes. In animal models of dystrophin-deficient dystrophy there is increased damage to muscle using eccentric contractions, which particularly stress these cytoskeletal elements.[32–34] Maximal eccentric contractions appear to damage the cytoskeletal framework with myofibrillar disruption, which clinically is associated with transient muscle weakness, elevation of serum creatine kinase, and delayed-onset muscle soreness.[35,36] In NMDs that affect the integrity of the muscle-cell membrane, it is possible that eccentric contractions may hasten the progression of muscle degeneration.

Dystrophinopathies

Several theories have been proposed to explain the pathogenesis of muscles from individuals with dystrophinopathies. Dystrophin deficiency destabilizes the dystrophin-glycoprotein complex, impairing localization of the dystroglycan and sarcoglycans to the muscle membrane, and compromising the structural integrity of the sarcolemma membrane. Dystrophin is a high molecular weight cytoskeleton protein localized at the inner surface of the muscle membrane, and is part of a dystrophin-glycoprotein complex that also includes dystroglycan and sarcoglycans. This dystrophin-glycoprotein complex provides a bridge across the muscle membrane; dystrophin couples F-actin in the cytoplasm with dystroglycan, which binds to merosin (laminin-2) in the extracellular matrix. Excessive mechanical stress creates micro- and macroinjuries to the sarcolemma membrane which, in turn, causes excessive calcium ion influx, phospholipase activation, oxidative muscle injury, and, ultimately, necrosis of the muscle fiber.[31] As muscle damage progresses, connective tissue and fat replace the damaged muscle fibers.[37,38] Disruption of the dystrophin complex downregulates neuronal nitric oxide synthase (nNOS), which disrupts the exercise-induced cell-signaling pathway that regulates blood flow to the muscle and results in functional muscle ischemia.[39] Recent studies have shown that when nNOS is not present at its normal location on the muscle membrane, the blood vessels that supply active muscles do not relax normally and show signs of fatigue.[40] Thus, the pathophysiology of the disease may significantly affect its response to exercise. Exercise, especially exercise that places a large amount of stress on the muscle fibers, such as high-resistive and eccentric exercise, damages skeletal muscle in the dystrophinopathies. Even mild exercise has been implicated in causing functional muscle ischemia and fatigue in dystrophinopathy patients, resulting from disruptions in nNOS signaling.[39,40]

Strengthening exercises

Very few randomized studies have systematically examined the effect of strengthening resistive exercise or aerobic exercise in persons with Duchenne muscular dystrophy and/or Becker muscular dystrophy. Most of the randomized controlled trials have been small in size, and the methodologies and results have been inconsistent.

Studies regarding the effect of exercise in individuals on skeletal muscles of individuals with Duchenne muscular dystrophy have produced conflicting results. Some investigations have demonstrated that low-intensity resistance or aerobic exercise maintains or even slightly improves strength in Duchenne muscular dystrophy.[41–44] However, others have presented case-study evidence that exercise induces weakness in dystrophinopathies. Garrood and colleagues[45] noted that individuals with Duchenne muscular dystrophy increase their physical activity after steroid treatment, and suggest that this increased activity places their dystrophin-deficient muscles under greater mechanical stress, which predisposes them to muscle-fiber damage and consequent myoglobinuria. A case study of a boy who had both spina bifida and Becker muscular dystrophy revealed that the dystrophic changes in the muscle biopsy were less severe in the lower extremities immobilized by spina bifida than in the unaffected upper extremities.[46] The investigators suggested that this adds to the evidence that excessive exercise causes muscle damage in dystrophinopathies, and should be restricted.

Respiratory muscle training

Studies that have examined the effect of respiratory muscle training on patients with dystrophinopathies have also produced conflicting results, depending on initial muscle strength. Several investigators have reported increased ventilatory strength and endurance following inspiratory and/or expiratory resistance training,[47–51] whereas others have shown no changes.[52,53] Koessler and colleagues[49] demonstrated an improvement in maximum inspiratory pressure and 12-second maximal voluntary ventilation after 24 months of inspiratory muscle training in 18 patients with Duchenne muscular dystrophy and 9 with spinal muscular atrophy whose forced vital capacity was greater than 25% predicted. However, inspiratory muscles that were very weak or near their fatigue threshold showed no improvement after respiratory training.[48,54]

Aerobic exercise training

Sveen and colleagues[55] studied the effect of endurance training (30 minutes of aerobic cycling 3–4 times per week at 65% of their Vo_{2max} for 12 weeks) in 11 ambulatory patients with mild Becker muscular dystrophy and 7 matched, healthy subjects. Aerobic endurance training increased Vo_{2max} by 47%, maximal workload by 80%, and muscle strength by 13% to 40%, without causing muscle damage as indicated by muscle abnormality and increased serum creatine kinase. These studies suggest that exercise is contraindicated in subjects with dystrophinopathies who have very weak muscles and are very susceptible to exercise-induced damage. Further short-term and long-term studies regarding the effect of endurance exercise and mild-resistance exercise is warranted for individuals who still have adequate strength, but these studies need to be well controlled and should be monitored with great care to prevent adverse effects from the exercise.

Limb-Girdle Muscular Dystrophies

Before the advent of genetic testing, patients commonly sharing a slowly progressive pattern of proximal greater than distal muscular weakness and classified as being of either autosomal recessive (type 2) or autosomal dominant (type 1) inheritance were termed as having LGMDs. Recent advances in molecular and genetic analyses have now identified several distinct genetic abnormalities with mutations in these patients. At present at least 22 subtypes of LGMD are recognized, and the list continues to grow.[57] Eight have autosomal dominant inheritance (LGMD type 1, A–H) and 14 have autosomal recessive inheritance (LGMD type 2, A–N). It is now known that

LGMD comprises many distinct diseases with genetic defects in genes that encode for sarcolemmal, sarcomeric, and sarcoplasmic proteins. The most common LGMDs include LGMD2A (calpainopathy), LGMD2B (dysferlinopathy), LGMD2C (γ-sarcoglycanopathy), LGMD2D (α-sarcoglycanopathy), LGMD2E (β-sarcoglycanopathy), LGMD2F (δ-sarcoglycanopathy), and LGMD2I.

The defects or loss of proteins encoded by these genes leads to a loss of sarcolemmal integrity and a progressive pattern of proximal greater than distal muscular weakness that is similar to that of the dystrophinopathies. Defects in these proteins render muscle fibers more susceptible to exercise-induced damage and the development of myoglobinuria. The reduction of nNOS levels in the sarcolemma of LGMD subjects alters their cell-signaling response to exercise and makes them more susceptible to injury and fatigue, in both humans and the dystrophin-deficient (mdx) and α-sarcoglycan deficient (Sgca) mouse.[40]

The effect of exercise in LGMD subjects is mixed. Sveen and colleagues[56] examined the effect of aerobic cycling in adults with mild LGMD2I, which is caused by a defect in fukutin-related protein, a sarcoplasmic enzyme that glycosylates dystroglycan needed for appropriate binding of the dystrophin-glycoprotein complex to laminin-2. The LGMD2I patients reported a 21% increase in Vo_{2max} and a 27% increase in work capacity, as well as a self-reported increase in strength and endurance without any evidence of muscle damage, as observed by serum creatine kinase and muscle biopsy. Yeldan and colleagues[57] reported that progressive resistance exercise improved respiratory function in 17 individuals with genetically confirmed LGMD and 6 with Becker muscular dystrophy.[57] However, muscle response of respiratory muscles was specific to the training protocol. Deep-breathing exercises improved maximal expiratory pressure while inspiratory muscle training improved maximal inspiratory pressure; however, neither regimen significantly altered spirometry results. Böhme and Arnold[58] examined the effect of intensive physical therapy in 156 patients with an LGMD and noted an improvement in functional parameters. The rarity of individuals with specific LGMDs and the lack of adequate genetic confirmation confound the difficulties in performing studies to determine the effect of exercise in these patients. As is true for the dystrophinopathies, high-resistance exercise training should be avoided in LGMD patients, especially those who are very weak.[59]

Facioscapulohumeral Dystrophy

FSHD was clinically categorized by its characteristic progressive muscular weakness in the facial and shoulder girdle musculature and onset of symptoms in adolescence or early adulthood. More recent studies have shown that FSHD is an autosomal dominant disorder resulting from a chromosomal abnormality identified at the 4q35 gene locus that causes reduced DNA fragment size at the telomere region[60] and epigenetic changes in the chromatin structure regulated by DUX4.[61,62] In contrast to the other muscular dystrophies, there are few distinctive findings on muscle biopsy, with histology frequently demonstrating mild findings of atrophied fibers along with hypertrophied fibers; they do not undergo necrosis and regeneration as do those in dystrophinopathies and sarcoglycanopathies.[63]

A randomized clinical trial was performed to assess the effect of progressive resistance strength training (3 times a week for 52 weeks) with and without albuterol in 65 FSHD subjects.[64] No muscle damage was observed as a result of the training. Whereas the isometric strength of the elbow flexors did not increase between the exercised and nonexercised group, the dynamic strength increased more in the exercised group. Lindeman and colleagues[65] suggested that different responses were due to the specificity of the training effect on dynamic strength. These results reiterate the need to develop proper outcome measures that are responsive to a specific type of exercise regimen. Because the weight training performed by van der Kooi and colleagues[64] used isokinetic exercise, it is not surprising that the training resulted in larger increases in isokinetic strength compared with isometric strength. Whereas the elbows responded to the exercise training, the ankle dorsiflexors showed no significant changes as a result of the weight training. The lack of response in the ankle dorsiflexors may be attributed to an ineffective training regimen. However, the investigators noted that the dorsiflexors may not have been able to move against gravity and therefore might have been too weak to respond to the training regimen. The amount of weight used for training the dorsiflexors may have been insufficient to cause a training effect. The conflicting responses observed by the various muscles examined by van der Kooi and colleagues[64] demonstrate the difficulties researchers face in developing an exercise prescription for each of the NMDs. The training needs to be optimized according to the initial strength of the patient, type of exercise, frequency of exercise, intensity of exercise, and the desired change, which are likely to differ depending on the muscle group that is being trained, the strength of the muscle, and the desired outcome (whether it is a change in isometric strength, isokinetic strength, or fatigue). Olsen and colleagues[66] reported that low-intensity aerobic cycling at a heart rate corresponding to a work intensity of 65% of Vo_{2max} for 35 minutes, 5 times a week for 12 weeks significantly increased the maximal oxygen uptake and workload in 8 subjects with FSHD, with no signs of muscle damage. Perhaps the most important outcome is not strength or Vo_{2max}, but whether the exercise changes function, improves quality of life, and alters future health outcomes.

Myotonic Muscular Dystrophy (DM1 and DM2)

There are 2 subtypes of myotonic muscular dystrophy, DM1 and DM2 (dystrophia myotonica types 1 and 2). DM1 is caused by abnormal expansion of the CTG trinucleotide repeats in the Dystrophia Myotonica Protein Kinase (DMPK) gene on chromosome 19q13.3, whereas DM2 is caused by an abnormal expansion of the CCTG repeats in the Zinc Finger protein 9 (ZNF9) gene on chromosome 3q21. The expansion of the gene is thought to trigger an RNA-mediated process that creates a toxic RNA that modulates other transcripts, including the chloride channel. As a result, DM1 and DM2 are multisystem disorders affecting skeletal muscle, smooth muscle, myocardium, brain, and ocular structures. This condition may manifest clinically with cataracts, cardiac conduction defects, endocrine abnormalities, swallowing dysfunction, and skeletal muscle weakness and myotonia. As opposed to the dystrophinopathies and sarcoglycanopathies, which are characterized as being necrotic muscle diseases with regeneration, myotonic muscular dystrophy necrosis is rare. In DM1 and DM2, atrophy leads to progressive reduction in muscle mass and weakness.[63]

Moderate-resistance exercise and aerobic training have been shown to be safe in patients with myotonic muscular dystrophy, although the benefits of these exercise programs are mixed. Lindeman and colleagues[65] found few significant effects of progressive resistance exercise in a group of clinically diagnosed ambulatory subjects with myotonic dystrophy. Aldehag and colleagues[67] reported that progressive resistance exercise of the hand function 3 times per week for 12 weeks significantly increased motor function and self-rated occupational performance in 5 patients with DM1. Orngreen and colleagues[68] reported that 12 weeks of moderate aerobic training increased Vo_{2max} by 14% and workload by 11% in patients with DM1, without any muscle damage as observed by serum creatine kinase or muscle pathology. The DM1 subjects had a self-reported increase in strength, endurance, and walking.

OTHER MYOPATHIES
Prototypical Metabolic Myopathy: McArdle Disease (Glycogen Storage Disease Type V)

McArdle disease (glycogen storage disease type V) is a metabolic myopathy that results from absence of the muscle glycolytic enzyme, myophosphorylase. This enzyme deficiency results in the muscle's inability to break down glycogen for energy (adenosine triphosphate) generation during anaerobic metabolism. In addition, lack of myophosphorylase also affects energy generation during aerobic metabolism because of decreased substrate generation (pyruvate) for the tricarboxylic acid cycle. Glycogen is the most important source of energy for the muscle during early exercise and at high exercise intensities. The oxidative capacity of McArdle disease muscle is less than half that of normal muscle in the first few minutes of moderate exercise, and a more vigorous activity triggers muscle cramps, pain, and myoglobinuria. Because of the risk for severe and potentially dangerous rhabdomyolysis associated with exercise, many patients with McArdle disease have traditionally been advised to avoid exercise. However, a sedentary and inactive lifestyle for these patients often results in deconditioning, which can further complicate and worsen the disease by decreasing their cardiovascular and circulatory capacity. With deconditioning and decline in circulatory capacity, the delivery of glucose and free fatty acids from blood to muscle becomes impaired, and the problem becomes compounded by blockage of glycogen breakdown. Deconditioning also reduces levels of muscle mitochondria and mitochondrial enzymes that are necessary for metabolizing energy sources. Thus, avoidance of physical activity and adoption of an inactive lifestyle in patients with McArdle disease may result in a downward spiral of decreased exercise tolerance and aerobic capacity, which in turn further lowers the threshold of physical activity, producing muscle injury and cramps. Given these issues, recent studies have looked into whether exercise training and aerobic conditioning can help in ameliorating the symptoms of McArdle disease. Haller and colleagues[69] have reported that cycle ergometer for 30 to 40 minutes per day, 4 days per week for 14 weeks, at an intensity of approximately 60% to 70% maximal heart rate, improved average work capacity by 36%, oxygen uptake by 14%, cardiac output by 15%, citrate synthase by 80%, and β-hydroxyacyl coenzyme A dehydrogenase by 62%, without causing pain, cramping, or increases in serum creatine kinase. An 8-month aerobic exercise training program was also well tolerated and showed similar beneficial results.[70] Other case reports and studies also support the use of moderate-intensity aerobic exercise and activity programs for McArdle disease.[71–73] These aerobic exercise programs improve exercise tolerance, work capacity, and overall health status by increasing cardiovascular fitness, improving circulatory delivery capacity, increasing mitochondrial enzyme levels, and improving metabolic efficiency of individuals with McArdle disease.

Mitochondrial Myopathies

Mitochondrial myopathies are a heterogeneous group of metabolic muscle disorders associated with abnormal structure and function of mitochondria. Brain and skeletal muscles are particularly susceptible to mitochondrial dysfunction because of their high requirement for oxidative energy metabolism. Mitochondrial myopathies often begin with fatigue, exercise intolerance, or muscle weakness during physical activity, and their symptoms range from mild to disabling. The clinical presentation ranges from single-organ to multisystem disorders that may cause muscle weakness or exercise intolerance, heart failure or rhythm disturbances, dementia, movement disorders, stroke-like episodes, deafness, blindness, droopy eyelids, limited mobility of the eyes, vomiting, and seizures. The underlying molecular defect in the mitochondrial myopathies involves a mutation in either nuclear or mitochondrial DNA (mtDNA), both of which ultimately impair electron transport and oxidative phosphorylation. The majority of known mutations are in the mtDNA. In most patients, mtDNA mutations coexist with wild-type mtDNA, a condition known as heteroplasmy. It appears that individuals with mild phenotypes have relatively higher proportions of wild-type mtDNA than individuals with more disabling phenotypes.

Therapeutic exercise has been suggested as a means to improve muscle oxidative capacity and reduce the proportion of mutant mtDNA in patients with mitochondrial myopathies.[74–78] Resistance training has been proposed as a therapy for mitochondrial myopathy patients who have single large-scale mtDNA deletions and sporadic mtDNA point mutations, and exhibit a high degree of mitochondrial heteroplasmy in skeletal muscle. Mature muscle cells of these patients often have a high degree of mtDNA mutations, whereas the level of mutations is low or undetectable in satellite cells. Because resistance exercise is known to serve as stimulus for satellite-cell induction within skeletal muscle, a series of experiments have been performed to determine whether it would lead to a shifting of normal mitochondrial genes from satellite cells to mature muscle, lowering the level of mutant mtDNA and improving oxidative capacity.[74–78] Murphy and colleagues[79] showed that 12 weeks of progressive overload resistance training caused myofiber damage and regeneration, increased neural cell adhesion molecule–positive satellite cells, improved muscle oxidative capacity, and increased muscle strength in 8 subjects with large-scale mtDNA mutations. Further work is needed to optimize the training effect and gene-shifting from mutant to wild-type mtDNA and to determine whether the training translates into long-term improvement.

Endurance training has also been hypothesized to induce mitochondrial biogenesis and capacity for oxidative phosphorylation and improve function of individuals with mitochondrial myopathies. In 1996, Taivassalo and colleagues[75] presented a case study demonstrating that aerobic training could improve exercise capacity and reverse the effects of deconditioning in a patient with a nuclear mutation causing cytochrome oxidase deficiency. Subsequent studies by these investigators have shown that that mild endurance exercise (30 minutes per day, 3–4 times per week for 8–14 weeks at 70% maximal heart rate) significantly increases aerobic capacity and oxygen efficiency, decreases resting heart rate, and decreases lactate in a group of patients with mitochondrial myopathies caused by both nuclear and mtDNA mutations.[76–78,80] However, it appeared that subjects with nuclear DNA mutations had a greater improvement than subjects with mtDNA improvements. Endurance training by 8 patients with a single large-scale mtDNA mutation and 20 patients with a variety of mutations in their mtDNA increased physiologic and biochemical markers of mitochondrial function, without any changes in the level of mutant mtDNA.[81,82] These patients showed a loss of endurance-training gains in exercise and mitochondrial capacity following the cessation of training, confirming the maladaptive effects of deconditioning. Overall, the beneficial effects of endurance training have been reported by several researchers, with no adverse effects.[74–78,80–83] However, it must be emphasized that these studies were short term ($\leq$14 weeks), had small numbers of subjects ($\leq$20), and were not randomized controlled trials. Nevertheless, the results are intriguing, and warrant further studies of both endurance exercise and resistance exercise in individuals with mitochondrial myopathies.

Inflammatory Myopathies

Most exercise studies in patients with acquired myopathies have been conducted in patients with inflammatory myopathies. The hallmark of an inflammatory myopathy is the predominance of inflammatory cells on muscle biopsy. There are 3 primary types of inflammatory myopathy: polymyositis (PM), dermatomyositis (DM), and sporadic inclusion body myositis (IBM). In addition, there at least 4 hereditary forms of IBM. Although each is distinct, this group of myopathies is thought to involve immune-mediated processes possibly triggered by environmental factors in genetically susceptible individuals. DM and PM may be associated with disorders of the heart and lung, as well as neoplasms. In addition, an inflammatory myopathy may be present as part of a multisystem disorder in other connective tissue diseases, most commonly scleroderma, systemic lupus erythematosus, mixed connective tissue disease, and Sjögren syndrome. In DM and PM, corticosteroids alone are often highly effective in both inducing a remission and preventing a recurrence, and can usually be gradually withdrawn. Adults with DM do not respond to corticosteroids quite so predictably, and other immunosuppressive agents are often required. IBM, which is distinguished by the presence of inflammatory cells and vacuolated muscle fibers with nuclear and cytoplasmic fibrillary inclusions, has distinctive involvement of both proximal and distal musculature.[84] Sporadic IBM is relentlessly progressive in most cases, sometimes to the point of requiring a wheelchair for mobility. Unfortunately, it has not been responsive to immunosuppressive medications, and treatment primarily involves appropriate assistive devices.

Until the early 1990s patients with inflammatory myopathies were discouraged from physical activity because of the fear of exacerbating muscle inflammation. Although sample sizes are small, more recent work suggests that moderate-intensity resistance exercise may improve strength and function without signs of increased muscle inflammation.[85–90] Response to exercise may vary depending on disease activity, medications, and degree of disability. Patients with stable, chronic inflammatory myopathy may be able to tolerate more intensive strengthening regimens (10 maximal muscle contractions 3 days per week) without untoward effects.[87] Decreased aerobic capacity compared with controls has been demonstrated in patients with adult inflammatory myositis[91] and juvenile DM.[92] A home exercise program consisting of 15 minutes of progressive resistive exercise and a 15-minute walk 5 times per week for 12 weeks did not significantly improve muscle function in patients with IBM, and no adverse effects were found on histopathology and inflammation.[93]

MOTOR NEURON DISEASES
Amyotrophic Lateral Sclerosis

ALS is a fatal, progressive, degenerative disease of the upper and lower motor neuron. Symptoms of weakness and muscle atrophy typically present asymmetrically in the distal regions of the upper or lower extremity or in the bulbar muscles. Although the pathogenesis of ALS has not been delineated, approximately 20% of the patients with hereditary ALS have a defect in the gene encoding copper-zinc superoxide dismutase.[94] Evidence from studies of exercise on superoxide dismutase–deficient transgenic mice suggests that endurance exercise training at moderate intensities slows disease progression and increases life span,[95–97] whereas high-intensity exercise showed no improvement or hastened symptoms and death.[98] Exercise has been shown to induce changes in motor neuron morphology, muscle-nerve interaction, glial activation, and altering levels of gene expression of antiapoptotic proteins and neurotropic factors in active tissue in these mice.[99]

The number of exercise studies that have been performed in humans with ALS is sparse. A randomized controlled trial examined the effects of a twice-daily exercise program of moderate-load endurance exercise versus usual activities in 25 persons with ALS.[100] ALS subjects performing the exercise showed less deterioration on the ALS functional rating scale (ALSFRS) and Ashworth scales after 3 months of exercise, but there was no significant difference at 6 months. Too many patients dropped out for the effect to be further evaluated at 9 and 12 months. Bello-Haas and colleagues[101] randomly assigned 27 ALS subjects with forced vital capacity greater than 90% predicted to a daily resistance exercise and stretching program, or to usual care. After 6 months the 8 subjects randomized to exercise had significantly higher ALSFRS cores, SF-36 functional subscale scores, and greater maximum voluntary isometric contraction scores than the 10 subjects in the nonexercise group. One nonrandomized study found that 8 ALS subjects who performed aerobic exercise to anaerobic threshold on treadmills coupled with noninvasive bi-level positive airway pressure ventilation for 1 year improved their functional independent mobility and lowered the rate in decline of respiratory function and muscle strength in comparison with a control group of 12 ALS subjects. After analyzing the results of these studies, a Cochrane review determined that the small number of randomized controlled trials combined with the small sample sizes preclude determination as to whether exercise is beneficial for individuals with ALS.[29]

Peripheral Neuropathies

Peripheral neuropathies consist of a heterogeneous group of genetic and acquired disorders affecting the peripheral nerves. Damage to the nerves can affect the axons, myelin, or both. Patients with peripheral neuropathies develop symptoms of numbness, pain, sensory defects, muscle weakness, and fatigue, which often lead to reduced physical activity, psychological dysfunction, and poor social adjustment. The natural history of the disease is largely dependent on the underlying pathophysiology. Some, such as Guillain-Barré syndrome, have acute onset and reach their greatest symptoms in a couple of weeks, then slowly recover. In the hereditary peripheral neuropathies, such as the hereditary motor and sensory neuropathies, individuals typically experience a slow onset and gradually deteriorate over many years.

Charcot-Marie-Tooth Disease

CMT, or hereditary motor sensory neuropathy (HMSN), encompasses a group of more than 40 clinically and genetically heterogeneous peripheral neuropathies that were initially characterized by their mode of inheritance and their nerve-conduction velocities, and were labeled as CMT1, CMT2, CMT3, and CMT4. Approximately 60% to 80% of CMT patients have an autosomal dominant mutation that causes demyelination and results in slow nerve-conduction velocities (10–35 m/s), and are labeled as CMT1.[102] Of these, approximately 70% are due to a mutation in the PMP22 protein and are labeled CMT1A, while 10% to 15% are due to a mutation in myelin protein zero and are labeled CMT1B.[103] Approximately 20% to 40% also have an autosomal dominant inheritance pattern, but with have normal nerve-conduction velocities (>38 m/s) because the mutation causes an axonopathy, and has been labeled as CMT2. Because CMT subjects exhibit muscle weakness, fatigue, and deconditioning, 3 studies have examined whether exercise could improve symptoms and quality of life in these patients. Lindeman and colleagues[65] randomized 29 CMT subjects randomized to 24 weeks of progressive resistance exercise of their lower extremity muscles and reported a significant increase in knee torque without adverse effects, but few functional changes in comparison with the control group. A home-based progressive strength-training program (3 days per week for 12 weeks using ankle and wrist weights) was performed by 18 CMT1A and 2 CMT2 patients with and without creatine supplementation.[104] Because there was no significant change as a result of creatine on these subjects, the groups were combined to assess the effect of exercise. Although there were several methodological problems including lack of randomization and lack of a control group, the investigators reported that the combined exercise group showed improved functional measures, increased tension of the knee and elbow, and an increase in type 1 fiber diameter after the exercise training. El Mandhi and colleagues[105] demonstrated that subjective pain and fatigue, Vo_{2max}, isokinetic knee torque, and functional abilities improved after aerobic cycling training (3 days per week for 24 weeks at 70% of maximum heart rate) in 4 CMT1A and 4 CMT2 male subjects, compared with their values before training.

Postpolio Syndrome

Halsted and Rossi[106] first described PPS as a condition that affects individuals who had a confirmed case of polio, had partial or fairly complete neurologic and functional recovery after the acute episode, had a period of at least 15 years with neurologic and functional stability, gradual or abrupt onset of new muscle weakness, muscle atrophy, and muscle pain, and fatigue that persists for more than 1 year. Before 1996, PPS patients were advised to avoid physical activity and intensive exercise because of concerns about overwork weakness.[107,108] Systematic reviews have differed as to whether aerobic training and progressive resistance exercise training has been shown to be beneficial for individuals with PPS.[28,109] Several studies[110-117] examined the effect of resistance strengthening with various types, intensities, and durations of exercise training on patients with PPS. One randomized controlled trial,[118] one clinical controlled trial,[119] and 2 other designs[120-122] examined the effect of aerobic training in PPS patients. These studies reported that aerobic training improved cardiovascular fitness and functional abilities in individuals with PPS. However, there is disagreement as to whether the methodology and data presented in these studies are adequate enough to draw any conclusions regarding the benefits of aerobic exercise for PPS patients.

SUMMARY

In the past decade, several international consensus conferences have been convened to develop recommendations regarding exercise in individuals with NMDs.[3,28,123,124] Although research regarding the use of exercise in NMDs is limited and is a consensus of expert opinion using evidence levels II to IV, these groups were able to make the following general recommendations[3,28,122,123]:

1. Because there are so many potential benefits from exercise, such as restoration of energy, and reductions in fatigue, depression, pain, social isolation, and loneliness, individuals with NMDs should adopt an active lifestyle for its physical and psychological benefits.
2. Stretching and range-of-motion exercises may be helpful in decreasing the discomfort attributable to the limited mobility of the joints secondary to muscle weakness.
3. Moderate resistance exercise (repeated repetitions at <30% of a 1-repetition maximum) should be given to patients with antigravity strength or better to maintain strength, and moderate aerobic exercise should be given to prevent deconditioning and loss of cardiopulmonary fitness. However, the effects of exercise should be closely monitored, as individuals with NMDs will have a variable response to

training depending on pathophysiology of their disease, their degree of weakness and fatigue, their rate of progression, and their level of conditioning;
4. High-intensity exercises relative to an individual's strength should be avoided. Significant muscle pain or myoglobinuria following an exercise activity is a sign of overexertion, and the activity should be modified.

Producing reliable evidence regarding the use of exercise in NMDs will require a long-term multicenter effort and a sustained research agenda, as well as an infrastructure capable of performing these studies. To determine the type, frequency, duration, and intensity of exercise for each of the specific NMDs will require the necessary funding to conduct multicenter trials that achieve the numbers of subjects required for adequate statistical power, and the achievement of reliable and valid results.

REFERENCES

1. Chamberlain JS, Rando TA. Duchenne muscular dystrophy: advances in therapeutics. Neurological disease and therapy. New York: Taylor & Francis; 2006. xxii, p. 461.
2. Fowler WM Jr. Management of musculoskeletal complications in neuromuscular diseases: weakness and the role of exercise. Phys Med Rehabil 1988;2: 489–504.
3. Fowler WM Jr. Role of physical activity and exercise training in neuromuscular diseases. Am J Phys Med Rehabil 2002;81:S187–95.
4. Fowler WM Jr, Taylor M. Rehabilitation management of muscular dystrophy and related disorders: I. The role of exercise. Arch Phys Med Rehabil 1982;63: 319–21.
5. Matheson GO, Klügl M, Dvorak J, et al. Responsibility of sport and exercise medicine in preventing and managing chronic disease: applying our knowledge and skill is overdue. Br J Sports Med 2011;45(16):1272–82 [Epub 2011 Sep 26].
6. Tremblay MS, Warburton DE, Janssen I, et al. New Canadian physical activity guidelines. Appl Physiol Nutr Metab 2011;36(1):36–46, 47–58.
7. Pate RR, Pratt M, Blair SN, et al. Physical activity and public health. A recommendation from the Centers for Disease Control and Prevention and the American College of Sports Medicine. JAMA 1995;273:402–7.
8. Zinna EM, Yarasheski KE. Exercise treatment to counteract protein wasting of chronic diseases. Curr Opin Clin Nutr Metab Care 2003;6:87–93.
9. Yarasheski KE. Exercise, aging, and muscle protein metabolism. J Gerontol A Biol Sci Med Sci 2003;58(10):M918–22.
10. Grutel M. The sarcomere and the nucleus: functional links to hypertrophy, atrophy and sarcopenia. Adv Exp Med Biol 2008;642:176–91.
11. Favier FB, Benoit H, Freyssenet D. Cellular and molecular events controlling skeletal muscle mass in response to altered use. Pflugers Arch 2008;456:587–600.
12. Kottke FJ, Stillwell GK, Lehman JF, editors. Krusen's handbook of physical medicine and rehabilitation. 3rd edition. Philadelphia: W.B. Saunders Co; 1982.
13. Pieterse AJ, Luttikhold TB, de Laat K, et al. Falls in patients with neuromuscular disorders. J Neurol Sci 2006;251(1–2):87–90 [Epub 2006 Nov 9].
14. Aitkens S, Kilmer DD, Wright NC, et al. Metabolic syndrome in neuromuscular disease. Arch Phys Med Rehabil 2005;86(5):1030–6.
15. Skalsky AJ, Abresch RT, Han JJ, et al. The relationship between regional body composition and quantitative strength in facioscapulohumeral muscular dystrophy (FSHD). Neuromuscul Disord 2008;18(11):873–80 [Epub 2008 Sep 24].

16. Miller TD, Balady GJ, Fletcher GF. Exercise and its role in the prevention and rehabilitation of cardiovascular disease. Ann Behav Med 1997;19:220–9.

17. Fowler WM Jr. Importance of overwork weakness. Muscle Nerve 1984;7(6): 496–9.

18. Bennett RL, Knowlton GC. Overwork weakness in partially denervated skeletal muscle. Clin Orthop 1958;12:22–92.

19. Johnson EW, Braddom R. Over-work weakness in facioscapulohumeral dystrophy. Arch Phys Med Rehabil 1971;52:333–62.

20. Pöche H, Kattner E, Hopfenmüller W. Myoglobinuria in hereditary progressive muscular dystrophies. Clin Physiol Biochem 1988;6(6):334–9.

21. Doriguzzi C, Palmucci L, Mongini T, et al. Exercise intolerance and recurrent myoglobinuria as the only expression of Xp21 Becker type muscular dystrophy. J Neurol 1993;240(5):269–71.

22. Figarella-Branger D, Baeta Machado AM, Putzu GA, et al. Exertional rhabdo-myolysis and exercise intolerance revealing dystrophinopathies. Acta Neuropathol 1997;94(1):48–53.

23. Minetti C, Tanji K, Chang HW, et al. Dystrophinopathy in two young boys with exercise-induced cramps and myoglobinuria. Eur J Pediatr 1993;152(10): 848–51.

24. Aitkens SG, McCrory MA, Kilmer DD, et al. Moderate resistance exercise program: its effect in slowly progressive neuromuscular disease. Arch Phys Med Rehabil 1993;74:711–5.

25. Kilmer DD, Aitkens S, Wright NC, et al. Response to high-intensity eccentric muscle contractions in persons with myopathic disease. Muscle Nerve 2001; 24:1181–7.

26. Milner-Brown HS, Miller RG. Muscle strengthening through high-resistance weight training in patients with neuromuscular disorders. Arch Phys Med Rehabil 1988;69:14–9.

27. van der Kooi EL, Lindeman E, Riphagen I. Strength training and aerobic exercise training for muscle disease. Cochrane Database Syst Rev 2005;(1):CD003907.

28. Cup EH, Pieterse AJ, Ten Broek-Pastoor JM, et al. Exercise therapy and other types of physical therapy for patients with neuromuscular diseases: a systematic review. Arch Phys Med Rehabil 2007;88:1452–64.

29. Dal Bello-Haas V, Florence JM, Krivickas LS. Therapeutic exercise for people with amyotrophic lateral sclerosis or motor neuron disease. Cochrane Database Syst Rev 2008;(2):CD005229.

30. White CM, Pritchard J, Turner-Stokes L. Exercise for people with peripheral neuropathy. Cochrane Database Syst Rev 2004;(4):CD003904.

31. Ervasti JM. A role for the dystrophin-glycoprotein complex as a transmembrane linker between laminin and actin. J Cell Biol 1993;122:809–23.

32. Franco A Jr, Lansman JB. Calcium entry through stretch-inactivated ion channels in mdx myotubes. Nature 1990;344:670–3.

33. Turner PR, Fong PY, Denetclaw WF, et al. Increased calcium influx in dystrophic muscle. J Cell Biol 1991;115:1701–12.

34. Stedman HH, Sweeney HL, Shrager JB, et al. The mdx mouse diaphragm reproduces the degenerative changes of Duchenne muscular dystrophy. Nature 1991;352:536–9.

35. Clarkson PM, Nosaka K, Braun B. Muscle function after exercise-induced muscle damage and rapid adaptation. Med Sci Sports Exerc 1992;24: 512–20.

36. Friden J, Lieber RL. Structural and mechanical basis of exercise-induced muscle injury. Med Sci Sports Exerc 1992;24:521–30.
37. Pasternak C, Wong S, Elson EL. Mechanical function of dystrophin in muscle cells. J Cell Biol 1995;128:355–61.
38. Petrof BJ. The molecular basis of activity-induced muscle injury in Duchenne muscular dystrophy. Mol Cell Biochem 1998;179(1–2):111–23.
39. Sander M, Chavoshan B, Harris S, et al. Functional muscle ischemia in neuronal nitric oxide synthase-deficient skeletal muscle of children with Duchenne muscular dystrophy. Proc Natl Acad Sci U S A 2000;97:13818–23.
40. Kobayashi YM, Rader EP, Crawford RW, et al. Sarcolemma-localized nNOS is required to maintain activity after mild exercise. Nature 2008;456(7221): 511–5, 26.
41. Vignos PJ Jr, Watkins MP. Effect of exercise in muscular dystrophy. JAMA 1966; 197:843–8.
42. Dubowitz V, Hyde SA, Scott OM, et al. Controlled trial of exercise in Duchenne muscular dystrophy. In: Serratrice G, editor. Neuromuscular diseases. New York: Raven Press; 1984. p. 571–5.
43. Scott OM, Hyde SA, Goddard C, et al. Effect of exercise in Duchenne muscular dystrophy: controlled six-month feasibility study of effects of two different regimes of exercises in children with Duchenne dystrophy. Physiotherapy 1981;67:174–6.
44. DeLateur BJ, Giaconi RM. Effect on maximal strength of submaximal exercise in Duchenne muscular dystrophy. Am J Phys Med 1979;58:26–36.
45. Garrood M, Eagle P, Jardine K, et al. Myoglobinuria in boys with Duchenne muscular dystrophy on corticosteroid therapy. Neuromuscul Disord 2008;18: 71–3.
46. Kimura S, Ikezawa M, Nomura K, et al. Immobility reduces muscle fiber necrosis in dystrophin deficient muscular dystrophy. Brain Dev 2006;28:473–6.
47. Vilozni D, Bar-Yishay E, Gur I, et al. Computerized respiratory muscle training in children with Duchenne muscular dystrophy. Neuromuscul Disord 1994;4: 249–55.
48. Wanke T, Toifl K, Merkle M, et al. Inspiratory muscle training in patients with Duchenne muscular dystrophy. Chest 1994;105:475–82.
49. Koessler W, Wanke T, Winkler G, et al. 2 years' experience with inspiratory muscle training in patients with neuromuscular disorders. Chest 2001;120: 765–9.
50. Martin AJ, Stern L, Yeates J, et al. Respiratory muscle training in Duchenne muscular dystrophy. Dev Med Child Neurol 1986;28(3):314–8.
51. Gozal D, Thiriet P. Respiratory muscle training in neuromuscular disease: long-term effects on strength and load perception. Med Sci Sports Exerc 1999;31:1522–7.
52. Rodillo E, Noble-Jamieson CM, Aber V, et al. Respiratory muscle training in Duchenne muscular dystrophy. Arch Dis Child 1989;64:736–8.
53. Stern LM, Martin AJ, Jones N, et al. Training inspiratory resistance in Duchenne dystrophy using adapted computer games. Dev Med Child Neurol 1989;31: 494–500.
54. Smith PE, Calverley PM, Edwards RH, et al. Practical considerations of respiratory care of patients with muscular dystrophy. N Engl J Med 1987;316:1197–205.
55. Sveen ML, Jeppesen TD, Hauerslev S, et al. Endurance training improves fitness and strength in patients with Becker muscular dystrophy. Brain 2008; 131:2824–31.

56. Sveen ML, Jeppesen TD, Hauerslev S, et al. Endurance training: an effective and safe treatment of patients with LGMD2I. Neurology 2007;68:59–61.

57. Yeldan I, Gurses HN, Yuksel H. Comparison study of chest physiotherapy home training programmes on respiratory functions in patients with muscular dystrophy. Clin Rehabil 2008;22(8):741–8.

58. Böhme P, Arnold C. Limb-girdle muscular dystrophy—results of physical therapy under stationary conditions. Aktuelle Neurologie 2004;1:1–5.

59. Ansved T. Muscular dystrophies: influence of physical conditioning on the disease evolution. Curr Opin Clin Nutr Metab Care 2003;6:435–9.

60. Wijmenga C, Frants RR, Hewitt JE, et al. Molecular genetics of facioscapulohumeral muscular dystrophy. Neuromuscul Disord 1993;3:487–91.

61. Tawil R. Facioscapulohumeral muscular dystrophy. Neurotherapeutics 2008; 5(4):601–6.

62. Lemmer R, van der Vliet PJ, Klooster R, et al. A unifying genetic model for facioscapulohumeral muscular dystrophy. Science 2010;329(5999):1650–3.

63. Karpati G, Molnar M. Muscle fibre regeneration in skeletal muscle diseases. In: Schiaffino S, Partridge T, editors. Skeletal muscle repair and regeneration. A.A. Dordrecht (The Netherlands): Springer Science; 2008. p. 199–216.

64. Van der Kooi EL, Vogels OJ, Van Asseldonk RJ, et al. Strength training and albuterol in facioscapulohumeral muscular dystrophy. Neurology 2004;63(4):702–8.

65. Lindeman E, Leffers P, Spaans F, et al. Strength training in patients with myotonic dystrophy and hereditary motor and sensory neuropathy: a randomized clinical trial. Arch Phys Med Rehabil 1995;76:612–20.

66. Olsen DB, Orngreen MC, Vissing J. Aerobic training improves exercise performance in facioscapulohumeral muscular dystrophy. Neurology 2005;64:1064–6.

67. Aldehag AS, Jonsson H, Ansved T. Effects of a hand training programme in five patients with myotonic dystrophy type 1. Occup Ther Int 2005;12:14–27.

68. Orngreen MC, Olsen DB, Vissing J. Aerobic training in patients with myotonic dystrophy type I. Ann Neurol 2005;57:754–7.

69. Haller RG, Wyrick P, Taivassalo T, et al. Aerobic conditioning: an effective therapy in McArdle's disease. Ann Neurol 2006;59:922–8.

70. Maté-Muñoz JL, Moran M, Pérez M, et al. Favorable responses to acute and chronic exercise in McArdle patients. Clin J Sport Med 2007;17(4):297–303.

71. Pérez M, Foster C, González-Freire M, et al. One-year follow-up in a child with McArdle disease: exercise is medicine. Pediatr Neurol 2008;38(2):133–6.

72. Pérez M, Maté-Muñoz JL, Foster C, et al. Exercise capacity in a child with McArdle disease. J Child Neurol 2007;22(7):880–2.

73. Ollivier K, Hogrel JY, Gomez-Merino D, et al. Exercise tolerance and daily life in McArdle's disease. Muscle Nerve 2005;31(5):637–41.

74. Taivassalo T, Haller RG. Exercise and training in mitochondrial myopathies. Med Sci Sports Exerc 2005;37:2094–101.

75. Taivassalo T, Matthews PM, De Stefano N, et al. Combined aerobic training and dichloroacetate improve exercise capacity and indices of aerobic metabolism in muscle cytochrome oxidase deficiency. Neurology 1996;47(2):529–34.

76. Taivassalo T, De Stefano N, Argov Z, et al. Effects of aerobic training in patients with mitochondrial myopathies. Neurology 1998;50:1055–60.

77. Taivassalo T, De Stefano N, Chen J, et al. Short-term aerobic training response in chronic myopathies. Muscle Nerve 1999;22:1239–43.

78. Taivassalo T, Shoubridge EA, Chen J, et al. Aerobic conditioning in patients with mitochondrial myopathies: physiological, biochemical, and genetic effects. Ann Neurol 2001;50(2):133–41.

79. Murphy JL, Blakely EL, Schaefer AM, et al. Resistance training in patients with single, large-scale deletions of mitochondrial DNA. Brain 2008;131:2832–40.
80. Siciliano G, Manca ML, Renna M, et al. Effects of aerobic training on lactate and catecholaminergic exercise responses in mitochondrial myopathies. Neuromuscl Disord 2000;10:40–5.
81. Taivassalo T, Gardner JL, Taylor RW, et al. Endurance training and detraining in mitochondrial myopathies due to single large-scale mtDNA deletions. Brain 2006 Dec;129(Pt 12):3391–401 [Epub 2006 Nov 3].
82. Jeppesen TD, Schwartz M, Olsen DB, et al. Aerobic training is safe and improves exercise capacity in patients with mitochondrial myopathy. Brain 2006;129:3402–12.
83. Trenell MI, Sue CM, Kemp GJ, et al. Aerobic exercise and muscle metabolism in patients with mitochondrial myopathy. Muscle Nerve 2006;33:524–31.
85. Askanas V, Engel WK. Inclusion body myositis, a multifactorial muscle disease associated with aging: current concepts of pathogenesis. Curr Opin Rheumatol 2007;19(6):550–9.
85. Alexanderson H, Stenstrom CH, Lundberg I. Safety of a home exercise programme in patients with polymyositis and dermatomyositis: a pilot study. Rheumatology 1999;38:608–11.
86. Alexanderson H, Lundberg IE. The role of exercise in the rehabilitation of idiopathic inflammatory myopathies. Curr Opin Rheumatol 2005;17:164–71.
87. Alexanderson H, Stenstrom CH, Jenner G, et al. The safety of a resistive home exercise program in patients with recent onset active polymyositis or dermatomyositis. Scand J Rheumatol 2000;29:295–301.
88. Alexanderson H, Dastmalchi M, Esbjornsson-Liljedahl M, et al. Benefits of intensive resistance training in patients with chronic polymyositis or dermatomyositis. Arthritis Rheum 2007;57:766–77.
89. Alexanderson H. Exercise in inflammatory myopathies, including inclusion body myositis. Curr Rheumatol Rep 2012;14(3):244–51.
90. Alexanderson H, Lundberg IE. Exercise as a therapeutic modality in patients with idiopathic inflammatory myopathies. Curr Opin Rheumatol 2012;24(2): 201–7.
91. Wiesinger GF, Quittan M, Nuhr M, et al. Aerobic capacity in adult dermatomyositis/polymyositis patients and healthy controls. Arch Phys Med Rehabil 2000; 81:1–5.
92. Hicks JE, Drinkard B, Summers RM, et al. Decreased aerobic capacity in children with juvenile dermatomyositis. Arthritis Rheum 2002;15:118–23.
93. Arnardottir S, Alexanderson H, Lundberg IE, et al. Sporadic inclusion body myositis: pilot study on the effects of a home exercise program on muscle function, histopathology and inflammatory reaction. J Rehabil Med 2003;35:31–5.
94. Rosen DR, Siddique T, Patterson D, et al. Mutations in Cu/Zn superoxide dismutase gene are associated with familial amyotrophic lateral sclerosis. Nature 1993;362(6415):59–62.
95. Kaspar BK, Frost LM, Christian L, et al. Synergy of insulin-like growth factor-1 and exercise in amyotrophic lateral sclerosis. Ann Neurol 2005;57:649–55.
96. Kirkinezos IG, Hernandez D, Bradley WG, et al. Regular exercise is beneficial to a mouse model of amyotrophic lateral sclerosis. Ann Neurol 2003;53(6): 804–7.
97. Veldink JH, Bär PR, Joosten EA, et al. Sexual differences in onset of disease and response to exercise in a transgenic model of ALS. Neuromuscl Disord 2003; 13(9):737–43.

98. Mahoney DJ, Rodriguez C, Devries M, et al. Effects of high-intensity endurance exercise training in the G93A mouse model of amyotrophic lateral sclerosis. Muscle Nerve 2004;29(5):656–62.

99. McCrate ME, Kaspar BK. Physical activity and neuroprotection in amyotrophic lateral sclerosis. Neuromolecular Med 2008;10(2):108–17.

100. Drory VE, Goltsman E, Reznik JG, et al. The value of muscle exercise in patients with amyotrophic lateral sclerosis. J Neurol Sci 2001;191:133–7.

101. Bello-Haas VD, Florence JM, Kloos AD, et al. A randomized controlled trial of resistance exercise in individuals with ALS. Neurology 2007;68:2003–7.

102. Jani-Acsadi A, Krajewski K, Shy ME. Charcot-Marie-Tooth neuropathies: diagnosis and management. Semin Neurol 2008;28:185–94.

103. Shy ME, Chen L, Swan ER, et al. Neuropathy progression in Charcot-Marie-Tooth disease type 1A. Neurology 2008;70(5):378–83.

104. Chetlin RD, Gutmann L, Tarnopolsky M, et al. Resistance training effectiveness in patients with Charcot-Marie-Tooth disease: recommendations for exercise prescription. Arch Phys Med Rehabil 2004;85:1217–23.

105. El Mhandi L, Millet GY, Calmels P, et al. Benefits of interval-training on fatigue and functional capacities in Charcot-Marie-Tooth disease. Muscle Nerve 2008; 37:601–10.

106. Halsted LS, Rossi CD. New problems in old polio patients: results of a survey of 530 polio survivors. Orthopedics 1985;8:845–50.

107. Halstead LS, Gawne AC. NRH proposal for limb classification and exercise prescription. Disabil Rehabil 1996;18:311–6.

108. March of Dimes. March of dimes international conference on post polio syndrome. Identifying best practices in diagnosis and care. White Plains (NY): March of Dimes; 2000.

109. Farbu E, Gilhus NE, Barnes MP, et al. EFNS guideline on diagnosis and management of post-polio syndrome. Report of an EFNS task force. Eur J Neurol 2006;13:795–801.

110. Chan KM, Amirjani N, Sumrain M, et al. Randomized controlled trial of strength training in post-polio patients. Muscle Nerve 2003;27:332–8.

111. Klein MG, Whyte J, Esquenazi A, et al. A comparison of the effects of exercise and lifestyle modification on the resolution of overuse symptoms of the shoulder in polio survivors: a preliminary study. Arch Phys Med Rehabil 2002;83:708–13.

112. Agre JC, Rodriquez AA, Franke TM, et al. Low-intensity, alternate-day exercise improves muscle performance without apparent adverse affect in postpolio patients. Am J Phys Med Rehabil 1996;78:50–62.

113. Prins JH, Hartung H, Merritt DJ, et al. Effect of aquatic exercise training in persons with poliomyelitis disability. Sports Med Train Rehabil 1994;5:29–39.

114. Agre JC, Rodriquez AA, Franke TM. Strength, endurance, and work capacity after muscle strengthening exercise in postpolio subjects. Arch Phys Med Rehabil 1997;78:681–6.

115. Einarsson G. Muscle conditioning in late poliomyelitis. Arch Phys Med Rehabil 1991;72:11–4.

116. Fillyaw MJ, Badger GJ, Goodwin GD, et al. The effects of long-term non-fatiguing resistance exercise in subjects with post-polio syndrome. Orthopedics 1991;14:1253–6.

117. Spector SA, Gordon PL, Feuerstein IM, et al. Strength gains without muscle injury after strength training in patients with postpolio muscular atrophy. Muscle Nerve 1996;19:1282–90.

118. Jones DR, Speier J, Canine K, et al. Cardiorespiratory responses to aerobic training by patients with postpoliomyelitis sequelae. JAMA 1989;261:3255–8.
119. Willén C, Sunnerhagen KS, Grimby G. Dynamic water exercise in individuals with late poliomyelitis. Arch Phys Med Rehabil 2001;82(1):66–72.
120. Ernstoff B, Wetterqvist H, Kvist H, et al. Endurance training effect on individuals with postpoliomyelitis. Arch Phys Med Rehabil 1996;77:843–8.
121. Kriz JL, Jones DR, Speier JL, et al. Cardiorespiratory responses to upper extremity aerobic training by postpolio subjects. Arch Phys Med Rehabil 1992;73:49–54.
122. Dean E, Ross J. Effect of modified aerobic training on movement energetics in polio survivors. Orthopedics 1991;14:1243–6.
123. Eagle M. Report on the muscular dystrophy campaign workshop: exercise in neuromuscular diseases Newcastle, January 2002. Neuromuscul Disord 2002;12(10):975–83.
124. Bushby K, Finkel R, Birnkrant DJ, et al, DMD Care Considerations Working Group. Diagnosis and management of Duchenne muscular dystrophy, part 2: implementation and multidisciplinary care. Lancet Neurol 2010;9(2):177–89 [Epub 2009 Nov 27].

Prevention and Management of Limb Contractures in Neuromuscular Diseases

Andrew J. Skalsky, MD[a], Craig M. McDonald, MD[b],*

KEYWORDS

- Contractures • Range of motion • Static positioning • Splinting • Bracing
- Stretching • Therapy • Surgery

KEY POINTS

- Known contributing extrinsic factors include decreased ability to actively move a limb through its full range of motion, static positioning for prolonged periods of time, and agonist-antagonist muscle imbalance.
- Known intrinsic factors contributing to contractures include fibrotic changes to the muscle resulting in reduced extensibility and disruption of muscle fiber architecture; thus, myopathic conditions are associated with more severe limb contractures compared with neuropathic disorders.
- A major rationale for controlling lower-limb contractures is to minimize their adverse effects on independent ambulation; however, the major cause of wheelchair reliance in neuromuscular diseases is generally weakness and not contracture formation.
- Static positioning of upper and lower limbs is an important cause of contracture formation.
- The primary focus of surgery has been on the management of lower-limb contractures to achieve a braceable lower extremity or plantigrade foot or because contractures of the arm and hand cause little functional deficit until the late stages of neuromuscular disease.

INTRODUCTION

Limb contractures are a common impairment in neuromuscular diseases (NMDs). They contribute to increased disability from decreased motor performance, mobility

This work was supported by Grant# H133B0900001 from the National Institute of Disability and Rehabilitation Research.

Disclosures. The authors take full responsibility for the contents of this paper, which do not represent the views of the National Institute of Disability and Rehabilitation Research or the United States Government.

[a] Rady Children's Hospital, Division of Pediatric Rehabilitation, MC 5096, 3020 Children's Way, University of California San Diego School of Medicine, San Diego, CA 92123, USA;
[b] Department of Physical Medicine and Rehabilitation, University of California Davis School of Medicine, Suite 3850, 4860 Y Street, Sacramento, CA 95817, USA
* Corresponding author.
E-mail address: cmmcdonald@ucdavis.edu

limitations, reduced functional range of motion (ROM), loss of function for activities of daily living, and increased pain. The pathogenesis of contractures is multifactorial. Known contributing extrinsic factors include decreased ability to actively move a limb through its full ROM, static positioning for prolonged periods of time, and agonist-antagonist muscle imbalance.[1] Intrinsic factors include fibrotic changes to the muscle resulting in reduced extensibility.[2–9] Contracture prophylaxis is important to maintain function, ROM, and skin integrity.[10–14] Lower-limb contractures are much more prevalent than upper-limb contractures. Myopathic conditions are associated with more severe limb contractures compared with neuropathic disorders. The rate of NMD progression is also related to the frequency and severity of contractures with more rapidly progressive conditions resulting in earlier and more severe contracture formation.[6] Bracing, stretching programs, and surgery have all been used in the prophylaxis and treatment of limb contractures.

PATHOGENESIS

A limb contracture is the lack of full passive ROM because of joint, muscle, or soft tissue limitations. Contractures in NMDs develop from intrinsic myotendinous structural changes and extrinsic factors.

Static Positioning

Weakness and inability to achieve active joint mobilization throughout the full normal range is the single most frequent factor contributing to the occurrence of fixed contractures. For example, less than antigravity knee extension strength places an individual at risk for knee flexion contractures, particularly if the patient no longer ambulates and spends most of their time seated with the knee joint positioned in flexion. The position in which a joint is statically positioned influences the number of sarcomeres present in any given muscle. A shortened muscle length may result in up to a 40% loss of sarcomeres.[1] A statically positioned limb developing fibrotic changes within the muscle develops contracture formation in the position of immobilization. Contractures rapidly develop in many NMDs after transitioning to a wheelchair.[9] The static nature of wheelchair mobility compared with the dynamic movement associated with gait contributes to the development of limb contractures. Compensatory strategies used to biomechanically stabilize joints to accommodate for muscle paresis result in reduced active ROM. For example, individuals with NMD resulting in proximal hip and knee extension weakness exhibit lumbar lordosis, diminished stance phase knee flexion, and equinus posturing at the ankle during stance and gait. The equinus posturing at the ankle is a compensation to keep the weight line and ground reaction force line anterior to the knee. The increased lumbar lordosis moves the weight line and ground reaction force line posterior to the hip. These compensations stabilize the lower limbs by creating a knee extension moment and a hip extension moment. However, these same compensations result in reduced active ROM of the same joints. This is likely why ankle plantar flexion contractures develop in Duchenne muscular dystrophy (DMD) before the onset of wheelchair reliance.[10]

Imbalance of Agonist and Antagonist Muscles

Asymmetries of strength are an important determinant of contracture formation. The imbalance between flexor and extensor muscle groups has not been shown to be a major factor leading to contracture formation, but contractures are frequently observed when major muscle imbalance is present. This is likely caused by reduced active ROM because the movement is dominated by the stronger muscle group.

For example, in several NMDs there is more pathologic involvement of the ankle dor-siflexors and evertors than the ankle plantarflexors and invertors. This imbalance in combination with intrinsic muscle changes leads to the frequently observed equinoca-vovarus foot deformities,[10] which become exacerbated if the patient loses ambulation and is no longer weight bearing.

Fibrosis and Fatty Tissue Infiltration

Intrinsic muscle tissue alterations in dystrophic myopathies contribute to contracture formation. The most significant histologic changes are those of muscle fiber loss; abnormal residual dystrophic muscle fibers; segmental necrosis of muscle fibers; and increased amounts of adipose tissue, connective tissue, and fibrosis. Replace-ment of functioning muscle fibers with collagen and fatty tissue in concert with chron-ically shortened resting muscle length results in contracture formation. The collagen fibers undergo rearrangement and proliferation causing muscle fibrosis and resistance to passive stretch. Neurogenic atrophy typically results in a diminished degree of fibrosis, which lowers the risk of severe contracture formation.[2–7]

CONTRACTURES IN SPECIFIC NMDS
Duchenne and Becker Muscular Dystrophies

The most common contractures observed in dystrophinopathies in the order of frequency are ankle plantar flexion, knee flexion, hip flexion, hip abduction, elbow flexion, and wrist flexion contractures.[9,15] Proximal lower-extremity contractures are rare while subjects with DMD are ambulatory, but develop soon after they transition to a sitting posi-tion in a wheelchair for most of the day. The occurrence of elbow flexion contractures also seems to be directly related to prolonged static positioning of the limb flexed because these contractures develop soon after full-time wheelchair reliance (**Fig. 1**). The relationship between wheelchair reliance and hip and knee flexion contractures has been noted by multiple authors.[5,9,16,17] Given the tremendous replacement of muscle by fibrotic tissue in individuals with DMD, it is not surprising that a muscle with less than antigravity strength statically positioned in a wheelchair would develop a contracture. Although 20% of subjects with DMD in the study by McDonald and colleagues[9] devel-oped ankle plantar flexion contractures of greater than 5 degrees before wheelchair reli-ance, there was a rapid acceleration in severity of these contractures after transition to wheelchair reliance (see **Fig. 1**). Ankle plantar flexion contractures were not likely a signif-icant cause of wheelchair reliance because less than 10% of subjects had plantar flexion contractures of greater than or equal to 15 degrees before their transition to the wheel-chair. The natural history data for DMD was described by McDonald and colleagues.[9] The cause and frequency of contractures in Becker muscular dystrophy is similar to DMD when comparing individuals of similar function. As a result, contractures are rare in ambulatory boys with Becker muscular dystrophy with exception to ankle plantar flexion. As they transition to a wheelchair, the prevalence of contractures increases.[15]

Emery-Dreifuss Muscular Dystrophy

Emery-Dreifuss muscular dystrophy (EMD) is a group of muscular dystrophies with early and extreme contracture formation disproportional to the degree of muscle weakness and immobility. EMD deserves special attention because of the notorious presence of limb contractures despite the presence of functional strength. EMD results from a group of genes that encode for nuclear proteins. The exact mechanisms of such profound contracture formation in EMD are not fully understood. The condition usually presents in adolescence or early adult life, and many clinical features may be

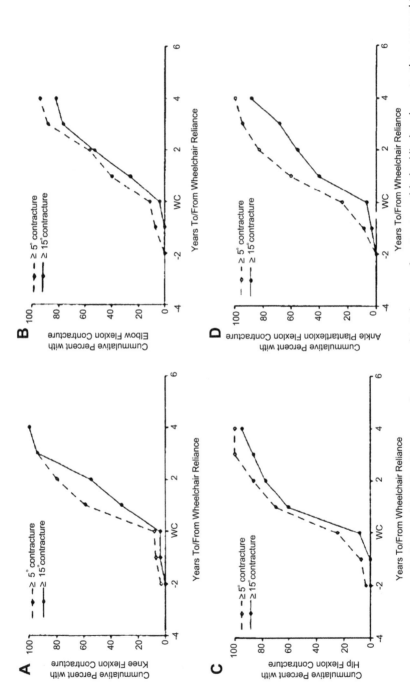

Fig. 1. Cumulative percentages of subjects with DMD with greater than or equal to 15 degrees of contractures (*dashed line*) and greater than or equal to 5 degrees of contractures (*solid line*) versus years to and from wheelchair reliance. (*A*) Knee flexion. (*B*) Elbow flexion. (*C*) Hip flexion. (*D*) Ankle plantarflexion. (*From* McDonald CM, Abresch RT, Carter GT, et al. Profiles of neuromuscular diseases. Duchenne muscular dystrophy. Am J Phys Med Rehabil 1995;74(Suppl 5):S70–92; with permission.)

seen in early childhood. An associated cardiomyopathy usually presents with arrhythmia and may lead to sudden death in early adult life. A hallmark of EMD type 1 is the early presence of contractures of the elbow flexors with limitation of full extension. Patients often have striking wasting of the upper arms accentuated by sparing of the deltoids and forearm muscles. The early presence of contractures of the elbow flexors is contrasted by focal wasting of the biceps brachii muscles. Heel cord tightness may be present early in the disorder concomitant with ankle dorsiflexion weakness and toe walking. Unlike DMD, the toe walking in EMD usually is secondary to ankle dorsiflexion weakness and contracture formation, and it is not a compensatory strategy to stabilize the knee because of proximal limb weakness. Tightness of the cervical and lumbar spinal extensor muscles or rigid spine results in limitation of neck and trunk flexion.[19]

Slowly Progressive Muscular Dystrophies

The slowly progressive muscular dystrophies are a heterogeneous group of muscular dystrophies with a slower progression, with a life expectancy into later adulthood. Limb-girdle muscular dystrophies, facioscapulohumeral muscular dystrophy, and myotonic muscular dystrophy types 1 and 2 can all be associated with contracture formation. The severity of contractures coincides with the degree of muscle weakness. Severe contractures are infrequent in ambulators but are more prevalent in full-time wheelchair users.[18,20–22] Contractures in congenital myotonic dystrophy are common affecting greater than 70% of individuals and most commonly affect the ankle but rarely the knees or hips. Patients with congenital myotonic muscular dystrophy may be born with clubfoot deformities. Scoliosis is also commonly observed.[23]

Congenital Muscular Dystrophies and Congenital Myopathies

Congenital muscular dystrophies and congenital myopathies represent groups of congenital or infant-onset myopathies. These disorders present with hypotonia and early presence of contractures. Subjects with congenital muscular dystrophies or myopathies often exhibit early contractures including ankle plantarflexion, knee flexion, hip flexion, wrist flexion, and long finger flexion. These myopathies have been reported to be fairly slowly progressive or relatively static; however, the contractures become more severe over time with prolonged static positioning and lack of active ROM.[19] Patients with Ullrich congenital muscular dystrophy have a primary defect in collagen VI in addition to a dystrophic myopathy. These patients have the unique combination of distal ligamentous laxity with hypermobile joints and proximal contractures.

Arthrogryposis

Arthrogryposis is a symptom complex characterized by congenital rigidity of the joints and is not a specific diagnostic entity. By definition, arthrogryposis involves multiple joints, with distal joints more often affected than proximal joints. The feet, ankles, hands, and wrists are most commonly affected. A variety of central nervous system disorders, such as chromosomal syndromes, developmental disorders, and congenital malformations of the central nervous system, may result in arthrogryposis. Alternatively, focal and segmental vascular insufficiency during embryonic development may lead to a focal loss of anterior horn cells and hypomyoplasia or amyoplasia. Arthrogryposis caused by amyoplasia leads to embryonic strength imbalance around joints, which results in congenital contractures.

Spinal Muscular Atrophy

Spinal muscular atrophy (SMA) is a term used to describe a varied group of inherited disorders characterized by weakness and muscle wasting secondary to degeneration of both anterior horn cells of the spinal cord and brainstem motor nuclei without pyramidal tract involvement. The most common SMA syndrome is predominantly proximal, autosomal-recessive, and linked to chromosome 5q. Contractures are problematic in patients with SMA who have lost ambulation or never obtained ambulation. One study found reductions in ROM by more than 20 degrees among 22% to 50% of subjects with SMA II depending on the joint. Hip, knee, and wrist contractures were most common.[21] Lower-extremity contractures have been found to be rare in ambulatory patients with SMA.[24] Patients with SMA perceive their elbow flexion contractures to hinder one or more daily functions, and the contractures were reported to be associated with greater discomfort.[25] Contractures are very common in SMA II. In the lower limbs, the knees are most affected followed by the hips and ankles.[26] The shoulders are the most severely affected in the upper limbs followed by the elbows and wrists.[27]

Amyotrophic Lateral Sclerosis

Amyotrophic lateral sclerosis is a rapidly progressive motor neuron disorder that results in profound appendicular, bulbar, and respiratory muscle weakness, but only mild joint contractures. In one study, only 26% of subjects with amyotrophic lateral sclerosis had ankle plantar flexion contractures, 13% had shoulder contractures, and 20% had contractures of any joint measuring greater than or equal to 20 degrees by goniometry.[6] The low prevalence and mild severity of contractures in amyotrophic lateral sclerosis is likely caused by the neurogenic nature of the muscle wasting with less severe fibrosis and fatty tissue infiltration.

Charcot-Marie-Tooth Disease

Multiple subtypes of Charcot-Marie-Tooth (CMT) or hereditary motor sensory neuropathy exist with genetic heterogeneity among the primarily demyelinating forms and the primarily axonal forms. In a study of 53 subjects, reduction in ROM by 20 degrees or more was seen in 9% at the ankle, 8% at the knee, 2% at the elbow, 14% at the hip, and 19% at the wrist. Focal wasting of intrinsic foot and hand musculature is common, and the most common lower-limb contracture is an equinocavovarus deformity.[28] Cavus foot deformities associated with hindfoot varus and a variety of complex foot deformities caused by muscle imbalance is common in CMT with disease progression.

MANAGEMENT OF CONTRACTURES

Although the evidence supporting interventions to improve ROM in NMDs is lacking,[29–31] there are generally accepted principles that may minimize the impact or disability from the contractures in NMD. Contractures in NMD conditions should be managed with the following concepts in mind:

1. Prevention of contractures requires early diagnosis and initiation of physical medicine approaches, such as passive ROM and splinting before contractures are present or while contractures are mild.
2. Contractures are inevitable in some NMD conditions.
3. Advanced contractures become fixed and show little response to conservative interventions, such as stretching or splinting programs, and may require surgical intervention.

4. A major rationale for controlling lower-limb contractures is to minimize their adverse effects on independent ambulation; however, the major cause of wheelchair reliance in NMD is generally weakness and not contracture formation.
5. Static positioning of upper and lower limbs is an important cause of contracture formation.
6. Mild upper-limb contractures may not negatively impact function.

Rehabilitation Management of Lower-Limb Contractures

Four principal physical therapy modalities must be regularly performed to prevent or delay the development of lower-limb contractures for those at risk for musculoskeletal deformity. These include (1) regularly prescribed periods of daily standing or walking; (2) passive stretching of muscles and joints; (3) positioning of the limbs to promote extension and oppose flexion; and (4) splinting, which is a useful measure for the prevention or delay of contractures.[32]

A minimum of 2 to 3 hours of daily standing or walking is necessary in addition to passive stretching for the control of contracture formation in myopathies. Passive stretching to maintain or improve ROM is an enormously important component of the program to prevent contractures. Such passive ROM has been documented to be efficacious in slowing the development of contractures in DMD.[32–38]

A program of passive stretching should be started as early as possible in the course of NMD and become part of a regular morning and evening routine. Proper technique is essential for passive stretching to be effective. With each stretch, the position should be held for a count of 15, and each exercise should be repeated 10 to 15 times during a session.[39] Stretching should be performed slowly and gently. An overly strenuous stretch may cause discomfort and reduce cooperation. Written instructional materials should be provided to the patient and family as a supplement to verbal instructions and demonstrations by the physical therapist. The specific anatomic focus of stretching exercises prescribed for lower-limb contractures varies with the type of NMD. Lower-limb positioning may be a useful adjunct for preventing contracture formation. The limb should be placed in a resting position that opposes or minimizes flexion. The prone lying position is an effective method to stretch the hip flexors.

Splinting is another adjunctive measure used to slow the development of contractures in NMDs. Ankle-foot orthotics (AFOs) or nighttime resting splints have been used to maintain a 90-degree angle of the foot relative to the tibia. Some authors indicate that such splinting is effective for reducing heel cord contractures in DMD; however, other investigators do not believe that AFOs change the natural history of heel cord contracture formation.[39,40] Foot deformities are common in peripheral neuropathies, such as CMT, and distal myopathies, such as myotonic dystrophy type 1. Treatment of foot deformities depends on the patient's age, flexibility of the foot, bony deformity, and muscle imbalance. A nighttime or full-time AFO in a neutral ankle position custom molded to the foot deformity may decrease the tendency toward further development of the deformity. A supple foot can be managed nonoperatively by a solid AFO in the neutral position.

Few randomized controlled trials have evaluated the efficacy of bracing. One such study found no benefit in nocturnal bracing in CMT, but the duration of treatment was only 6 weeks; however, the same group did report benefit from serial night casting.[41,42] Crosbie and Burns[43] found no benefit from the use of an AFO in CMT in regards to functional outcomes and pain.

Any splinting program must be used in conjunction with passive stretching and standing or ambulation. Splinting for prevention of equinus deformity generally has been used at night. However, AFOs may be worn while in the wheelchair throughout the day. Long leg knee-ankle-foot orthoses (KAFO), which immobilize the knee in extension, may be worn for ambulation, for standing, or as a night resting brace. Most patients with tight hamstrings generally do not tolerate long leg bracing. Stretching, positioning, and splinting have limited roles in the management of hip and knee contractures in patients who primarily use a wheelchair.

Bracing of contractures for prolonged ambulation in NMD conditions with proximal weakness, such as DMD, was first reported by Spencer and Vignos in 1962.[44] Lightweight polypropylene KAFOs with a neutral solid ankle, drop-lock knee joints, and ischial weight-bearing polypropylene upper thigh component have been used in DMD. The ischial seating gives a more upright standing posture with reduction in lordosis. Patients with DMD who have had excellent stretching programs can be placed immediately into KAFO bracing without surgical interventions. There are some experts who believe the use of KAFOs prolongs ambulation in DMD by 1 to 3 years.[45,46] Although the literature to support this is poor,[47] the greater reason why fewer patients are using KAFO bracing in recent years is because of the efficacy of corticosteroids in prolonging ambulation. In addition, the compliance of patients with DMD with KAFO bracing is variable.[47–50] The disadvantages of braced ambulation with KAFOs center on the excessive energy cost of such ambulation and safety concerns in the event of falls. Subjects with DMD prescribed long leg braces (ie, KAFOs) need gait training by physical therapy, and they need to be taught fall techniques with locked knees.

Surgical Management of Lower-Limb Contractures

While subjects with DMD are still ambulating independently, they use the ankle equinus posturing from the gastrocnemius soleus group to create a knee extension moment to stabilize the knee because of weak knee extensors. Several authors have cautioned against isolated tendo Achillis lengthening (TAL) while patients with DMD are still ambulating independently.[51–53] TAL without simultaneous bracing above the knee can lead to loss of walking ability unless the quadriceps are grade 3+ to 4 or better. Overcorrection (overlengthening) of the heel cord contracture in a patient with DMD may result in immediate loss of the ability to walk.[37]

Surgery before the loss of ambulation in DMD has not been shown to prolong ambulation and some studies have suggested that early surgery may have deleterious effects on ambulation.[48] Some surgeons have performed early prophylactic TAL and posterior tibialis lengthening surgery years before anticipated loss of ambulation in patients with relatively mild contractures. In a randomized trial, Manzur and colleagues[52] showed no benefit from early surgical treatment of distal lower-extremity contractures in DMD. After braced ambulation ceases, surgical heel cord lengthening may have the benefit of better foot positioning on the wheelchair leg rests and occasionally allows improved shoe wear. Although surgery may improve the ankle ROM and positioning of the foot on the wheelchair footrest in DMD after transitioning to full-time wheelchair use, it does not usually impact shoe wear, pain, hypersensitivity, or self-perceived cosmesis in a significant manner.[53]

Distal lower-limb surgical interventions in ambulatory patients with slowly progressive NMD, particularly in such neuropathies as CMT, are often used. If a fixed deformity is present, surgical intervention may be required to obtain a plantigrade foot. The Coleman block test is commonly used in cavovarus feet to determine whether the contracture involves the forefoot, hindfoot, or both.[54–56] The patient stands on a wood block 2.5 to 4 cm thick with the heel and lateral border of the foot on the block with the first three metatarsals hanging freely over the block. This negates the effect the forefoot may have on the hindfoot stance. The hindfoot should be bearing the patient's full weight. The correction of hindfoot varus with the patient standing on the block suggests the hindfoot is flexible and surgical intervention should be directed to correct the forefoot position. If the hindfoot varus does not correct while standing on the block, correction of the forefoot and hindfoot are likely needed to obtain a more plantigrade foot.[57] Rarely is TAL needed to correct a cavovarus foot because the calcaneus is already in calcaneus or dorsiflexion (**Fig. 2**).[54–56] TAL may worsen the cavus deformity by tilting the hindfoot into more calcaneus and the forefoot into more equinus to maintain ground contact. A dorsal closing wedge osteotomy of the midfoot at the apex of the cavus foot deformity is often performed in CMT (**Fig. 3**). The osteotomy improves the forefoot position in relation to the hindfoot. This improves weight-bearing biomechanics and can reduce pain.[54,55]

Rehabilitation Management of Upper-Limb Contractures

The primary focus in the literature has been on the management of lower-limb contractures because contractures of the arm and hand cause little functional deficit until the late stages of NMD. Upper-limb contractures rarely develop when there is functional strength of upper-limb musculature with the exception of EMD. Elbow flexion contractures in DMD occur soon after full-time wheelchair reliance and are likely secondary to the static positioning of the arms in elbow flexion on the arm rests of the wheelchair (see **Fig. 1**).[9] In DMD, deterioration in upper-limb function lags approximately 2 years behind the loss of lower-limb function. Other common upper-limb contractures include forearm pronation and wrist flexion with ulnar deviation in the later stages of NMD. Although mild elbow flexion contractures of 15 degrees or less are of minimal functional consequence, elbow flexion contractures greater than 30 degrees can interfere with effective gait aid use in ambulatory patients with NMD. Severe elbow flexion contractures greater than 60 degrees decreases distal upper-limb function by reducing the reachable workspace, and makes dressing difficult.[58] Shoulder contractures are less problematic in patients with profound proximal muscle weakness. Combined shoulder adduction contractures and elbow flexion contractures may interfere with independent feeding. Severe shoulder adduction contractures complicate dependent dressing and can lead to hygiene difficulties including skin breakdown in the axilla.

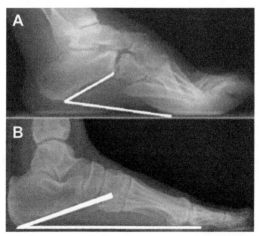

Fig. 2. (*A*) The calcaneal inclination angle is increased in the cavus foot because the hindfoot is already calcaneus despite the forefoot equinus. (*B*) Normal calcaneal inclination angle.

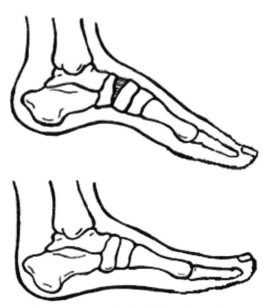

Fig. 3. The dorsal osteotomy improves the forefoot equinus without worsening the hind-foot calcaneus.

Prophylactic occupational therapy management of wrist and hand ROM is recommended to slow the development of contractures and to maintain fine motor skills for functional tasks, such as power wheelchair control. Nighttime resting splints, which promote wrist extension, metacarpophalangeal extension, and proximal interphalangeal flexion, are recommended to maintain active ROM as late as possible. Daytime positioning should emphasize wrist and finger extension, but any splinting should not compromise sensation or hand function. Passive stretching of the elbow flexors may be combined with passive stretch into forearm supination.

Patients with NMD with proximal shoulder girdle weakness have been managed with mobile arm supports; however, in the authors' experience, these often are prescribed but rarely accepted and used long term. A raised tray placed on the existing wheelchair lap tray or an elevating hospital bedside table can support the upper limbs in the same plane as the head. This allows the hand to still be brought to the mouth when less than antigravity strength of the elbow flexors is present. Alternatively, some patients choose to eat meals at higher counters or tables.

Surgical Management of Upper-Limb Contractures

Upper-limb contractures rarely require surgical intervention.[58] Release of elbow flexion contractures in EMD is not usually performed because of the high rate of contracture recurrence. Surgical intervention may be warranted if the reduced upper-limb ROM is impeding care and hygiene. This is especially important if the contracture is leading to skin breakdown or intolerable pain.

SUMMARY

Contractures are exceedingly common impairments in NMD, but weakness more often leads to disability. Less than antigravity strength produces an inability to achieve full active ROM. Static positioning of limbs and lack of active ROM result in progressive contractures. Aggressive rehabilitation interventions including stretching, positioning, and splinting in addition to orthopedic surgical interventions may help minimize the degree of disability caused by contractures in NMD.

REFERENCES

1. Spector SA, Simard CP, Fournier M, et al. Architectural alterations of rat hind-limb skeletal muscles immobilized at different lengths. Exp Neurol 1982;76(1):94–110.
2. Brooke MH, Fenichel GM, Griggs RC, et al. Duchenne muscular dystrophy: patterns of clinical progression and effects of supportive therapy. Neurology 1989;39(4):475–81.
3. Johnson EW. Walter J. Zeiter Lecture: pathokinesiology of Duchenne muscular dystrophy: implications for management. Arch Phys Med Rehabil 1977;58(1):4–7.
4. Sutherland DH, Olshen R, Cooper L, et al. The pathomechanics of gait in Duchenne muscular dystrophy. Dev Med Child Neurol 1981;23(1):3–22.
5. Archibald KC, Vignos PJ Jr. A study of contractures in muscular dystrophy. Arch Phys Med Rehabil 1959;40(4):150–7.
6. Johnson ER, Fowler WM Jr, Lieberman JS. Contractures in neuromuscular disease. Arch Phys Med Rehabil 1992;73:807–10.
7. Hsu JD, Furumasu J. Gait and posture changes in the Duchenne muscular dystrophy child. Clin Orthop Relat Res 1993;(288):122–5.
8. D'Angelo MG, Berti M, Piccinini L, et al. Gait pattern in Duchenne muscular dystrophy. Gait Posture 2009;29(1):36–41.
9. McDonald CM, Abresch RT, Carter GT, et al. Profiles of neuromuscular diseases. Duchenne muscular dystrophy. Am J Phys Med Rehabil 1995;74(Suppl):S70–92.
10. Dubowitz V. Progressive muscular dystrophy: prevention of deformities. Clin Pediatr (Phila) 1964;3:323–8.
11. Dubowitz V. Prevention of deformities. Isr J Med Sci 1977;13(2):183–8.
12. Fowler WM Jr. Rehabilitation management of muscular dystrophy and related disorders: II. Comprehensive care. Arch Phys Med Rehabil 1982;63(7):322–8.
13. Vignos PJ Jr. Physical models of rehabilitation in neuromuscular disease. Muscle Nerve 1983;6(5):323–38.
14. Siegel IM, Weiss LA. Postural substitution in Duchenne's muscular dystrophy. JAMA 1982;247(5):584.
15. McDonald CM, Abresch RT, Carter GT, et al. Profiles of neuromuscular diseases. Becker's muscular dystrophy. Am J Phys Med Rehabil 1995;74(Suppl 5):S93–103.
16. Scott OM, Hyde SA, Goddard C, et al. Quantitation of muscle function in children: a prospective study in Duchenne muscular dystrophy. Muscle Nerve 1982;5(4):291–301.
17. Vignos PJ Jr. Management of musculoskeletal complications in neuromuscular disease: limb contractures and the role of stretching, braces and surgery. Phys Med Rehabil: State of the Art Reviews. 1988;2:509–15.
18. Johnson ER, Abresch RT, Carter GT, et al. Profiles of neuromuscular diseases. Myotonic dystrophy. Am J Phys Med Rehabil 1995;74(Suppl 5):S104–16.
19. Dubowitz V. Muscle disorders in childhood. 2nd edition. Philadelphia: WB Saunders; 1995.
20. Kilmer DD, Abresch RT, McCrory MA, et al. Profiles of neuromuscular diseases. Facioscapulohumeral muscular dystrophy. Am J Phys Med Rehabil 1995;74(Suppl 5):S131–9.
21. Carter GT, Abresch RT, Fowler WM Jr, et al. Profiles of neuromuscular diseases. Spinal muscular atrophy. Am J Phys Med Rehabil 1995;74(Suppl 5):S150–9.

22. McDonald CM, Johnson ER, Abresch RT, et al. Profiles of neuromuscular diseases. Limb-girdle syndromes. Am J Phys Med Rehabil 1995;74(Suppl 5): S117–30.

23. Canavese F, Sussman MD. Orthopaedic manifestations of congenital myotonic dystrophy during childhood and adolescence. J Pediatr Orthop 2009;29(2): 208–13.

24. Iannaccone ST, Browne RH, Samaha FJ, et al. Prospective study of spinal muscular atrophy before age 6 years. DCN/SMA Group. Pediatr Neurol 1993; 9(3):187–93.

25. Willig TN, Bach JR, Rouffet MJ, et al. Correlation of flexion contractures with upper extremity function and pain for spinal muscular atrophy and congenital myopathy patients. Am J Phys Med Rehabil 1995;74(1):33–8.

26. Fujak A, Kopschina C, Gras F, et al. Contractures of the lower extremities in spinal muscular atrophy type II. Descriptive clinical study with retrospective data collection. Ortop Traumatol Rehabil 2011;13(1):27–36.

27. Fujak A, Kopschina C, Gras F, et al. Contractures of the upper extremities in spinal muscular atrophy type II. Descriptive clinical study with retrospective data collection. Ortop Traumatol Rehabil 2010;12(5):410–9.

28. Carter GT, Abresch RT, Fowler WM Jr, et al. Profiles of neuromuscular diseases. Hereditary motor and sensory neuropathy, types I and II. Am J Phys Med Rehabil 1995;74(Suppl 5):S140–9.

29. Rose KJ, Burns J, Wheeler DM, et al. Interventions for increasing ankle range of motion in patients with neuromuscular disease. Cochrane Database Syst Rev 2010;(2):CD006973.

30. Sackley C, Disler PB, Turner-Stokes L, et al. Rehabilitation interventions for foot drop in neuromuscular disease. Cochrane Database Syst Rev 2009;(3): CD003908.

31. Young P, De Jonghe P, Stögbauer F, et al. Treatment for Charcot-Marie-Tooth disease. Cochrane Database Syst Rev 2008;(1):CD006052.

32. Scott OM, Hyde SA, Goddard C, et al. Prevention of deformity in Duchenne muscular dystrophy. A prospective study of passive stretching and splintage. Physiotherapy 1981;67(6):177–80.

33. Abramson AS, Rogoff J. An approach to rehabilitation of children with muscular dystrophy, Proceedings of the First and Second Medical Conferences of the MDAA, Inc. New York: Muscular Dystrophy Association of America; 1953. p. 122–245.

34. Allsop KG, Ziter FA. Loss of strength and functional decline in Duchenne's dystrophy. Arch Neurol 1981;38(7):406–11.

35. Harris SE, Cherry DB. Childhood progressive muscular dystrophy and the role of physical therapy. Phys Ther 1974;54(1):4–12.

36. Seeger BR, Caudrey DJ, Little JD. Progression of equinus deformity in Duchenne muscular dystrophy. Arch Phys Med Rehabil 1985;66(5):286–8.

37. Williams EA, Read L, Ellis A, et al. The management of equinus deformity in Duchenne muscular dystrophy. J Bone Joint Surg Br 1984;66(4):546–50.

38. Vignos PJ Jr. Rehabilitation in the myopathies. In: Vinken PJ, Bruyn GW, editors. Handbook of clinical neurology. Amsterdam: North Holland Publishing; 1980. p. 457–500.

39. Vignos PJ Jr, Archibald KC. Maintenance of ambulation in childhood muscular dystrophy. J Chronic Dis 1960;12:273–90.

40. Vignos PJ Jr, Spencer GE, Archibald KC. Management of progressive muscular dystrophy in childhood. JAMA 1963;184:89–96.

41. Refshauge KM, Raymond J, Nicholson G, et al. Night splinting does not increase ankle range of motion in people with Charcot-Marie-Tooth disease: a randomised, cross-over trial. Aust J Physiother 2006;52(3):193–9.

42. Rose KJ, Raymond J, Refshauge K, et al. Serial night casting increases ankle dorsiflexion range in children and young adults with Charcot-Marie-Tooth disease: a randomised trial. J Physiother 2010;56(2):113–9.

43. Crosbie J, Burns J. Predicting outcomes in the orthotic management of painful, idiopathic pes cavus. Clin J Sport Med 2007;17(5):337–42.

44. Spencer GE, Vignos PJ Jr. Bracing for ambulation in childhood progressive muscular dystrophy. J Bone Joint Surg Am 1962;44:234–42.

45. Pardo AC, Do T, Ryder T, et al. Combination of steroids and ischial weight-bearing knee ankle foot orthoses in Duchenne's muscular dystrophy prolongs ambulation past 20 years of age: a case report. Neuromuscul Disord 2011;21(11):800–2.

46. Heckmatt JZ, Dubowitz V, Hyde SA, et al. Prolongation of walking in Duchenne muscular dystrophy with lightweight orthoses: review of 57 cases. Dev Med Child Neurol 1985;27(2):149–54.

47. Bakker JP, de Groot IJ, Beckerman H, et al. The effects of knee-ankle-foot orthoses in the treatment of Duchenne muscular dystrophy: review of the literature. Clin Rehabil 2000;14(4):343–59.

48. Garralda ME, Muntoni F, Cunniff A, et al. Knee-ankle-foot orthosis in children with Duchenne muscular dystrophy: user views and adjustment. Eur J Paediatr Neurol 2006;10(4):186–91.

49. Eyring EJ, Johnson EW, Burnett C. Surgery in muscular dystrophy. JAMA 1972; 222(8):1056–7.

50. Siegel IM, Miller JE, Ray RD. Subcutaneous lower limb tenotomy in the treatment of pseudohypertrophic muscular dystrophy. Description of technique and presentation of twenty-one cases. J Bone Joint Surg Am 1968;50(7):1437–43.

51. Spencer GE Jr. Orthopaedic care of progressive muscular dystrophy. J Bone Joint Surg Am 1967;49(6):1201–4.

52. Manzur AY, Hyde SA, Rodillo E, et al. A randomized controlled trial of early surgery in Duchenne muscular dystrophy. Neuromuscul Disord 1992;2(5–6): 379–87.

53. Leitch KK, Raza N, Biggar D, et al. Should foot surgery be performed for children with Duchenne muscular dystrophy? J Pediatr Orthop 2005;25(1):95–7.

54. Johnson BM, Child B, Hix J, et al. Cavus foot reconstruction in 3 patients with Charcot-Marie-Tooth disease. J Foot Ankle Surg 2009;48(2):116–24 PubMed PMID: 19232961.

55. Tullis BL, Mendicino RW, Catanzariti AR, et al. The Cole midfoot osteotomy: a retrospective review of 11 procedures in 8 patients. J Foot Ankle Surg 2004; 43(3):160–5.

56. Krause FG, Wing KJ, Younger AS. Neuromuscular issues in cavovarus foot. Foot Ankle Clin 2008;13(2):243–58.

57. Coleman SS, Chesnut WJ. A simple test for hindfoot flexibility in the cavovarus foot. Clin Orthop Relat Res 1977;(123):60–2.

58. Do T. Orthopedic management of the muscular dystrophies. Curr Opin Pediatr 2002;14(1):50–3.

Augmentative and Alternative Communication for People with Progressive Neuromuscular Disease

Laura J. Ball, PhD, CCC/SP[a],*, Susan Fager, PhD, CCC/SP[b],
Melanie Fried-Oken, PhD, CCC/SP[c]

KEYWORDS

- AAC • Amyotrophic lateral sclerosis • Duchenne muscular dystrophy
- Myotonic muscular dystrophy • Spinal muscular atrophy • Communication
- Assistive technology

KEY POINTS

- Augmentative and alternative communication (AAC) is considered standard practice in interventions for individuals with progressive neuromuscular disease.
- Individuals with progressive neuromuscular disease can maintain effective, functional communication by implementing AAC when natural speech no longer meets their needs.
- AAC strategies and systems may be customized to accommodate for individual needs by exploiting intact abilities (eg, spinal muscular atrophy distal movements, amyotrophic lateral sclerosis eye movements).
- New technologies under development promise access to communication systems for individuals with progressive neuromuscular diseases who previously were considered locked-in and unable to retain effective interactions (ie, brain-computer interface).

The purpose of this article was to (1) profile frequently occurring communication impairments associated with neuromuscular disease, (2) identify communication needs within an augmentative and alternative communication (AAC) framework, and (3) identify options for AAC supports. Four neuromuscular diseases are examined: amyotrophic

Funding sources: None.

Conflict of interest: None.

[a] Massachusetts General Hospital Institute of Health Professions, Communication Sciences and Disorders, 36 First Avenue, Charlestown Navy Yard, Boston, MA 02129-4557, USA; [b] Communication Center, Institute for Rehabilitation Science and Engineering, Madonna Rehabilitation Hospital, 5401 South Street, Lincoln, NE 68506, USA; [c] Neurology, Pediatrics, ENT, BME, Oregon Health & Science University, Portland, OR 97239-3098, USA

* Corresponding author.

E-mail address: ljball9134@gmail.com

lateral sclerosis (ALS), Duchenne muscular dystrophy (DMD), myotonic muscular dystrophy (MMD), and spinal muscular atrophy (SMA). Electronic databases including CINAHL, MEDLINE (PubMed), OVID, and EBM Reviews from January 1995 through March 2012 were queried. Search terms included the name(s) and acronyms of the disease (eg, for ALS: amyotrophic lateral sclerosis, ALS, Lou Gehrig's disease, motor neuron disease; for DMD: Duchenne muscular dystrophy, DMD, Duchenne, pseudohypertrophic; for MMD: myotonic muscular dystrophy, MMD, Steinert disease) AND dysarthria, communication disorder, speech, speech disorder, speaking, communication device, speech generating device, augmentative and alternative communication, technology/computer access, and assistive technology.

The review for ALS (amyotrophic lateral sclerosis, motor neuron disease, Lou Gehrig's disease and dysarthria, communication disorder, speech, speech disorder, speaking, communication device, speech-generating device, augmentative and alternative communication, and technology/computer access, assistive technology) yielded 122 different references and articles. There were no randomized controlled trials identified. Among those reporting data on ALS and AAC, 36 were published in peer-reviewed journals and presented outcome research and individual cohort studies (ie, levels 2b and 2c); these are presented in this document. Additionally, the literature review yielded no results for Duchenne, myotonic, or spinal muscular atrophy related to AAC.

AMYOTROPHIC LATERAL SCLEROSIS

Amyotrophic lateral sclerosis is a rapidly progressive paralyzing disease. Most individuals with ALS die within 2 to 5 years of onset.[1] No cure exists, and limited treatments are available; clinical management consists primarily of symptom management. Many people diagnosed with ALS participate in multidisciplinary clinics where they receive coordinated care from a neurologist and/or physiatrist, physical therapist, occupational therapist, speech-language pathologist, dietitian, social worker, respiratory therapist, and nurse case manager. In general, participation in multidisciplinary clinics is supported by evidence indicating increased use of effective interventions including riluzole, percutaneous endoscopic gastrostomy, and noninvasive ventilation, resulting in fewer hospitalizations.[2] The impact of ALS on a person's participation patterns will vary depending on the individual's life stage, ALS type, and life-extending decisions (eg, gastrostomy, ventilator).[3]

Communication Impairments in ALS

Because of the involvement of both upper and lower motor neurons in ALS, motor speech impairments result in a mixed spastic-flaccid dysarthria. Initial speech symptoms among people with ALS (pALS) vary, but a general pattern is often apparent. Initially, speaking rate slows, followed by moderate and then more severe reductions in intelligibility that affect overall communication effectiveness, and continued progression ultimately leaves the person with no functional speech (ie, anarthric).[4] Because there have been no controlled studies examining communication in ALS,[1] the American Academy of Neurology notes that there are insufficient data to support or refute treatment to optimize communication in ALS.[5] Still, because of progressive loss of natural speech, the standard of care for individuals with ALS indicates treatment emphasizing strategies for optimizing natural speech ("communication for as long as possible") and focusing on an individual's expressive language capabilities as well as communication effectiveness among various partners.

Although respiratory failure is the most common cause of death in ALS, mechanical ventilation can prolong life expectancy, but will not halt the relentless progression of paralysis. Noninvasive ventilation is often the initial treatment to alleviate respiratory symptoms and invasive ventilation via tracheostomy is proposed when noninvasive ventilation is no longer effective owing to disease progression, low tone in bulbar musculature, or difficulty with secretions.[6] When a pALS accepts mechanical ventilation, the clinician must be aware of and resolve incongruent decisions (ie, accepts mechanical ventilation to prolong life but refuses a speech-generating device [SGD] to provide communication even with ongoing functional decline). Similarly, when a pALS accepts ventilation, she or he requires ongoing intervention to ensure appropriate access accommodations to the SGD to maintain effective communication.

Customized AAC systems should be designed for each pALS that include means to communicate basic medical messages as well as new information for daily conversation; a way to "chat" or just casually interact; a means to access and use the telephone; options to call attention for assistance; and ways to express affection, humor, and emotions.[7] The AAC system should change as dysarthria progresses in ALS, with system components ranging from basic alphabet or symbol boards to computer-based SGDs.[6] One key indication for the use of AAC by pALS is that "functional communication is an essential component to improved quality of life for persons with severe physical limitations, such as those experienced by persons with ALS."[8(p377)] Although outcomes have not been studied systematically, individuals often comment on the value of the AAC system: "My computer has many functions. It is my writing system; my communication system (e-mail, fax), especially for family farther away; my information system; my database for addresses and other lists; my financial and legal organizer; my entertainment system; and, lastly, my speech system."[9(p124)]

AAC Acceptance in ALS

Caregivers who support individuals with ALS report very positive attitudes toward AAC technology, indicating greater rewards associated with caregiving and increased social closeness to the person with ALS.[7] AAC has a high level of acceptance among pALS, with nearly 96% accepting AAC technology (90% on initial recommendation, 6% following a delay) when provided with options in a timely manner.[10] One departure from this acceptance may be individuals with ALS who have co-occurring severe frontotemporal lobar dementia or accompanying severe health issues, as these may have a higher rejection rate of AAC technology and therefore require careful consideration.[10] Individuals who reject AAC technology may, however, implement strategies that do not rely on technology to support their communication, such as partner-supported scanning, hierarchical yes/no responses, and eye gaze to direct interactions.[4]

AAC Use in ALS

Individuals with ALS use AAC technology to sustain employment, program computers, access word processing to write documents, provide accounting services, and interact on the telephone and Internet.[11] Advances in technology promise greater access to interactions that support social, recreational, educational, commercial, volunteer, and employment activities.[12] Duration of AAC technology use may be dependent on factors including life expectancy, nutritional status, timelines for AAC provision, and decisions for life-prolonging procedures. In one report, individuals with ALS who acquire and use AAC technology continue to communicate using the same device for a mean duration of 28.4 months, with those who presented with spinal ALS having a mean duration of 32.1 months and those with bulbar ALS having a mean duration of 25.2 months.[8] Individuals with ALS who acquire AAC technology to support their communication continue to use the devices until the end of life, or within a couple weeks before death.[8]

ALS case study

Gil is a 39-year-old man who works at a large regional hospital as a data entry specialist in the Information Technology Department. Recently diagnosed with bulbar-onset ALS, Gil hopes to continue working as long as possible. At his most recent ALS clinic visit, the speech-language pathologist completed a brief evaluation and identified slowed speaking rate and mild dysarthria; she then referred him for an AAC evaluation. During the AAC evaluation, Gil had the opportunity to examine and try a variety of SGDs and together with his wife and teenage daughter, planned for his communication strategy. He already was using an iPad to keep his schedule, plan meetings, surf the Web/e-mail, and for entertainment. To minimize out-of-pocket expense but remain functionally communicative, his initial plan was to add a communication app (eg, Verbally [Intuary, Inc, San Francisco, CA, USA]) with an onscreen keyboard and synthesized voice output to his existing iPad. He purchased a small external speaker that was embedded in an iPad case so that the voice output would be loud enough to be heard in most of his communication situations. He used this system to interact with others at work, to participate in religious services, and when he went out to play cards with his friends. As Gil's ALS progressed, he began having difficulty using his hands to access the iPad keyboard and relied on a walker to steady himself while ambulating. At that point, his respiratory function had declined and he made the decision with his family to proceed with mechanical ventilation; subsequently, he also acquired a dedicated SGD to provide more access options. As he was also in the process of acquiring a power wheelchair (eg, Permobil [Permobil, Inc, Lebanon, TN, USA]), he selected a large-format SGD with eye gaze access (eg, Dynavox Eyemax [DynaVox Mayer-Johnson, Pittsburgh, PA, USA]) that could be mounted to the wheelchair and easily moved to another mount in his home. He used the SGD to communicate with coworkers until he resigned (10 months from initial iPad implementation) and continued using the SGD until approximately 1 week before death. During the final days of life, Gil used the SGD intermittently, but also used a partner-supported hierarchy of questions to which he responded *yes* by looking up and *no* by looking down.

DUCHENNE MUSCULAR DYSTROPHY

DMD is an X-linked recessive degenerative disease caused from absence of the dystrophin protein that stabilizes and protects muscle fibers.[13] Standards of care were recently developed by the DMD Care Considerations Working Group under the auspices of the US Centers for Disease Control and Prevention.[14] Among others, the recommendations included the multidisciplinary approach and the multidisciplinary team, including a speech-language pathologist, as a key aspect of care.

Communication Impairments in DMD

Speech intelligibility decreases because of deteriorating respiratory support. Compensatory strategies, speech amplification, and AAC become appropriate as communication becomes increasingly limited.[14]

DMD case study

RJ is a 26-year-old man with DMD who resides in an adult foster home in a rural community. RJ graduated from the local high school 5 years ago without any means to control his environment, no computer for writing, recreation, or employment. He did not have a means to explore the Internet for information. He is currently quadriplegic with strained respiration. He can move his head and has control of his eye movements and eye blinks. He does have a significant head tilt to the right, which affects his face-to-face eye contact for conversation. RJ uses a wheelchair for mobility that is pushed by his caregivers. He leans forward in his chair to facilitate respiration. RJ relies on speech with significantly reduced volume for spontaneous personal communication (Melanie Fried-Oken, 2010), as well as for calling attention, talking on a speakerphone, and managing his medical needs. When he is travelling in his adapted van, he does not have an effective means to speak with the driver or other passengers. RJ came to the AAC clinic looking for a means to control his computer to surf the Internet and write. Language and cognitive testing indicated that this young man had receptive and expressive language skills that were within normal limits for adults. He was an adequate speller and enjoyed reading magazines when someone held them up and turned pages for him. With assistance from a clinical consultant at Words+, RJ tried to use an SGD accessed through advanced eye gaze technology. A computer with a low-voltage USB camera (EyePro GS [Words+, Inc, Lancaster, CA, USA]) was set up in front of him, and he learned how to use his eyes to control a mouse and select letters from an on-screen keyboard. After an initial evaluation, RJ worked with the consultant through remote training sessions. The consultant and RJ would meet on Skype, where she could watch RJ practice eye control with different computer applications over multiple sessions. He learned how to set up an e-mail account, surf the Internet, and compose text with specialized word processing software (called E Z Keys [Words+, Inc, Lancaster, CA, USA]) that provided keystroke enhancement techniques for word prediction, macros, and text storage. RJ acquired the necessary technology through his medical insurance. He now has an effective AAC system that includes an SGD for writing and environmental control, head nods, facial expression, and smiles for face-to-face communication, and a simple voice amplifier (the Chattervox, Indian Creek, IL, USA) for increasing his speaking volume when he is in a room alone and needs medical assistance or is in the van with a driver or other passengers. He still relies on caregivers to set up the computer and EyePro so that he can use it for different tasks, but his access to the world, his acquisition of new knowledge through the Internet, and his quality of life have been enhanced by current assistive technology.

MYOTONIC MUSCULAR DYSTROPHY

MMD is an autosomal dominant disease that may be evident at birth (the congenital form is more severe) or more commonly in teenage or adult years.[15] Myotonia is characterized by slow relaxation of muscles following voluntary contraction that may require repeated attempts to ultimately return to a neutral position (ie, prolonged muscle contractions).[16] Cognitive impairment, executive dysfunction, and avoidant personality traits, eventually deteriorating with age, have been described.[17]

Communication Impairments in MMD

In addition to the motor deficits, up to 51% of children with MMD may demonstrate symptoms of autism spectrum disorder, 83% to 95% have moderate to severe learning disability, and 94% to 100% have problems with social interaction. The relationship between MMD type and cognitive function illustrate that with more severity, the IQ (ie, Wechsler Intelligence Scale for Children–III full-scale IQ [severe M = 40.3, mild M = 27.9]) and adaptive skill scores (ie, Vineland Adaptive Behavior Scales; severe M = 36.5, mild M = 44.8) may be lower.[18] Although impaired, children with MMD have relative strengths with verbal understanding (eg, vocabulary, similarities) and receptive language.[18] For AAC, it is important to consider that the myotonia may influence an individual with MMD regarding access, particularly direct access that requires muscle contraction and release. AAC systems should be programmed to support expressive communication and exploit stronger receptive language abilities.

SPINAL MUSCULAR ATROPHY

SMA is a recessively inherited neuromuscular disease characterized by degeneration of spinal cord (ie, lower) motor neurons, resulting in progressive muscular atrophy and weakness. There is a broad spectrum of severity ranging from early infant death to normal adult life span with only mild weakness. There are unique clinical features of each SMA type and heterogeneous clinical features are used to classify various phenotypes. Some features of SMA that may affect communication include impaired head control, tongue atrophy, weakness and hypotonia in limbs and trunk, typical cognitive and emotional development, delayed motor milestones (proximal more than distal), and severe respiratory weakness.[19]

Communication Impairments in SMA

Flaccid dysarthria and swallowing impairments occur among individuals with SMA, the severity of which will vary based on the SMA type and overall disease severity.[20] The natural history of SMA involves inspiratory, expiratory, and bulbar weakness that may affect communication, particularly in types 1 and 2. Because strength tends to be preserved in distal (eg, extremities) more than proximal structures (eg, head/neck), a focus on access to AAC via distal body movements (eg, hands, fingers, toes) may be recommended. The young age of the most severe forms of SMA also implies a need for adapting AAC for preliterate children by using transparent symbols and photographs that are readily associated with the item.

AAC TECHNOLOGIES FOR COMPLEX COMMUNICATION NEEDS

Because the progressive nature of neurodegenerative disorders often ultimately results in the complete loss of functional upper extremity and lower extremity skills, access to traditional AAC systems can become challenging. Although the preponderance of research in AAC for people with neuromuscular diseases has focused on ALS, the technologies described may be used to provide support to people with other neuromuscular impairments (eg, DMD, MDD, SMA).

Eye Gaze Tracking

Because of the ongoing progression of ALS and subsequent loss of upper extremity function, direct access to AAC technology is most commonly accomplished using eye gaze technologies at present.[21] Eye movements of individuals with ALS are typically spared but occasional impairments are identified (eg, oculomotor apraxia, reduced saccade velocity, eyelid opening/closure) making trial use of eye gaze–based AAC technology essential in determining effectiveness.[22] Previous studies have examined eye movement in ALS and identified decreased saccadic velocity and some abnormal saccadic patterns (eg, overlapping, low velocity, long duration) along with fewer eye movements.[23] Assessment of eye fatigue has been limited in ALS research, but reports indicate that eye gaze can be an effective means of AAC input.[24]

Infrared eye-tracking technology projects a safe, invisible infrared light that causes a reflection on the pupil of the person's eye. Paired with the infrared light, AAC technology uses software to triangulate eye movement to track items on screen. When the person's eye(s) dwells on a location, the system selects the item and thereby assembles a message; which, when paired with synthesized voice output will "speak." Compared with scanning through items on screen and selecting the desired item with a switch, eye control has been found to produce faster messages with reduced error rates for people with ALS.[25]

Head Movement Tracking

Tracking of head movements may be accomplished by infrared or video cameras, with the most common application using infrared technologies. Head movement tracking uses similar methods of capture, but track movement of a reflective surface (eg, dot, sphere) instead of eye movements. Essentially, this technology allows the head movements to "take over" the computer mouse and operate the AAC technology. Selections, as with eye tracking, are made using a dwell function or a secondary switch.[26]

A second form of head tracking is accomplished using laser pointers mounted to the head or other body part (eg, headband, glasses frame, cap, sock, hand). The laser beam is directed to the item for communicating a message. With concerns regarding the eye safety of laser beams, a Safe-Laser was developed. The Safe-Laser System (Invotek, Inc, Alma, AR, USA.) operates at a low, eye-safe level until directed uninterrupted at a laser safe surface. The surface can then be programmed with AAC technology for message formulation and may be an effective strategy for some individuals with ALS.[27]

Gesture Tracking

Currently, eye-tracking and head-tracking technology uses a dwell function to select items on a screen to assemble messages. Gesture input strategies are now emerging that allow more precise targeting and activation of items on a display, but typically require touchscreen access (eg, SWYPE [Nuance Communications, Inc, Burlington, MA, USA]).[28] Recently, a prototype (ie, Gesture-Enhanced Word Prediction [Invotek, Inc, Alma, AR, USA]) has been developed to take head and hand movement tracking and translate it into the gesture interface for faster, more accurate message assembly and production by reducing the number of precise dwells that are required to generate text.[29]

Speech Recognition

Use of speech recognition has increased and has been incorporated into mainstream technologies (eg, smart phones, tablets); however, commercially available speech recognition has been developed for a market of typical (nondisabled) users. For individuals with dysarthria, this technology remains largely inaccessible, as it does not recognized moderate to severely dysarthric speech[30–32]; however, technology is being developed that uses speech recognition based on models of dysarthric speech.[33–37] Applications include environmental control and specific software programs with limited recognition vocabulary sets. Others have investigated the use of dysarthric speech recognition along with electromyography signals to increase accuracy,[38] or the use of alphabet supplementation and language modeling to develop a functional writing and communication system for individuals with moderate and severe dysarthria.[39] As researchers and developers begin to look at speech recognition as part of an "input" system to computerized technology, individuals with neuromuscular conditions will be able to functionally use the technology to support writing and communication.

Brain-Computer Interface

Another input system that is receiving considerable research attention for individuals with severe neuromuscular impairments is the novel brain-computer interface (BCI).[40]

The technology for BCI relies on a signal detection system that translates neuronal activity into device demands. The components necessary for functional BCI have matured sufficiently that we can imagine devices that are powered by mere thoughts. There are 3 recognized categories for BCI: the invasive BCI records neuronal action potentials (spikes) or local field potentials when a circuit board is actually placed directly on to the cortex.[41] One publicized invasive BCI is the Braingate Neural Interface System where intracortical microelectrode sensors read control signals directly from the motor cortex.[42] Noninvasive BCI relies on recording sites at the scalp for electroencephalography or on magnetic brain forces: magnetoencephalography. A final technique is a "partially invasive" BCI: electrocorticography, which uses sensors placed within the skull but outside gray matter. The noninvasive methods must filter artifact from a signal that is far from its source, but filtering techniques are improving rapidly so that the advantages of lower cost, portability, lack of concern for infection, avoiding surgery, and faster application are improving their appeal.

BCI for communication is being examined worldwide. Reports of functional use for daily tasks are beginning to appear for individuals with ALS or spinal cord injuries as a means to significantly improve quality of life and productivity.[43,44] The RSVP Keyboard (under development by Cognitive Systems Laboratory, Northeastern University, Boston, MA, USA) is one noninvasive system that incorporates language models into signal acquisition to monopolize on word prediction and completion for spelling.[45] The P300 speller is another noninvasive BCI that has been used by individuals with ALS.[46] BCI will one day be a clinically available tool for increasing independent daily function. It has much to offer as a promising access method for people with severe neuromuscular impairment as a tool to improve quality of life and support participation for communication, environmental control, and computer access.

SUMMARY

Individuals with progressive neuromuscular disease often develop complex communication needs and consequently find that interaction using their natural speech may not sufficiently meet their daily needs. Increasingly, assistive technology advances provide accommodations for and/or access to communication. Although research evaluating the use of AAC across all neuromuscular disease is severely lacking, studies in ALS suggest that use of an AAC is generally well accepted and improves quality of life. AAC systems continue to be designed and implemented to provide targeted assistance based on an individual's changing needs. Advanced technologies using BCI are becoming more readily available and have the potential to extend access to communication to even the most severely disabled patient with neuromuscular disease.

REFERENCES

1. Miller R, Jackson C, Kasarskis E, et al. Practice parameter update: the care of the patient with amyotrophic lateral sclerosis (an evidence-based review). Report of the Quality Standards Subcommittee of the American Academy of Neurology. Neurology 2009;73(15):1227–33.
2. Chio A, Bottacci E, Buffa C, et al. Positive effects of tertiary centres for amyotrophic lateral sclerosis on outcome and use of hospital facilities. J Neurol Neurosurg Psychiatr 2006;77:948.
3. Beukelman DR, Fager S, Ball L, et al. AAC for adults with acquired neurological conditions: a review. Augment Altern Commun 2007;23(3):230–42.
4. Ball LJ, Beukelman DR, Bardach L. Amyotrophic lateral sclerosis. In: Beukelman DR, Garrett KL, Yorkston KM, editors. Augmentative communication

strategies for adults with acute or chronic medical conditions. Baltimore (MD): Paul H. Brookes; 2007. p. 87.

5. Miller R, Rosenberg J, Gelinas D, et al. Practice parameter: the care of the patient with amyotrophic lateral sclerosis (an evidence-based review): report of the Quality Standards Subcommittee of the American Academy of Neurology. Neurology 1999;52(7):1311.

6. Andersen PM, Borasio G, Dengler R, et al. Good practice in the management of amyotrophic lateral sclerosis: clinical guidelines. An evidence-based review with good practice points. EALSC Working Group. Amyotroph Lateral Scler 2007;8(4):195.

7. Fried-Oken M, Fox L, Rau MT, et al. Purposes of AAC device use for persons with ALS as reported by caregivers. Augment Altern Commun 2006;22(3): 209–21.

8. Ball LJ, Beukelman DR, Anderson E, et al. Duration of AAC technology use by persons with ALS. J Med Speech Lang Pathol 2007;15(4):371–81.

9. Houston S. Reflections on a kayak expedition in Scotland. In: Fried-Oken M, Bersani H, editors. Speaking up and spelling it out. Baltimore (MD): Paul H. Brookes Publishing; 2006. p. 209.

10. Ball LJ, Beukelman DR, Pattee GL. Acceptance of augmentative and alternative communication technology by persons with amyotrophic lateral sclerosis. Augment Altern Commun 2004;20(2):113–22.

11. McNaughton D, Light J, Groszyk L. "Don't give up": employment experiences of individuals with amyotrophic lateral sclerosis who use augmentative and alternative communication. Augment Altern Commun 2001;17(3):179–95.

12. Shane HC, Blackstone S, Vanderheiden G, et al. Using AAC technology to access the world. Assist Technol 2012;24:3.

13. Richman S, Schub T. Quick lesson about. Duchenne's muscular dystrophy. Glendale (CA): Cinahl Information Systems; 2011.

14. Bushby K, Finkel R, Birnkrant DJ, et al. Diagnosis and management of Duchenne muscular dystrophy, part 2: implementation of multidisciplinary care. Lancet Neurol 2010;9:77.

15. Muscular Dystrophy Association, 2011. Facts about myotonic muscular dystrophy. Available at www.mdausa.org.

16. National library of medicine. Myotonic dystrophy. 2010. Available at: http://ghr. nlm.nih.gov/condition/myotonic-dystrophy. Accessed May 17, 2012.

17. Modoni A, Silvestri G, Vita MG, et al. Cognitive impairment in myotonic dystrophy type 1 (DM1): a longitudinal follow-up study. Arch Neurol 2008;61:1943.

18. Ekström A, Hakenas-Plate L, Tulinius M. Cognition and adaptive skills in myotonic dystrophy type 1: a study of 55 individuals with congenital and childhood forms. Dev Med Child Neurol 2009;51:982.

19. Wang CH, Finkel RS, Bertini ES, et al. Consensus statement for standard of care in spinal muscular atrophy. J Child Neurol 2007;22:1027.

20. Duffy JR. Flaccid dysarthrias. In: Motor speech disorders: substrates, differential diagnosis and management. 2nd edition. Philadelphia: Elsevier Mosby; 2005. p. 112–413.

21. Ball LJ, Nordness AS, Fager SK, et al. Eye-gaze access to AAC technology for people with amyotrophic lateral sclerosis (augmentative and alternative communication) (Report). J Med Speech Lang Pathol 2010;18(3):9.

22. Zadikoff C, Lang AE. Apraxia in movement disorders. Brain 2005;128:1480.

23. Leveille A. Eye movements in amyotrophic lateral sclerosis. Arch Neurol 1982; 39:684.

24. Calvo A, Chio A, Castellina W, et al. Eye tracking impact on quality-of-life of ALS patients. In: Miesenberger K, editor. Computers helping people with special needs. Berlin: Springer-Verlag; 2008. p. 70.

25. Gibbons C, Beneteau E. Functional performance using eye control and single switch scanning by people with ALS. Perspect Augment Altern Commun 2010; 19(3):64–9.

26. Fager S, Beukelman DR, Fried-Oken M, et al. Access interface strategies. Assist Technol 2012;24(1):25.

27. Fager S, Beukelman DR, Karantounis R, et al. Use of Safe-Laser access technology to increase head movement in persons with severe motor impairment: a series of case reports. Augment Altern Commun 2006;22(3):222.

28. Kushler C, Marsden R. Swype. Computer access software. 2002.

29. Fager S, Jakobs T, Beukelman DR. New AAC access strategy for gesture tracking: a technical note. Perspect Augment Altern Commun 2011;21(1):11.

30. Young V, Mihailidis A. Difficulties in automatic speech recognition of dysarthric speakers and implications for speech-based applications used by the elderly: a literature review. Assist Technol 2010;22:99.

31. Raghavendra P, Rosengren E, Hunnicutt S. An investigation of different degrees of dysarthric speech as input to speaker-adaptive and speaker-dependent recognition systems. Augment Altern Commun 2001;17:265.

32. Magnuson T, Blomberg M. Acoustic analysis of dysarthric speech and some implications for automatic speech recognition. TMH-QPSR 2000;41:19.

33. Hawley M, Enderby P, Green P, et al. A speech-controlled environmental control system for people with severe dysarthria. Med Eng Phys 2007;29(5):586.

34. Judge S, Robertson Z, Hawley M, et al. Speech-driven environmental control systems—a qualitative analysis of users' perceptions. Disabil Rehabil Assist Technol 2009;4:151.

35. Development of an automatic recognizer for dysarthric speech. Proceedings of the RESNA Annual Conference. Phoenix (AZ): RESNA; 2007.

36. Omar S, Morales C, Cox S. Modeling errors in automatic speech recognition for dysarthric speakers. EURASIP J Adv Signal Process 2009. Available at: http://www.hindawi.com/journals/asp/2009/308340.html. Accessed July 6, 2012.

37. Hamidi F, Baljko M, Livingston N, et al. CanSpeak: a customizable speech interface for people with dysarthric speech. Lect Notes Comput Sci 2010; 6179:605.

38. Deng Y, Patel R, Heaton J, et al. Disordered speech recognition using acoustic and sEMG signals. INTERSPEECH 2009;644.

39. Fager S, Beulekman D, Jakobs T, et al. Evaluation of a speech recognition prototype for speakers with moderate and severe dysarthria: a preliminary report. Augment Altern Commun 2010;26:267.

40. Daly J, Wolpaw J. Brain-computer interfaces in neurological rehabilitation. Lancet Neurol 2008;7:1032.

41. Wolpaw J, Birbaumer N. Brain-computer interfaces for communication and control. Textbook of neural repair and rehabilitation, vol. 1. Cambridge (United Kingdom): Cambridge University Press; 2006. p. 602.

42. Hochberg L, Bacher D, Jarosiewicz B, et al. Reach and grasp by people with tetraplegia using a neutrally controlled robotic arm. Nature 2012;285(7398):372.

43. Sellers E, Vaughan TM, Wolpaw JR. A brain-computer interface for long-term independent home use. Amyotroph Lateral Scler 2010;11(5):449.

44. Nijboer F, Sellers E, Mellinger J, et al. A P300-based brain-computer interface for people with amyotrophic lateral sclerosis. Clin Neurophysiol 2008;119:1909.

45. Orhan U, Erdogmus D, Roark B, et al. Fusion with language models improves spelling accuracy for ERP-based brain computer interface spellers. Boston: IEEE Engineering in Medicine and Biology Society; 2011:5774–7.

46. Sellers EW, Donchin E. A P300-based brain-computer interface: initial tests by ALS patients. Clin Neurophysiol 2006;117(3):538–48.

Robotics, Assistive Technology, and Occupational Therapy Management to Improve Upper Limb Function in Pediatric Neuromuscular Diseases

Tariq Rahman, PhD[a,b,*], Joseph Basante, MA, MS, OTR/L, CHT[c],
Michael Alexander, MD[d,c]

KEYWORDS

- Robotics • Occupational therapy management • Assistive technology
- Pediatric neuromuscular diseases

KEY POINTS

- Description of current occupational therapy assessment methods for children with neuromuscular disabilities is presented.
- Methods of occupational therapy treatment are provided for neuromuscular conditions.
- Homemade adaptive equipment descriptions and methods are provided.
- State-of-the-art robotics and orthoses, to improve function and mobility for neuromuscular conditions, are becoming more widely available. A review of these options is provided.

INTRODUCTION

In treating patients with neuromuscular conditions, occupational therapists (OT) are concerned with the patients' acquisition and maintenance of skills necessary to perform daily tasks, such as feeding, dressing, grooming, toileting, functional mobility, communication, and play. This article addresses primarily upper-extremity issues faced by people with neuromuscular disorders, such as Charcot Marie Tooth (CMT),

[a] Department of Biomedical Research, Nemours/Alfred I duPont Hospital for Children, 1600 Rockland Road, Wilmington, DE 19899, USA; [b] Department of Mechanical Engineering, University of Delaware, 126 Spencer Laboratory, Newark, DE 19716, USA; [c] Department of Occupational Therapy, Nemours/Alfred I duPont Hospital for Children, 1600 Rockland Road, Wilmington, DE 19899, USA; [d] Pediatrics and Physical Medicine and Rehabilitation, Thomas Jefferson University, 1020 Walnut Street, Philadelphia, PA 19107, USA
* Corresponding author. Department of Mechanical Engineering, University of Delaware, 126 Spencer Laboratory, Newark, DE 19107.
E-mail address: trahman@nemours.org

Phys Med Rehabil Clin N Am 23 (2012) 701–717
http://dx.doi.org/10.1016/j.pmr.2012.06.008
1047-9651/12/$ – see front matter © 2012 Published by Elsevier Inc.

brachial plexus palsy injuries, arthrogryposis multiplex congenita (AMC), spinal muscular atrophy (SMA), and muscular dystrophy (MD).

When treating patients with neuromuscular disorders, it is a particular challenge to the treating therapist because of the lack of homogeneity in physical, cognitive, perceptual, and emotional presentation within the same diagnosis. Smith[1] states, "the OTs view the child, the child's environment and the interaction between the child and the environment in a holistic way." She also states that the OT must determine whether limitations in performance are caused by the external environment (which is ever changing), intrinsic patient-centered factors, or a combination of extrinsic and intrinsic factors. The next statement by Smith clearly puts into focus the challenge for the practitioner in the treatment of the child with neuromuscular disorders when she states, "although functional performance can be divided into specific skills and skill components, it is the spirit of a child that holds these components together. The maturation of a child and the complexity of the interrelationships between mind and body and between physical and social development are beyond human analytic ability."[1]

Effective treatment techniques require a particular philosophy and groundwork in evidence-based research, but the treating therapist must also be willing to adapt and change therapeutic approaches as the patients' long- and short-term physical and emotional responses warrants. The variable presentation can manifest as weakness, which may or may not be progressive. This group may include conditions with sensory loss, such as in CMT, or alterations in sensory processing, systemic sequelae, and concomitant impairment in cognitive abilities.

Historical and current treatment techniques range from neurophysiological and developmental,[2] biomechanical,[3] cognitive and psychosocial,[4,5] and sensory integration.[6] These treatment strategies can be divided into 3 broad categories: remedial approaches, compensatory approaches, and a combination of both. The remedial approach concerns the restoration of physiologic, cognitive/perceptual, and emotional balance via improving strength, flexibility, coordination, cognition, visual perception and the integration of environmental stimuli. The compensatory approach focuses on the continual adaptation of the environment to the person and vice versa.

The use of assistive devices and assistive technology (AT) in environmental modification has been used in OT practice for many years.[7–9] This practice could include the use of low-technology devices, such as swivel spoons and button hook devices; adaptive equipment, such as a self-feeding apparatus and overhead slings; augmentative communication devices; and robots and exoskeletal systems.

Robots and therapy machines are increasingly finding their way into clinics and research facilities as a means to provide repetitive, labor-intensive therapy and AT to patients with neuromuscular disorders. Although this technology is still in its infancy and its effectiveness is still unproven, it is starting to demonstrate positive outcomes in patients with various types of broader neuromuscular conditions, including stroke,[10] cerebral palsy,[11–13] spinal cord injury (SCI), MD, and SMA.[14,15]

The next section discusses the upper-extremity presentation. This discussion is followed by OT technology, techniques, and evaluations that are currently used. The last section describes the use of robots and machines in the treatment of neuromuscular disorders.

UPPER-EXTREMITY PRESENTATION

Neuromuscular conditions present in 2 distinct motor patterns: (1) those that initially present with proximal weakness while sparing fine-motor muscles until later in the condition and (2) those that present with distal weakness first and are accompanied with a loss of position, kinesthetic, and proprioceptive awareness. The latter tend to affect fine-motor control, which makes simple tasks, like buttoning a shirt, arduous. The following neuromuscular conditions are considered in this article.

CMT is the most common of the hereditary motor-sensory neuropathies and presents with distal intrinsic muscle wasting and sensory disturbances.

Brachial plexus palsy injuries fall into the traumatic and obstetric category. The most common being the obstetric upper-nerve trunk injury, termed Erb palsy. Upper-trunk injuries result in weakness about the shoulder that affects arm placement, taking away a stable platform for using the distal arm, which is rich in sensory feedback. Additionally, brachial plexus injuries of the lower trunk can result in an insensate hand with no hand intrinsic muscle function.

AMC is a consequence of an intrauterine loss of movement, which results in joint contractures. Most commonly, it is the result of an intrauterine loss of anterior horn cells and, in most cases, a sparing of sensation and proprioception.

SMA is the result of a progressive loss of anterior horn cells caused by genetic mutations. It is characterized by a loss of motor power, initially affecting proximal, then progressing to distal musculature with sensory sparing.

MD is a group of hereditary muscle disorders that present with a progressive loss of muscle fibers with a resultant loss of strength proximally at first and then progressing distally. This condition also benefits from sensory and proprioceptive sparing.

OT ASSESSMENT

The purpose of OT assessments in neuromuscular disorders is to objectively identify those deficit areas that negatively impact occupational performance. An excellent compendium of hand therapy/upper-extremity assessment measures can be found in Goldfarb and colleagues.[16] They identify and give a brief summary regarding general descriptions and citations for each evaluation. The evaluations are divided between criterion based with normative ranges and self-report scales. Richardson[17] reviewed criteria for the underlying rationale for all standard assessments and standardized tests that have uniform procedures for administration and scoring. Tests can either be criterion referenced or norm referenced. Norm referenced tests refer to how the child performs relative to standard scores for age and gender. Criterion referenced tests refer to how the child's performance relates to an expected level of performance or set criterion.

The results of the standardized assessments are important for establishing a therapeutic baseline of performance by identifying deficits in functional performance. They are also extremely helpful in establishing a rationale for the payment of services by second-party payers, therapy program efficacy, and in the establishment of treatment goals. Some of the limitations of these standardized tests are in the construct and content validity, that is, their ability to accurately assess a true relationship between score and limitation in occupational performance. The validity and reliability of a great number of these evaluations have not been studied in many populations with rare neuromuscular disorders. More systematic reviews into the reliability and construct validity of various upper-extremity assessment tools are available as references.[18,19]

Although the importance of standardized testing and assessment has been established, it is by no means the only method of assessment of performance deficits in children with a neuromuscular disease. In fact, a combination of standardized testing, interpretation of skilled clinical observations, ecological assessments (contextual interaction between the child and her environment), and subjective interview of patients or caregivers[20] are all used to capture the intricacy and nuance of functional occupational performance deficits in these patients. A comprehensive neuromuscular examination for the OT practitioner must be custom tailored for each child based on both physiologic and psychosocial variables along with the patients' or parent's expectations and social customs regarding the course.

The interview portion of the OT assessment is integrally important. It should assess whether the child's symptomology has improved, stabilized, or worsened and, if so, over what time frame. It should also ascertain subjective concerns of the patients or parents. It is an opportunity to give the patients or parents an opportunity to candidly discuss contextually relevant developmental and occupational performance concerns.

In addition to the aforementioned standardized assessment tools, an OT assessment for the child may include the following parameters when applicable:

1. Assessment of the pain level at rest and with normal activities: numeric rating or visual analog scale for patients old enough or cognitively aware enough to conceptualize and verbalize the continuum of pain (graded from 0 [no pain] to 10 [excruciating pain]) (Other scales used to assess pain in the pediatric population can be found at the National Institutes of Health (NIH) Pain Consortium Website.[21] Some of the scales are appropriate for children and adults and others are used for infants. Researchers at the NIH Clinical Center use the following: Wong-Baker Faces, COMFORT Scale, Crying, Requires O2, Increased vital signs, Expression, Sleeplessness [CRIES] Pain Scale, and the Faces, Legs, Activity, Cry, Consolability [FLACC] scale).
2. Postural analysis: cervical, thoracic, and lumbar alignment in standing, sitting, supine, prone, and quadruped positions; scapular arthrokinematics (winging, tipping, elevation at rest and in loaded positions, dyskinesis); and trunk control
3. Upper-extremity active and passive range of motion
4. Joint deformities: fixed contractures with interpretation of joint end feel, swan-neck deformities, Boutonniere deformities, Jeanne's sign related to hyperlaxity of the thumb metacarpal phalangeal joint, intrinsic wasting, thenar wasting, hypothenar wasting, intrinsic plus or minus positioning
5. Assessment of sensibility: Semmes-Weinstein monofilament, 2-point discrimination, stereognosis
6. Coordination: dysmetria, proprioception, kinesthesia, stereognosis, static and dynamic sitting, and standing balance
7. Assessment of tonicity: hypotonia, hypertonia, rigidity, spasticity, mixed patterns, choreiform, athetoid (use of Ashworth scale to assess tonicity)[22]
8. Assessment of reflexive integration/automatic reactions; assessment for primitive reflexive patterns present past expected age of integration or absence or delays in equilibrium and protective reactions[20]
9. Transitional movement patterns: rolling, sit to prone and prone to sit, supine to sit, pull to stand and stand to sit with and without rotation[20]
10. Ocular and ocular motor screening: visual focus, tracking, esotropia, exotropia, nystagmus,[20] ptosis, enophthalmos
11. Functional fine-motor skills: prehension patterns, hand preference, writing and cutting skills[20]
12. Strength: grip, pinch,[23] manual muscle testing[24]

OCCUPATIONAL THERAPY TREATMENT

Occupational therapy treatment techniques for children with musculoskeletal are based on a multitude of factors as detailed previously in the section on assessment.

One important concept when working with children with neuromuscular disorders is to determine whether the intervention implemented is to restore function and/or adapt to the environment. For those conditions that are classified as lower motor neuron diseases with a subtype of anterior horn involvement, such as SMA, care must be taken to avoid excessive fatigue during strength-training exercises because of neural rather than muscular fatigue and the potential for sarcolemmal membrane injury in response to increased mechanical loads, especially in those with rapidly progressive disease.[25]

REMEDIATION TECHNIQUES

1. Range of motion: Poorer prognosis have been associated in those children who present impaired external rotation of the shoulder.[26]
2. Strength: Use Thera-Bands (The Hygenic Corporation, Akron, OH, USA), light weights, and manual resistance working proximal to distal whenever possible. There seems to be no benefit from high-resistance, low-repetition resistance training[25] because of a possibility of weakening with those with slowly progressing neuromuscular diseases. Care must be taken with individuals with rapidly progressing neuromuscular diseases because there may be a likelihood of weakening because of some strength-training exercises. However, there are no conclusive data that show an equivocal relationship between all types of strength training and the loss of strength within these populations. Prudence would dictate that all strength-training programs for both slowly progressing and rapidly progressing neuromuscular diseases are submaximal and function based (play, recreation) in nature. Light theraputty (Sammons Preston Roylan, Bolingbrook, IL, USA) can be used to enhance grip and pinch strength and light grippers during play and game activity can be used to manipulate game pieces and dice. Submaximal isometrics at varying joint angles may also be helpful as are place/hold exercises with varying degrees of gravitational offloading.
3. Sensory enhancement/desensitization: Techniques, such as fluidotherapy, transcutaneous electrical nerve stimulation at submotor threshold, retrograde massage, and gentle soft tissue mobilization, may be beneficial in decreasing neurogenic pain. Depending on the condition and current status of functioning sensibility, sensory retraining techniques may be beneficial.
4. Many remediation techniques have been used with a myriad of neuromuscular conditions in the past including the following:
   a. Bobath or neurodevelopmental treatment in which specialized neuromuscular handling techniques can be used to facilitate postural control and movement coordination are used.[27]
   b. Rood techniques are used to normalize tone through the use of certain appropriately applied sensory stimuli.[8]
   c. Brunnstrom techniques that use reflexes, associated proprioceptive facilitation or exteroreceptive facilitation to develop muscle tension in preparation for voluntary movement.[3]
   d. The OT task-oriented approach incorporates a client-centered approach influenced by developmental and motor learning theories.[23]
   e. The Carr and Shepherd theoretical framework includes the dynamic system theory of motor control and the plasticity of central nervous system.[28]
   f. Constraint-induced movement therapy[29] also uses the concept of neuroplasticity or the ability to cortically reorganize with focused concentrated therapy.

COMPENSATORY TECHNIQUES

Compensatory techniques can affect the use of assistive and adaptive equipment and alterations of the physical environment. It can have many considerations, including the following:

- What is the gadget tolerance of the children and parents?
- What is the weight, size, and balance of the equipment?
- What is the expense of the equipment?
- Is it easy to maintain and durable?
- Does it really help?
- Is it safe?
- Will it accommodate a growing child?
- Is it socially and culturally acceptable to patients, parents, or caregivers?
- Is it contextually relevant and adaptable to a multitude of changing environments at home and in the community?

There are excellent compendiums available[7] regarding environmental adaptations, stabilization procedures and applications, and developmental sequences.

Consideration must be given to the amount of other medical equipment the child may have when prescribing adaptive equipment. Examples of other equipment are wheelchairs, walkers, leg braces, thoracolumbosacral orthosis, nasogastric tubes, and percutaneous indwelling catheter lines. Care must be taken that any equipment given does not itself impair the use of existing equipment or be above the tolerance level of the patients or parents.

Listed later are some of the more common assistive devices and they are meant to give the reader a sense of the progression from simple to complex. Many of the assistive devices or adaptive equipment items are homemade and use simple household items, such as foam blocks and polyvinyl chloride (PVC) piping. In many cases, patients or family members give the OT many good ideas for developing and passing on assistive devices for other families with similar functional challenges.

Some of the more common types of adaptive equipment/assistive devices used are the following:

- Built up handles on feeding, writing, and grooming implements to decrease the amount of force needed to secure and maintain grasp
- The use of a universal cuff with feeding or writing implements when grip and pinch mechanics are impaired
- Purchase of specialized feeding equipment (eg, Dining With Dignity [Dining With Dignity Inc, Williamsburg, Virginia], which has regular silverware that is retrofitted with bendable finger rings to slide over fingers, decreasing the need for a strong grip)
- Attachment of feeding or writing implements onto a splint whereby gross arm movements are turned into functional tasks
- The use of scoop dishes (one edge of the dish is built up and angled gently back toward the plate to allow patients to push the food onto the feeding implement by pushing it up against the scooped edge)
- The use of swivel spoons (the distal portion of the spoon is attached to a swivel, allowing the spoon to be angled properly relative to the plate or bowl and be brought to the mouth without spilling if pronation or supination of the forearm is difficult)
- The use of a spork (a combination of a spoon and a fork to allow the implement to perform multiple functions)

- The use of Dycem (Dycem Limited, Warwick, Rhode Island) (a commercially available nonskid surface to place under eating containers, much like a place mat, to prevent the plates or bowls from sliding across table while feeding)
- The use of rocker knives to allow a rocking motion through the use of a curvilinear blade rather than a more difficult linear cutting pattern
- The use of a long-handled reacher to grasp objects outside of the functional range of motion (reachers with a forearm-bracing component are inherently more stable because they shift some of the load to the forearm and not directly to the radial side of the wrist)
- The use of leg lifters to allow arm bracing and trunk control to lift legs into a car or wheelchair
- The use of dressing sticks that have various hooks and or protrusions that enable patients to grasp and manipulate clothing items while dressing (An adjustable Swiffer [The Proctor & Gamble Company, Cincinnati, Ohio] handle with the cleaning end removed will also allow for easier manipulation of pants and other clothing items when grip is impaired [Marnie King, OT, Wilmington, Delaware, 2010, personal communication]; The handle extension can be compacted for easier storage and then extended as needed.)
- The use of Velcro (Velcro USA Inc, Manchester, NH) fasteners for shoes, pants, and other clothing items (The incorporation of a D-ring may allow for a child to use crude grip patterns more efficiently by hooking the ring along a hand web space to allow for a more gross arm movement to complete dressing tasks when grip and pinch are impaired.)
- The use of PVC piping to attach to the end of a faucet handle to act as an extension allowing the child to manipulate the control of water flow
- The attachment of a light dowel to a light switch to enable a child to manipulate the lights from his or her wheelchair
- Adaptations in seating and positioning using such devices as the Rifton Chair (Rifton Equipment, Rifton, NY, USA) and Trip Trap Chair (Chair Stokke LLC, Stamford, CT, USA), along with appropriate postural stability inserts for proper proximal stability enhancement through biomechanically proper posture

Many of these items may be combined to suit the patients' needs and may be fabricated by the innovative OT after careful analysis of functional deficits and patient goals.

Reducing the effects of gravity are exceptionally important concepts in the development of therapy programs for individuals with neuromuscular disorders. The reduction of gravity may facilitate function by allowing weakened muscles to contract to a fuller degree and allow for better joint excursion and function. The concept of gravitational grading could be considered to be remedial or compensatory, depending on the potential for recovery of each particular condition. There are several ways in which this could be accomplished:

1. Foam blocks or wedges on tabletops can be used to prop arms up and allow for active-assisted or passive shoulder flexion to assist in feeding or grooming and other tasks requiring hand-to-mouth movement patterns. Shoulder flexion or hand-to-mouth patterning are then achieved by incorporating trunk flexion.
2. The use of an adapted scooter board with pivoting wheels may be used to facilitate the range of motion in friction-reduced planes.[7] An excellent variation of this concept is to use a toy car or other toy with 4 wheels to replicate the scooter board. The car could be attached to the child's extremity with Velcro splint strapping.
3. Positioning the child in a side-lying position with the upper extremity placed on a smooth surface, such as 1/4 inch particleboard propped up on pillows or

fabricated into a sturdier bench configuration, will also enhance gravity and friction-reduced motion for shoulder forward flexion. Position the child in a supine position with the arm in horizontal abduction and external rotation on the particleboard. Shoulder abduction could then be performed. If the particleboard is supported at an oblique angle from the front axillary line, then shoulder motion could be performed in the scapular plane, which has been stated to be a more functional movement pattern for the shoulder than pure shoulder flexion or pure abduction. A pillowcase, towel, powder, or lotion could be also be used to further reduce friction (the last two methods are a bit messy). If shoulder motion is desired and there is a predominance of flexion at the biceps, then a lightweight static elbow splint, such as a pediwrap or an inflatable pneumatic cuff, may be used to keep the elbow in a static position, redirecting motion toward the shoulder. This offloading technique may be used for any functional movement pattern for the upper extremity. Depending on the potential for recovery and the existing level of strength, patients may be placed at an appropriate level within the gravity-reduction continuum that allows for maximal range of self-generated motion with minimal fatigue.

4. PVC pipe stands with a sturdy base can be easily fabricated and used in the bath or shower to prop arms and assist in hand-to-head bathing and grooming (Marnie King, OT, Wilmington, Delaware, 2010, personal communication). In addition, hooks and other types of securing devices can be added for storage of washrags, brushes, and so forth.

5. Aquatic therapy is a reasonable therapeutic medium for children who have neuromuscular diseases.[25] A person immersed to the symphysis has effectively offloaded 40% of his or her bodyweight. When further immersed to the umbilicus, approximately 50% is offloaded. Xiphoid-level immersion offloads bodyweight by 60% or more depending on whether the arms are overhead or beside the trunk.[30] Care must be taken, however, in incremental immersion above chest level secondarily to the effects of hydrostatic pressure and if patients have impaired respiration. The effects of water buoyancy will enable patients to contract muscles in a gravity-reduced plane and allow for range of motion and play activity.

6. Overhead slings can be fabricated from PVC piping. The slings can be fabricated from neoprene, fabric, or soft strapping material. They could be wrist based or forearm based depending on the level of stability desired. The slings are then connected to the PVC frame with the use of Thera-Bands and tubing, rubber bands, or other elastic medium. The patients' hands and forearms are then suspended by the slings to allow for gravity-reduced active-assisted movement.

7. Counterbalanced slings consist of an arm sling attached to a frame via a cable or string using series of pulleys and a counterbalance weight to offload the weight of the upper extremity. The purpose being to allow for functional active-assisted movement in gravity-reduced planes. The use of counterbalanced slings allows motion in multiple planes but they are attached to a large frame that is bulky and often difficult to properly maneuver into biomechanically correct alignment. Additionally, the method of counterbalance weight delivery may not be as precise as needed for a zero-balance effect for the upper extremity. The slings may also tend to slip off of the forearm.

8. Balanced forearm orthoses (BFO) consists of an adjustable forearm trough attached to a guidepost arm that articulates with a swivel. This assembly supports the weight of the forearm and arm against gravity and is used primarily in patients with high-level tetraplegia or severe proximal arm weakness or paralysis. It may be attached to a wheelchair or table; patients may be able to perform tabletop activities. Prerequisites for its use include a power source, such as neck or trunk

muscles (to shift the trunk center of gravity) or adequate scapular movement.[31] A limitation of the BFO is that it does not allow for shoulder flexion, shoulder abduction, or shoulder scapular plane movement.

Upper-extremity splints can be considered remedial or compensatory. In conditions whereby there is a reasonable expectation of recovery, splints can be used to substitute for lost function or protect against malpositioning and contracture until recovery occurs. For those conditions with a more guarded prognosis, splinting may help to substitute for lost function and be used on a more continual basis to augment function. Splinting design classifications include the following[32]:

1. Static splints place the anatomic structures at a nonmoveable maximally available length to enact soft tissue lengthening or a mobilizing effect. It can also be used to position a joint at a comfortable/stable angle for the stabilization of a joint to allow for improved function. Static splints may also be used to redirect forces from poorly moving joints to more efficiently moving joints to augment function or torque transmission.
2. Serial static splints require the serial remolding of a static splint to progressively increase the mobilization of tight and contracted structures. Serial static splinting techniques are effective in mobilization of tight and contracted joints.
3. Static progressive splints allow for a patient-controlled application of nonelastic mobilizing force and are used to illicit increased range of motion. It uses the stress-relaxation principal, which is how less force is required to maintain a tissue at a set length over time. Controlled, graded amounts of force are held at maximal tolerable tissue limits.[33]
4. Dynamic splints use dynamic forces to either elicit increased range of motion or to substitute for lost function. For a mobilizing effect, dynamic splints use the creep principle. This principle describes the ability of a tissue to elongate over time when a constant load is applied to it with the use of elastic components.[33]
5. Dropout splints allow motion in one direction while blocking motion in another. For example, a splint may be designed to enhance wrist extension while blocking wrist flexion.[32]

Splinting considerations can include patient cognitive status and developmental level, patient acceptance and willingness to wear a splint, skin integrity, weight, cosmetic appearance, and the gadget tolerance of patients or caregivers. Splints can be custom fabricated from low-temperature thermoplastic or neoprene or foam of varying thicknesses or they can be purchased prefabricated.

ROBOTICS

Robots were used in the better part of the twentieth century in a manufacturing environment, such as automobile assembly. These tasks were repetitive tasks that were labor intensive and required a high degree of accuracy. Toward the latter part of the century, the possibility of robots interacting with humans was becoming a possibility. These devices included advanced prosthetics, motorized feeding devices, and sentry robots.[34] These devices were starting to augment or replace mobility and manipulation functions for humans. As World War II was a big driver of improvements in prosthetics technology, the advancement of technology, such as miniaturization of the microprocessor, became a driver of the technology development for assistive devices. Another factor was the aging population because of the baby-boom generation entering old age. The graying of the population is a worldwide phenomenon, particularly in Japan where robotics technology in health care is more readily embraced than in many other developed countries.

Robots were first seen in research laboratories[35] as assistive devices to help people with paralysis of the upper extremity. Later, wheelchair-mounted and fixed robots were developed and also commercial industrial robots were adapted for health care.[36] These devices were used for a diverse set of motor disabilities, including neuromuscular diseases, such as MD and SMA. Although these devices had a profound effect on people with neuromuscular diseases, widespread commercial success was not seen. Several factors are thought to contribute to this, including weight, human-machine interface, and cost. In contrast, rehabilitation robotics has shifted emphasis in the last 10 to 15 years toward therapy robots, and the prime beneficiary is the stroke population. This emphasis has been driven by the large number of people with stroke, science showing the ability of the brain to adapt through neuroplasticity even in the chronic stage,[37] and the need to contain health care costs. The last few years have seen more projects looking at cerebral palsy and robots.[11–13] The following sections are broken up into assistive robots, therapeutic robots, and upper-extremity orthoses, with an emphasis on devices that currently exist in the market and that are used clinically and as consumer products.

ASSISTIVE ROBOTS AND ORTHOSES

This section describes the commercially available robots and orthoses including feeders.

A device that has been available for more than 20 years is the iARM (Assistive Innovations Corp, Newark, New Jersey; formerly known as the Manus) **Fig. 1**. This device

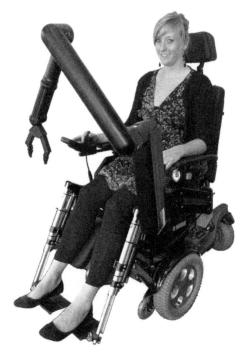

Fig. 1. The iArm wheelchair-mounted robot. (*Courtesy of* Assistive Innovations Corp, Newark, New Jersey; with permission.)

is a 7-jointed robot arm that is wheelchair mounted and allows people with neuromuscular conditions to access their environment and perform a subset of tasks their natural arm would. The iARM allows someone to get a drink or feed himself or herself. It can be controlled by a joystick or keypad. It can be controlled in joint mode, programmed mode, or Cartesian mode, which moves the gripper in an *xyz* configuration. The motors are powered by the wheelchair battery and the iARM sits alongside the wheelchair. The iARM[38] costs $20,000. It is used by people with MD, spinal MD, SCI, cerebral palsy and many other motoric disabilities. There are approximately 400 iARM units in use worldwide.

Upper-extremity exoskeletons are used for people who have some residual strength in their arms. This strength is often seen in people with neuromuscular disorders, such as MD, SMA, arthrogryposis, and other motor disorders, such as amyotrophic lateral sclerosis and SCI. These exoskeletons are generally passive, which means that they do not have external power, such as motors. They are often attached to wheelchairs and are lightweight. One such exoskeleton is the WREX (JAECO Orthopedic, Hot Springs, Arkansas; Wilmington Robotic EXoskeleton) (**Fig. 2**). The WREX is a mechanical linkage that can be attached to a wheelchair and is powered by elastic bands.[14,15] The device moves alongside the arm and makes antigravity movements effortless, which is particularly useful for people with MD and SMA whereby weakness in larger proximal muscles is evident, whereas distal muscles are less affected. The WREX allows them to navigate their hand in front of them and perform activities of daily living. The WREX comes in one size and can be adjusted to accommodate different sized individuals and the number of elastic bands can be changed depending on the weight of the individual. The WREX is sold through JAECO[39] and Patterson Medical (Bolingbrook, Illinois). The cost is approximately $2000.

The BFO or ball-bearing feeder is a mechanical linkage that hooks on to a wheelchair and allows people to move their arm in the horizontal plane. They are able to move their hand to their mouth by pivoting about a fulcrum at the midpoint of the forearm. There is also a version that allows elevation with an elastic band; however, this is rarely

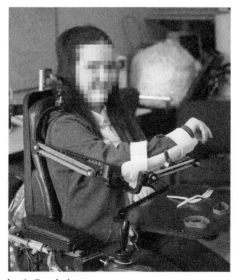

Fig. 2. Wilmington Robotic Exoskeleton.

used. The BFO was developed in the 1950s and is available through Patterson Medical for approximately $600.

The ARMON (Assistive Innovations Corp, Newark, NJ, USA) is available in Europe and is also a wheelchair-mounted passive exoskeleton that allows the arm to move against gravity. It uses adjustable springs as the power source and is used for people with neuromuscular conditions, such as MD and SMA. The ARMON has a different configuration to the WREX in that it is not a true exoskeleton as it originates from the base of the wheelchair. It allows a large range of gravity free motion. It costs about $3000.[38]

Another commercially available device is called the DAS (Dynamic Arm Support, [Assistive Innovations Corp, Newark, NJ, USA]).[38] This device is also a spring-loaded upper-extremity orthosis for people with arm weakness. It also attaches to a wheelchair and is available in Europe.

FEEDERS

Task-specific devices exist for feeding, such as the Winsford feeder (sold through Patterson Medical for approximately $3800). This device is a motorized device intended for people without available arm function. They activate a chin switch, which sends a signal to scoop up food off a mechanized plate and present it to the user. The Neater Eater (Neater Solutions, Buxton, United Kingdom) is a table-mounted feeding device that comes in 2 versions. The first is a motorized feeding arm that can be controlled by a user with little arm function and retails for about $4000. It is attached to a tabletop and can be controlled by a foot switch. A manual version is also attached to a tabletop and is for someone with some arm movement, which may be erratic or tremulous. The arm has a built-in damper that filters out unwanted movement.

ASSISTIVE ORTHOTICS RESEARCH

A cable-driven upper-extremity orthosis is being developed at the University of Delaware.[40] The goals are to develop a motorized lightweight device that manipulates the arm through cables. A.I. duPont hospital for Children/Nemours is developing a power-assisted upper-extremity assistive orthosis to help people with neuromuscular disabilities. A powered device is required if the individual is profoundly weak and retains minimal strength and sensation.[41] Also if they wish to pick up an item, a passive device would not be sufficient. The Scuola Superiore Sant' Anna in Pisa Italy is conducting research in many aspects of rehabilitation robotics for the upper extremity.[42]

THERAPY ROBOTS

In the last few years, several therapy robots have become commercially available primarily geared toward the stroke population. The MIT (Massachusetts Institute of Technology) Manus is among the earliest of the upper-extremity therapy robots. It is a multiple degree of freedom impedance-controlled device. It is capable of moving the user's arm to specific locations or provides partial assistance in moving their arm. It has a video monitor and guides the user to locations visually. It has been shown to be as good as manual therapy after a period of exercise.[10] The MIT Manus is sold through Interactive Motion Technologies, Cambridge, Massachusetts. It is ideal for repetitive delivery of upper-extremity therapy in an automated and measurable manner. Another similar device is the Motorika Reo (Motorika Medical Ltd, Caesarea, Israel). It is also an upper-extremity motorized device that takes a paretic arm through an exercise regimen controlled by a computer screen.

Hocoma AG, Volketwil, Switzerland makes a suite of upper-extremity therapy devices. Two of these are the ArmeoSpring and the ArmeoPower. The former is an offshoot of the WREX described earlier and uses springs to counter gravity. It is connected to a computer screen to provide an interactive environment for therapy. Hocoma AG has sold approximately 250 of these units to date. The newer Armeo-Power is a motorized upper-extremity exoskeleton that allows early rehabilitation of motor disorders, such as stroke, traumatic brain injury, and other neurologic disorders. It is based on the ARMIN technology developed at ETH (Swiss Federation Institute of Technology, Zurich, Switzerland).[43] The ArmeoPower provides assistance as needed and adapts to patients' capabilities.

There are a host of commercially available lower-extremity devices available. These devices are used for repetitive, body weight–supported movement. Some operate by propelling the legs through the gait cycle. The Locomat by Hocoma AG is perhaps the most prominent among these devices (**Fig. 3**). It is a multiple-degree-of-freedom robotic device that is treadmill based. It includes a partial weight-bearing feature.[44] Approximately 415 Locomat devices are currently in use worldwide.

Motorika offers the ReoAmbulator, which integrates body weight–supported treadmill therapy and a robotic device similar to the Locomat to promote neural recovery. An interactive display provides feedback and multiple scene modes to increase motivation. Kineassist[45] is an overground mobile base that provides body

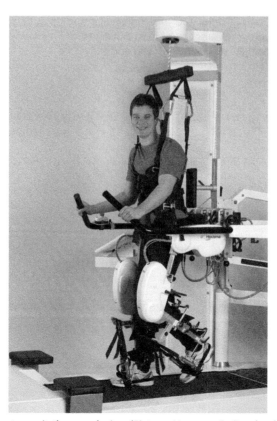

Fig. 3. The Locomat: a gait therapy device. (Picture: Hocoma, Switzerland.)

weight–supported treadmill training in a rehabilitation setting for assistive therapeutic exercises and gait training. It consists of various modes that allow patients
to relearn movements and postures by providing a stable and assistive environment
to provide overground walking. ZeroG (Aretech LLC, Ashburn, Virginia) is a new
overground body weight–supported system that uses a ceiling-mounted rail
system[46] to provide gait, posture, and balance activities. It allows patients to walk
on flat terrain or stairs. Rewalk (Argo Medical Technologies Ltd, Yokneam, Israel) is
a powered exoskeleton that assists people with walking impairments. It is a motorized device that straps on the legs and assists in hip and knee flexion. Movement of
the legs is initiated by tilting the torso back and forth. Currently, the Rewalk is undergoing clinical trials at various therapy centers and hospitals. It requires crutches or
a walker to insure balance during gait. Ekso Bionics (Point Richmond, California) has
developed a device called eLegs that offers a powered exoskeleton that propels the
legs during gait, similar to the Rewalk. The device is currently undergoing clinical
trials in various rehabilitation institutes in the United States. The projected price of
the eLegs is approximately $100,000.

SUMMARY

This article presents current occupational therapy techniques and assessment methodologies for children with neuromuscular disorders. Included is a section on homemade technical solutions to OT challenges. Also presented is the state of the art in
robotic and orthotic applications for neuromuscular and other conditions. As robots
and machines become more acceptable to clinicians and consumers, these devices
will become increasingly visible in the clinic and the home.

REFERENCES

1. Smith JC. An overview of occupational therapy with children. In: Smith JC,
   Allen A, Pratt PN, editors. Occupational therapy for children. St Louis (MO):
   Mosby; 1996. p. 3–17.
2. Trombly CA. Optimizing motor behavior using the Brunnstrom movement therapy
   approach. In: Occupational therapy for physical dysfunction. 5th edition.
   Baltimore (MD): Lippincott Williams & Wilkins; 2002. p. 543–84.
3. Jackson J, McLaughlin G, Zemke R. Optimizing abilities and capacities: range of
   motion, strength and endurance. In: Trombly CA, Radomsky MV, editors. Occupational therapy for physical dysfunction. 5th edition. Baltimore (MD): Lippincott
   Williams & Wilkins; 2002. p. 463–80.
4. Warren M. A hierarchical model for evaluation and treatment of visual perception
   dysfunction in adults with acquired brain injury, part 2. Am J Occup Ther 1993;47:
   55–66.
5. Toglia JP. Generalization of treatment. A multicontext approach to cognitive
   perceptual impairment in adults with brain injury. Am J Occup Ther 1991;45:
   505–16.
6. Parham LD, Mailloux Z. Sensory integration. In: Smith JC, Allen A, Pratt PN,
   editors. Occupational therapy for children. 3rd edition. St Louis (MO): Mosby;
   1996. p. 307–56.
7. Shepherd J, Procter S, Coley IL. Self-care and adaptations for independent living.
   In: Case-Smith J, Allen A, Pratt PN, editors. Occupational therapy for children. 3rd
   edition. St Louis (MO): Mosby; 1996. p. 461–503.

8. Trombly CA. Managing deficit of first level motor control capacities. In: Trombley CA, editor. Occupational therapy for physical dysfunction. 5th edition. Baltimore (MD): Lippincott Williams & Wilkins; 2002. p. 571–84.

9. Angelo J, Buning ME. High technology adaptations to compensate for disability. In: Occupational therapy for physical dysfunction. 5th edition. Baltimore (MD): Lippincott Williams & Wilkins; 2002. p. 389–584.

10. Lo AC, Guarino PD, Richards LG, et al. Robot-assisted therapy for long-term upper-limb impairment after stroke. N Engl J Med 2010;362:1772–83.

11. Fasoli SE, Fragala-Pinkham M, Hughes R, et al. Upper limb robotic therapy for children with hemiplegia. Am J Phys Med Rehabil 2008;87:929–36.

12. Fasoli SE, Fragala-Pinkham M, Hughes R, et al. Robotic therapy and botulinum toxin type A: a novel intervention approach for cerebral palsy. Am J Phys Med Rehabil 2008;87:1022–5.

13. Cioi D, Kale A, Burdea G, et al. Ankle control and strength training for children with cerebral palsy using the Rutgers Ankle CP: a case study. IEEE Int Conf Rehabil Robot 2011;2011:5975432.

14. Rahman T, Sample W, Seliktar R, et al. Design and testing of a functional arm orthosis in patients with neuromuscular diseases. IEEE Trans Neural Syst Rehabil Eng 2007;15:244–51.

15. Haumont T, Rahman T, Sample W, et al. Wilmington robotic exoskeleton: a novel device to maintain arm improvement in muscular disease. J Pediatr Orthop 2011; 31:e44–9.

16. Goldfarb CA, Calhoun VD, Dailey L, et al. Hand therapy evaluations/testing/questionnaires. In hand and upper extremity therapy. Congenital, Pediatric and Adolescent Patients – St. Louis Protocols. 2011.

17. Richardson P. Use of standardized tests in pediatric practice. In: Smith JC, Allen A, Pratt PN, editors. Occupational therapy for children. 3rd edition. St Louis (MO): Mosby; 1996. p. 200–24.

18. Ven-Stevens L, Munneke M, Spauwen P, et al. Assessment of activities in patients with hand injury: a review of instruments in use. Hand Ther 2007;12: 4–14.

19. Gilmore R, Sakzewski L, Boyd R. Upper limb activity measures for 5 to 16 year old children with congenital hemiplegia, a systematic review. Dev Med Child Neurol 2010;52:14–21.

20. Stewart K. Occupational therapy assessment in pediatrics, purposes, process, and methods of evaluation. In: Case-Smith J, O'Brien JC, editors. Occupational therapy for children. 3rd edition. St Louis (MO): Mosby; 1996. p. 165–99.

21. NIH pain consortium. Pain intensity scales. In: NIH pain consortium homepage. Available at: http://painconsortium.nih.gov/pain_scales/index.html. Accessed April 17, 2012.

22. Miller F. Upper extremity. In: Miller F, editor. Cerebral palsy. New York: Springer; 2004. p. 387–432.

23. Haugen JB, Mathiowetz V, Flinn N. Optimizing behavior using the occupational therapy task-oriented approach. In: Trombley CA, editor. Occupational therapy for physical dysfunction. 5th edition. Baltimore (MD): Lippincott Williams & Wilkins; 2002. p. 481–99.

24. Kendall FP, McCreary EK. Muscles testing and function. 4th edition. Baltimore (MD): Lippincott Williams and Wilkins; 1993.

25. McDonald CM. Neuromuscular diseases. In: Alexander MA, Matthews DJ, editors. Pediatric rehabilitation- principles and practice. 4th edition. New York: Demos Medical; 2010. p. 277–335.

26. Kozin SH. Correlation between external rotation of the glenohumeral joint after brachial plexus birth palsy. J Pediatr Orthop 2004;24(2):189–93.

27. Howle J. Neuro-developmental treatment approach. Theoretical foundations and principles of clinical practice. Laguna Beach (CA): Neuro-Developmental Treatment Association; 2007.

28. Sabari JS. Optimizing motor control using the Carr and Shepherd approach. In: Occupational therapy for physical dysfunction. 5th edition. Baltimore (MD): Lippincott Williams & Wilkins; 2002.

29. Taub E, Uswatte G, Pidikiti R. Constraint induced movement therapy: a new family of techniques with broad application to physical rehabilitation- a clinical review. J Rehabil Res Dev 1999;36:237–51.

30. Becker BE. Aquatic therapy: scientific foundations and clinical rehabilitation applications. PM R 2009;1:859–72.

31. Lansang R. Upper limb support devices. In: Medscape reference: drugs, diseases and procedures. Available at: http://emedicine.medscape.com/article/314774-overview. Accessed April 17, 2012.

32. Shultz-Johnson K. Splinting foundations. In: Coppard B, Lohman H, editors. Splinting-A clinical reasoning and problem-solving approach. St Louis (MO): Elsevier; 1996. p. 3–14.

33. Mallac C. A physiotherapist's view on flexibility. In: Brian Mackenzie's successful coaching, Issue 8. Available at: http://www.brianmac.co.uk/articles/scni8a3.htm. Accessed April 17, 2012.

34. Thring MW. Robots and telechairs: manipulators with memory, remote manipulators, machine limbs for the handicapped (Ellis Horwood series in engineering science). Chichester (United Kingdom): Halsted Pr; 1983.

35. LeBlanc M, Leifer L. Environmental control and robotic manipulation aids. IEEE Eng Med Biol Mag 1982;1:16–22.

36. Burgar CG, Lum PS, Shor PC, et al. Development of robots for rehabilitation therapy: the Palo Alto VA/Stanford experience. J Rehabil Res Dev 2000;37:863–73.

37. Krebs HI, Hogan N, Aisen ML, et al. Robot-aided neurorehabilitation. IEEE Trans Rehabil Eng 1998;6:75–87.

38. Assistive innovations. Assistive innovations product listing. In: Assistive innovations index page. Available at: www.assistive-innovations.com. Accessed April 17, 2012.

39. Jaeco Orthopedic. WREX: Wilmington Robotic Exoskeleton Arm. In: Jaeco orthopedic product listing. Available at: http://jaecoorthopedic.com/products/products/WREX%3A-Wilmington-Robotic-EXoskeleton-Arm.html. Accessed April 17, 2012.

40. Mao Y, Agrawal S. A cable driven upper arm exoskeleton for upper extremity rehabilitation. Proceedings of the IEEE International Conference on Robotics and Automation. ICRA 2011 IEEE International Conference 2011;2011:4163–8.

41. Ragonesi D, Agrawal S, Sample W, et al. Series elastic actuator control of a powered exoskeleton. Conf Proc IEEE Eng Med Biol Soc 2011;2011:3515–8.

42. Cavallo F, Aquilano M, Bonaccorsi M, et al. Multidisciplinary approach for developing a new robotic system for domiciliary assistance to elderly people. Conf Proc IEEE Eng Med Biol Soc 2011;2011:5327–30.

43. Brokaw EB, Murray T, Nef T, et al. Retraining of interjoint arm coordination after stroke using robot-assisted time-independent functional training. J Rehabil Res Dev 2011;48:299–316.

44. Westlake KP, Patten C. Pilot study of Lokomat versus manual-assisted treadmill training for locomotor recovery post-stroke. J Neuroeng Rehabil 2009;6:18.

45. Kinea Design. Portfolio: Kineassist walking & balance retraining. In: Kinea design product portfolio. Available at: http://www.kineadesign.com/portfolio/kineassist/. Accessed April 17, 2012.

46. Aretech, LLC. ZeroG Overview. In: Aretech, LLC homepage. Available at: http://www.aretechllc.com/overview.html. Accessed April 17, 2012.

Disease Burden in Neuromuscular Disease: The Role of Chronic Pain

Gregory T. Carter, MD, MS[a,b,*], Jordi Miró, PhD[c],
R. Ted Abresch, MS[b], Rima El-Abassi, MD[d], Mark P. Jensen, PhD[e]

KEYWORDS

- Neuromuscular disease • Chronic pain • Burden of disease • Quality of life
- Muscular dystrophy

KEY POINTS

- Assessing burden of disease is a complex process involving identifying the physical, psychological, and socioeconomic aspects that make up the totality of disease burden on patients, families, and caregivers, and society as a whole, with chronic pain affecting all of these aspects.
- It is the job of the physiatrist to identify disability and promote interventions to minimize it, including facilitating access to appropriate treatment for chronic pain, and ultimately easing disease burden.
- Chronic pain causes significant psychosocial dysfunction for patients with neuromuscular disease and contributes substantially to the overall disease burden.
- There are many psychosocial factors closely associated with pain and dysfunction in patients with neuromuscular disease, most notably a perception of inadequate psychosocial support.
- The assessment of children with neuromuscular disorders must include the parents or guardians as well, given that chronic pain in a child will affect the entire family.

This work was supported by Grant #H133B0900001 from the National Institute of Disability and Rehabilitation Research. The authors take full responsibility for the contents of this article, which do not represent the views of the National Institute of Disability and Rehabilitation Research or the United States Government.

[a] Olympia Physical Medicine, 410 Providence Lane, Building 2, Olympia, WA 98506, USA; [b] Department of Physical Medicine and Rehabilitation, University of California at Davis, 2315 Stockton Blvd., Sacramento, CA 95817, USA; [c] Unit for the Study and Treatment of Pain - ALGOS, Centre de Recerca en Avaluació i Mesura del Comportament, Institut d'Investigació Sanitària Pere Virgili, Universitat Rovira i Virgili, Sant Llorenç, 2143201 Reus, Catalonia, Spain; [d] Division of Neuromuscular Disorders, Department of Neurology, Louisiana State University Health Sciences Center, School of Medicine, New Orleans, LA 70112, USA; [e] Department of Rehabilitation Medicine, University of Washington School of Medicine, 1959 N.E Pacific Avenue, Box 356490, Seattle, WA 98195, USA
* Corresponding author. PO Box 1019, Centralia, WA 98531.
E-mail address: gtcarter@uw.edu

INTRODUCTION

Neuromuscular disorders (NMDs) include a variety of conditions that affect components of a motor unit, sensory and autonomic nerves, or their supportive structures, such as myopathies, disorders of the neuromuscular junction, and neuropathies. To date, there are no curative treatments available for any NMD. Most patients with NMD understand that they will have to reconcile themselves to rehabilitation or perhaps even simply palliative treatment, and dealing with chronic pain is part of that paradigm.

One important goal of a clinician treating someone with NMD is to lessen the disease burden by treating chronic pain. This is important, given the body of evidence indicating that chronic pain is a major part of the disease burden in NMD, and in most neuromuscular diseases in general.[1–16] Despite this, pain is often underdiagnosed and treatment is often overlooked. Although chronic pain is often very difficult to treat, there are at least some aspects than can potentially be ameliorated with treatment, which is unlike so many other aspects of NMD. The more difficult task might be defining how chronic pain affects burden of disease, which refers not only to the burden that ill health and risk factors place on the patient with NMD but on society as well. Measures of this burden include prevalence, mortality, life expectancy, economic costs, hospitalization rates, and specific measures of quality of life and disability.

The first investigations that defined chronic pain as a significant part of the disease burden in NMD resulted from a collaborative effort between the chronic pain research group at the University of Washington (UW), and the University of California, Davis (UCD) National Institute on Disability and Rehabilitation Research (NIDRR) Neuromuscular Research Training Center. This was done through a series of sequential program project grants initially funded by the NIDRR, the National Institutes of Health, the National Institute of Child Health and Human Development, and the National Center for Medical Rehabilitation Research. The funding for this research continues as a part of a Rehabilitation Research and Training Center on Aging with Disability at UW and the UCD Neuromuscular Research Training Center, both funded by NIDRR.

WHY IS PAIN OVERLOOKED IN NMD?

With respect to evaluating patients with NMD, most of this care is still centered on diagnosis and subsequent treatment, with the aim of treatment being disease modification, rather than palliation. In terms of diagnostic workup, this is appropriate. Most of the clinical care of patients with NMD is delivered by neurologists and physiatrists. Neurologists are trained to detect specific abnormal neurologic signs, such as motor weakness, lack of fine motor coordination, or a Babinski sign, and then use those findings to direct a workup that will arrive at the correct disease diagnosis. On the other hand, physiatrists are specifically trained to try, with as much structure as possible, to evaluate impairment and identify disability, such as not being able to climb the stairs, which then results in an inability to use public transport. It is the job of the physiatrist to identify disability and promote interventions to minimize it, including facilitating access to appropriate assistive devices, such as wheelchairs, hearing aids, orthoses, prostheses, and so forth. Indeed, any clinician, including neurologists, other physicians, and therapists can do this but may not be specifically trained or oriented toward providing this service. Ultimately, the overarching goal is to ease disease burden and help ensure the inclusion and participation of people with disabilities into mainstream society; however, evaluation and modification of disease burden is currently not included as part of any clinical algorithm.

Further, pain is a phenomenological experience rather than an objective sign. The International Association for the Study of Pain uses this definition: "an unpleasant sensory and emotional experience associated with actual or potential tissue damage, or described in terms of such damage" (http://www.iasp-pain.org). As such, many clinicians used to assessing symptoms via objective signs struggle with the idea of a symptom that is best assessed by asking, then listening to and relying on the report of the patient. Moreover, pain is influenced by a large number of biologic, psychological, and social contextual factors. Thus, chronic pain is best assessed and treated at a multidisciplinary pain treatment center. However, chronic pain needs to be identified as part of the patient's diagnoses before that referral would be undertaken.

The other barrier in the current health care algorithm is funding. Although there is some activism by organizations, such as the Muscular Dystrophy Association (MDA) to support the integration of rehabilitation services into the public health system, owing to economic issues, many Medicaid-sponsored and Medicare-sponsored health programs have little or no covered rehabilitation services. It will take ongoing collaborative efforts on the part of NMD physician specialists and other clinicians in both academia and the private sector, as well as nongovernmental organizations like the MDA, to keep pressure on federal and state governments to include comprehensive services for disabled people as a routine part of health care coverage. As it is now, the vast majority of patients with NMD are unemployed and, as such, are on state funding (Medicaid) with federal backup coverage (Medicare).[17] Fowler and colleagues[17] identified factors that limited employment opportunities for individuals with slowly progressive NMD. At the time of their study in the late 1980s, only 40% of subjects with NMD were employed in the competitive labor market, with 50% having been employed in the past, and 10% having never been employed. Strikingly, the major consumer barrier to employment was education. Physical impairment and disability were not associated with level of unemployment. Rather, psychological characteristics were associated with level of unemployment, including intellectual capacity, psychosocial adjustment, and the belief by most individuals that their physical disability was the only or major barrier to obtaining a job. The problem was compounded by a low level of referrals to the Department of Vocational Rehabilitation (DVR) by physicians, and ultimately a low acceptance rate into the DVR programs. The irony here is that a population of disabled patients with extensive medical problems ends up being unemployed, and thereby on the most restrictive form of health care coverage. This, in turns, leads to limited resources to evaluate and treat complex problems, such as chronic pain, in the disabled population.

There is also a need for better ways to assess chronic pain and determine its impact on functional status in patients with NMD. As mentioned previously, although function may be objectively measured with performance-based scales, such as the functional independence measure (FIM), Barthel index, and timed motor performance measures, among many others, pain is a personal experience that requires patient self-report for valid assessment.

Patient self-report measures have been shown to be reliable and valid in the NMD population,[18-25] and these scales retain that validity when tested in an NMD population with chronic pain.[10] For example, the internal consistency coefficients of the self-reported FIM (FIM-SR) scale ranges from adequate to excellent (Cronbach alpha range, 0.73–0.98; median, 0.96).[17] FIM-SR scales associated with motor function discriminate between those subjects who report being ambulatory and those who report requiring use of a wheelchair or other assistive device for mobility. Finally, FIM-SR scales discriminate between different types of NMDs, with patients with amyotrophic lateral sclerosis (ALS) showing significantly lower scores on the

FIM-SR self-care, motor, and total scores than all other NMD diagnostic groups, and showing significantly lower scores on the FIM-SR sphincter control, mobility, and locomotion scales than most of the other diagnostic groups. Thus, the FIM-SR scales appear to be reliable and valid measures of independence in 6 specific (self-care, sphincter control, mobility, locomotion, communication, social cognition) and 3 global (motor, cognition, total) areas of functioning in persons with NMD and chronic pain. Although no one wishes to diminish the personal suffering of anyone suffering from ill health, these measures can be used to compare levels of public health spending or levels of research funding and scientific interest. These comparisons can be useful and identify any large inequalities in funding that could lead to an increased societal burden of disease.

WHAT DO WE KNOW ABOUT PAIN IN NMD NOW? A BRIEF REVIEW OF THE LITERATURE

Recently, Jensen and colleagues[1] systematically reviewed the research findings regarding the associations between psychosocial factors and adjustment to chronic pain in persons with physical disabilities. They performed a comprehensive literature search on a number of major diagnostic groups, including muscular dystrophy, in addition to spinal cord injury, acquired amputation, cerebral palsy, and multiple sclerosis. Perhaps not surprisingly, psychosocial factors were shown to be significantly associated with pain and dysfunction in all disability groups, including muscular dystrophy. The psychosocial factors most closely associated with pain and dysfunction across the samples included (1) catastrophizing cognitions; (2) task persistence, guarding, and resting coping responses; and (3) perceived social support and solicitous responding social factors. Thus, psychosocial factors are clearly important predictors of pain and functioning in persons with physical disabilities, including muscular dystrophy, a subset of NMD.

The importance of psychosocial factors in chronic pain for patients with NMD has been confirmed in other studies as well. Nieto and colleagues[10] studied a sample of 107 adults with either myotonic muscular dystrophy (MMD) or facioscapulohumeral muscular dystrophy (FSHD). A sample of 107 adults with either MMD or FSHD reported pain in the past 3 months, completing assessments at 2 time points, separated by approximately 24 months. The results showed that changes in pain-related psychological variables were significantly associated with changes in psychological functioning, pain intensity, and pain interference. Specifically, increases in the belief that emotion influences pain and catastrophizing were associated with decreases in psychological functioning. Increases in the coping strategies of asking for assistance and resting, and the increases of catastrophizing were associated with increases in pain intensity. Finally, increases in pain intensity and asking for assistance were associated with increases in pain interference. These results further support the use of the biopsychosocial model of pain for understanding pain and its impact in individuals with MMD or FSHD.

Miró and colleagues[13] studied 182 persons with either FSHD or MMD in a similar fashion. They found that greater catastrophizing was associated with increased pain interference and poorer psychological functioning, pain attitudes were significantly related to both pain interference and psychological functioning, and coping responses were significantly related only to pain interference. In addition, greater perceived social support was associated with better psychological functioning. The results support the use of studying pain in persons with MMD/FSHD from a biopsychosocial perspective, and the importance of identifying psychosocial factors that may play a role in the adjustment to and response to pain secondary to MMD/FSHD.

Jensen and colleagues[5] used a cross-sectional, community-based survey on a convenience sample to determine the nature and scope of pain in working-aged adults with either MMD or FSHD. Results showed that more subjects with FSHD (82%) than with MMD (64%) reported pain. The most frequently reported pain sites for both diagnostic groups were lower back (66% MMD, 74% FSHD) and legs (60% MMD, 72% FSHD). Significant differences in pain intensity were found between the diagnostic groups in the hands, legs, knees, ankles, and feet, with patients with MMD reporting greater pain intensity at these sites than patients with FSHD. Age was related to the onset of pain (participants reporting pain were younger than those not reporting pain in the FSHD sample), but pain severity was not significantly associated with age in those reporting pain. Respondents with both diagnoses, who reported mobility limitations and used assistive devices (eg, wheelchair, cane), reported more pain severity than those with mobility limitations who did not use assistive devices, who, in turn, reported more pain severity than respondents who reported no mobility limitations at all. The treatments that were reported to provide the greatest pain relief were not necessarily those that were the most frequently tried or still used. The findings indicate that pain is a more common problem in persons with FSHD than in persons with MMD, although it is common in both populations. In addition, these pain problems are chronic, underscoring the need to identify and provide effective pain treatments for patients with these NMDs.

One of the few European studies assessing pain frequency, severity, location, treatment, and relief in adults with NMD was done by Tiffreau and colleagues.[26] Using a mailed in, self-completed questionnaire, 125 adults with a confirmed diagnosis of hereditary NMD participated (response rate = 45%). Outcome measures included self-reported motor function, anxiety and depression scores, pain intensity (on a 0–10 numeric scale) and location, frequency of pain-aggravating situations, and pain treatment and relief. Most (73%) respondents reported pain and 62% reported chronic pain (defined as pain for at least 3 months). Mean pain intensity was 6.1 of 10.0 with 40% reporting severe pain (a score of ≥ 7). Almost half (46%) reported anxiety, although only 16% of subjects reported depression. The most common pain-aggravating situations were "walking," "standing," and "muscle stretching." Walking was more frequently cited as a pain-aggravating situation by the chronic pain population than by the acute pain population. Analgesics were used by 70% of these patients, with massage being the most frequently prescribed physical treatment (45%). Interestingly, these patients did not report adequate relief from analgesics or massage.

Guy-Coichard and colleagues[27] published one of the largest studies to date, having mailed out 862 questionnaires to outpatients with NMD at 10 centers. A total of 511 subjects responded with answers suitable for analysis (300 men and 211 women; response rate: 59.3%). The questionnaire packet included numeric scales for pain intensity and relief, the Brief Pain Inventory, the Saint Antoine Pain Questionnaire, and a scale to assess disability. More than two-thirds of the 331 patients (67.3%) suffered pain during the last 3 months, with mean pain intensity being 4.8 ± 2.5. Pain was usually diffuse (153 patients, 44%) and intermittent (228, 71%). Pain intensity varied by the NMD diagnosis, with the most severe pain reported from patients with metabolic myopathy and myasthenia gravis.

Engel and colleagues[11] examined the prevalence and characteristics of pain in children with NMD. A total of 42 youths completed a comprehensive evaluation, including a detailed intake interview and structured questionnaire that included demographic and functional data. Youths who reported chronic pain were further queried about pain characteristics, locations, and intensity using an 11-point numerical rating scale and a modified Brief Pain Inventory (BPI). The sample consisted of 24 males (57%) and

18 females (43%), ages ranging from 9 to 20 years (mean = 14.8, SD = 2.96). Participants included 14 (37%) with Duchenne muscular dystrophy, 6 (14%) with MMD, 2 (5%) with Becker dystrophy, 2 (5%) with limb-girdle dystrophy, 2 (5%) with congenital muscular dystrophy, 1 (2%) FSHD, and 15 (36%) were classified as "other NMD." Twenty-one (50%) were ambulatory, whereas 26 (62%) used power wheelchairs/scooters and 9 (2%) used manual wheelchairs. A total of 23 (55%) of the youths reported having chronic pain, with pain intensity "over the past week" being 2.39 (range = 0–7). Pain in the legs was most commonly reported, and remarkably 83% reported using pain medications. This study indicates that chronic pain is also a significant problem in youths with NMD.

PAIN AND BURDEN OF DISEASE IN NMDS: A COMPLEX RELATIONSHIP

Assessing burden of disease is a complex process involving the identification of the physical, psychological, and socioeconomic aspects that make up the totality of disease burden on patients, families, and caregivers, and society as a whole. Chronic pain falls under this bracket, certainly having an impact that extends well beyond the affected individual with NMD. Thus, further strategies for further assessing NMD disease burden and appropriate modalities for management should include not only NMD clinicians and researchers, but also patients and their families, and patient registries and advocacy groups.

Given that health care reform, in one form or another, is on the horizon, it is expected that this will have a significant impact on the lives of individuals with NMD and chronic pain, and their families and caregivers.[28–32] Bridging the chasm between patients with NMD with chronic pain and the actual delivery of care in the setting of ever-shrinking health care finances will require inputs and opinions from all stakeholders. The degree of success will depend on whether there is a true and open exchange of ideas, as well as the synthesis of novel and ethically sound models of health care delivery and use. This means we must develop a system in which there is a seamless application of the research findings to solve the complex clinical problems faced by these patients. As discussed earlier, that will likely mean, in part, a paradigm shift away from emphasizing "cure" in terms of treatment and orienting it more toward improving care. This will pose challenges for clinicians, as there is still a tendency of patients with NMD with chronic pain to limit physical activity, often with the support of their providers. The evidence regarding activity and pain would orient toward a more physically active lifestyle.[32–37] This would be the preferred trend, when realistically possible, for patients with NMD, which would benefit their physical condition and limit their risk for comorbidity, including metabolic syndrome.[38,39] Indeed, inactivity is likely an independent risk factor for the development of chronic pain in the NMD population.

FUTURE CONSIDERATIONS AND DIRECTIONS
Mimic Established Models

The future of assessing the complex relationship between chronic pain and burden of disease in NMD must involve data collection, including tracking population trends, and monitoring the effects of changing health care policy. Ultimately, the goal is to establish research priorities and maintain longitudinal, dynamic communication with the NMD population over an extended period, as pain and disease burden are both ever-changing variables. This is the best way to accelerate the development of new therapies, yet it is also the most costly, as can be learned from studying the literature on chronic low back pain.[40–43] This point must be considered in an era of shrinking research monies.

Other challenges include the time and effort required to tap caregivers and patients to complete surveys at set intervals, as well as the need to strike a balance between getting too detailed and disease-specific data versus missing the intricacies and finer points by using broader measurements of pain that may be more comparable across the various NMDs. Again, looking at the low back pain model, this question is not yet clearly answered, particularly when it comes to changing clinician behavior and enhancing clinical treatment.[44,45] The situation becomes more complex when it comes to assessing children with NMD. In that setting, one is assessing both parents and children, and it becomes important to define pain and disease burden broadly enough to include the impact not only on the patients but parents as well, just as one should include families, caregivers, employers, and society, when pertinent, in adults with NMD and chronic pain.

There is a need to capture intangible burdens that patients with NMD face that contribute to pain, including the emotional impact of isolation experienced by many patients with NMD, as well as financial burdens from medical bills, costs of home and automobile adaptation, and assistive technologies, all in the specter of income lost. This follows an established, effective research model for chronic low back pain.[46–49]

Develop Better Measurement Tools

Currently, there are a very limited number of surveys designed specifically for studying any aspect of people with NMD, let alone chronic pain and disease burden. Most surveys used in NMD studies have previously been used for more common musculoskeletal diseases, such as chronic low back pain, and then modified to fit an NMD population. The only real exception to that would be neuropathic pain, which is common in some of the NMDs, most notably Charcot Marie Tooth Disease.[14,50–53] This became possible with the development of the Neuropathic Pain Scale by Galer and Jensen.[54] This allowed for an in-depth evaluation of the impact of neuropathic pain on disease burden and quality of life in many neuropathy disease states, including diabetes.[55–58]

Use NMD Registries

There now exist national registries for people with NMDs, including MMD, and FSHD, among others, worldwide. One example is the Canadian Neuromuscular Disease Registry (CNDR), a Canada-wide registry of people with a confirmed NMD diagnosis (www.cndr.org). The CNDR collects important medical information from patients with NMD across the entire country of Canada. Population-based data sets are useful for capturing all the people in a region who have a specific condition, expanding into cross-regional studies via multicenter collaboration. Contrast this to doing research via clinics and hospitals; there is added value of gathering data that are not based on the International Classification of Diseases, Ninth Revision (ICD-9) coding system. Basing inclusion into a study solely based on an ICD-9 code is limited because the different types of muscular dystrophies, having no distinct codes, must be studied as a whole. The use of NMD registries is somewhat of a necessity when studying many of the individual NMDs, owing to the low incidence of these diseases. Population-based studies also allow the economic costs of the disease to be estimated.

SUMMARY

There is now good evidence indicating that chronic pain is a common problem among patients with NMDs, across the age span. Although there are many similarities in the nature, scope, and impact of pain, there are also important differences between NMD diagnostic groups. The available studies indicate that chronic pain is associated with significant physical and psychosocial dysfunction, negatively affecting quality of life for patients with NMD. Despite this, there is very little information on the relationship of chronic pain and burden of disease in the NMD patient population. Future studies addressing the psychosocial aspects of chronic pain, including clinical trials to test the efficacy of psychosocial treatments for pain, are warranted. Studies to determine the extent to which chronic pain contributes to disease burden and the degree to which psychosocial factors influence pain disease burden are also warranted. Strategies to achieve this include the development of better measurement instruments for chronic pain, quality of life, and burden of disease, as well as use of NMD registries.

ACKNOWLEDGMENTS

This research was supported by the National Institutes of Health, National Institute of Child Health and Human Development, National Center for Rehabilitation Research (grant no. P01HD33988), and the National Institute for Disability Rehabilitation Research (grant no. H133B0900001).

REFERENCES

1. Jensen MP, Moore MR, Bockow TB, et al. Psychosocial factors and adjustment to chronic pain in persons with physical disabilities: a systematic review. Arch Phys Med Rehabil 2011;92(1):146–60.
2. Jensen MP, Abresch RT, Carter GT, et al. Chronic pain in persons with neuromuscular disorders. Arch Phys Med Rehabil 2005;86(6):1155–63.
3. Suokas KI, Haanpää M, Kautiainen H, et al. Pain in patients with myotonic dystrophy type 2: a postal survey in Finland. Muscle Nerve 2012;45(1):70–4.
4. Abresch RT, Carter GT, Jensen MP, et al. Assessment of pain and health-related quality of life in slowly progressive neuromuscular disease. Am J Hosp Palliat Care 2002;19(1):39–48.
5. Jensen MP, Hoffman AJ, Stoelb BL, et al. Chronic pain in persons with myotonic and facioscapulohumeral muscular dystrophy. Arch Phys Med Rehabil 2008; 89(2):320–8.
6. Hirsch AT, Kupper AE, Carter GT, et al. Psychosocial factors and adjustment to pain in individuals with postpolio syndrome. Am J Phys Med Rehabil 2010; 89(3):213–24.
7. Molton I, Jensen MP, Ehde DM, et al. Coping with chronic pain among younger, middle-aged, and older adults living with neurologic injury and disease: a role for experiential wisdom. J Aging Health 2008;20:972–96.
8. Stoelb BL, Carter GT, Abresch RT, et al. Pain in persons with postpolio syndrome: frequency, intensity, and impact. Arch Phys Med Rehabil 2008;89(10): 1933–40.
9. Carter GT, Jensen MP, Stoelb BL, et al. Chronic pain in persons with myotonic muscular dystrophy, type 1. Arch Phys Med Rehabil 2008;89(12):2382.
10. Nieto R, Raichle KA, Jensen MP, et al. Changes in pain-related beliefs, coping, and catastrophizing predict changes in pain intensity, pain interference, and psychological functioning in individuals with myotonic muscular dystrophy and facioscapulohumeral dystrophy. Clin J Pain 2012;28(1):47–54.
11. Engel JM, Kartin D, Carter GT, et al. Pain in youths with neuromuscular disease. Am J Hosp Palliat Med 2009;26(5):405–12.

12. Engel JM, Kartin D, Jaffe KM. Exploring chronic pain in youths with Duchenne Muscular Dystrophy: a model for pediatric neuromuscular disease. Phys Med Rehabil Clin N Am 2005;16(4):1113–24.
13. Miró J, Raichle KA, Carter GT, et al. Impact of biopsychosocial factors on chronic pain in persons with myotonic and facioscapulohumeral muscular dystrophy. Am J Hosp Palliat Med 2009;26(4):308–19.
14. Carter GT, Jensen MP, Galer BS, et al. Neuropathic pain in Charcot Marie Tooth disease. Arch Phys Med Rehabil 1998;79:1560–4.
15. Abresch RT, Jensen MP, Carter GT. Health quality of life in peripheral neuropathy. Phys Med Rehabil Clin N Am 2001;12(2):461–72.
16. Hoffman AJ, Jensen MP, Abresch RT, et al. Chronic pain in persons with neuromuscular disorders. Phys Med Rehabil Clin N Am 2005;16(4):1099–112.
17. Fowler WM Jr, Abresch RT, Koch TR, et al. Employment profiles in neuromuscular diseases. Am J Phys Med Rehabil 1997;6(1):26–37.
18. McDonald CM, Abresch RT, Carter GT, et al. Profiles of neuromuscular disease: Duchenne muscular dystrophy. Am J Phys Med Rehabil 1995;74(5):S70–92.
19. McDonald CM, Abresch RT, Carter GT, et al. Profiles of neuromuscular disease: Becker muscular dystrophy. Am J Phys Med Rehabil 1995;74(5):S93–103.
20. Johnson ER, Carter GT, Kilmer DD, et al. Profiles of neuromuscular disease: myotonic muscular dystrophy. Am J Phys Med Rehabil 1995;74(5):S104–16.
21. McDonald CM, Abresch RT, Carter GT, et al. Profiles of neuromuscular disease: limb-girdle syndromes. Am J Phys Med Rehabil 1995;74(5):S117–30.
22. Kilmer DD, Abresch RT, Aitkens SG, et al. Profiles of neuromuscular disease: facioscapulohumeral dystrophy. Am J Phys Med Rehabil 1995;74(5):S131–9.
23. Carter GT, Abresch RT, Fowler WM, et al. Profiles of neuromuscular disease: hereditary motor and sensory neuropathy, types I and II. Am J Phys Med Rehabil 1995;74(5):S140–9.
24. Carter GT, Abresch RT, Fowler WM, et al. Profiles of neuromuscular disease: spinal muscular atrophy. Am J Phys Med Rehabil 1995;74(5):S150–9.
25. Jensen MP, Abresch RT, Carter GT. The reliability and validity of a self-reported version of the functional independence measure in persons with neuromuscular disease and chronic pain. Arch Phys Med Rehabil 2005;86(1):116–22.
26. Tiffreau V, Viet G, Thévenon A. Pain and neuromuscular disease: the results of a survey. Am J Phys Med Rehabil 2006;85(9):756–66.
27. Guy-Coichard C, Nguyen DT, Delorme T, et al. Pain in hereditary neuromuscular disorders and myasthenia gravis: a national survey of frequency, characteristics, and impact. J Pain Symptom Manage 2008;35(1):40–50.
28. Berger A, Dukes EM, Oster G. Clinical characteristics and economic costs of patients with painful neuropathic disorders. J Pain 2004;5:143–349.
29. Keeley P, Creed F, Tomenson B, et al. Psychosocial predictors of health-related quality of life and health service utilization in people with chronic low back pain. Pain 2008;135:142–50.
30. Niv D, Devor M. Chronic pain as a disease in its own right. Pain Pract 2004;4:179–80.
31. Blyth FM, March LM, Brnabic AJ, et al. Chronic pain and frequent use of health care. Pain 2004;111:51–8.
32. Ohayon MM, Schatzberg AF. Using chronic pain to predict depressive morbidity in the general population. Arch Gen Psychiatry 2003;60:39–47.
33. Houben RM, Ostelo RW, Vlaeyen JW, et al. Health care providers' orientations towards common low back pain predict perceived harmfulness of physical

activities and recommendations regarding return to normal activity. Eur J Pain 2005;9:173–83.

34. Cook AJ, Thomas MR. Pain and the use of health services among the elderly. J Aging Health 1994;6:155–72.

35. Bishop A, Thomas E, Foster NE. Health care practitioners' attitudes and beliefs about low back pain: a systematic search and critical review of available measurement tools. Pain 2007;132:91–101.

36. Poiraudeau S, Rannou F, Baron G, et al. Fear-avoidance beliefs about back pain in patients with subacute low back pain. Pain 2006;124:305–11.

37. Coudeyre E, Rannou F, Tubach F, et al. General practitioners' fear-avoidance beliefs influence their management of patients with low back pain. Pain 2006; 124:330–7.

38. Aitkens S, Kilmer DD, Wright NC, et al. Metabolic syndrome in neuromuscular disease. Arch Phys Med Rehabil 2005;86(5):1030–6.

39. Kilmer DD, Zhao HH. Obesity, physical activity, and the metabolic syndrome in adult neuromuscular disease. Phys Med Rehabil Clin N Am 2005;16(4): 1053–62.

40. Gross DP, Ferrari R, Russell AS, et al. A population-based survey of back pain beliefs in Canada. Spine 2006;31:2142–5.

41. Tait RC, Chibnall JT. Attitude profiles and clinical status in patients with chronic pain. Pain 1998;78:49–57.

42. Grimshaw JM, Shirran L, Thomas R, et al. Changing provider behavior: an overview of systematic reviews of interventions. Med Care 2001;39:112–45.

43. van Tulder MW, Croft PR, van Spulunteren P, et al. Disseminating and implementing the results of back pain research in primary care. Spine 2002;27:E121–7.

44. Fritz JM, Cleland A, Brennan GP. Does adherence to the guideline recommendation for active treatments improve the quality of care for patients with acute low back pain delivered by physical therapists? Med Care 2007;45:973–80.

45. Dahan R, Borkan J, Brown JB, et al. The challenge of using the low back pain guidelines: a qualitative research. J Eval Clin Pract 2007;13:616–20.

46. Dagenais S, Caro J, Haldeman S. A systematic review of low back pain cost of illness studies in the United States and internationally. Spine J 2008;8:8–20.

47. Rapoport J, Jacobs P, Bell NR, et al. Refining the measurement of the economic burden of chronic diseases in Canada. Chronic Dis Can 2004;25:13–21.

48. Ekman M, Jonhagen S, Hunsche E, et al. Burden of illness of chronic low back pain in Sweden. Spine 2005;30:1777–85.

49. Breivik H, Collett B, Ventafridda V, et al. Survey of chronic pain in Europe: prevalence, impact on daily life, and treatment. Eur J Pain 2006;10:287–333.

50. Ribiere C, Bernardin M, Sacconi S, et al. Pain assessment in Charcot-Marie-Tooth (CMT) disease. Ann Phys Rehabil Med 2012;55(3):160–73.

51. Padua L, Cavallaro T, Pareyson D, et al. Italian CMT QoL Study Group. Charcot-Marie-Tooth and pain: correlations with neurophysiological, clinical, and disability findings. Neurol Sci 2008;29(3):193–4.

52. Vinci P, Serrao M, Millul A, et al. Quality of life in patients with Charcot-Marie-Tooth disease. Neurology 2005;65(6):922–4.

53. Pazzaglia C, Vollono C, Ferraro D, et al. Mechanisms of neuropathic pain in patients with Charcot-Marie-Tooth 1 A: a laser-evoked potential study. Pain 2010;149(2):379–85.

54. Galer BS, Jensen MP. Development and preliminary validation of a pain measure specific to neuropathic pain: the Neuropathic Pain Scale. Neurology 1997;48(2): 332–8.

55. Rodriquez MJ, Garcia AJ. A registry of the aetiology and costs of neuropathic pain in pain clinics. Results of the Registry of Aetiologies and Costs (REC) in Neuropathic Pain Disorders Study. Clin Drug Investig 2007;27:771–82.
56. O'Connor AB. Neuropathic pain: quality-of-life impact, costs and cost effectiveness of therapy. Pharmacoeconomics 2009;27(2):95–112.
57. Galer BS, Gianas A, Jensen MP. Painful diabetic polyneuropathy: epidemiology, pain description, and quality of life. Diabetes Res Clin Pract 2000; 47(2):123–8.
58. Gore M, Brandenburg NA, Hoffman DL, et al. Burden of illness in painful diabetic peripheral neuropathy: the patients' perspectives. J Pain 2006;7(12):892–900.

Index

Note: Page numbers of article titles are in **boldface** type.

Phys Med Rehabil Clin N Am 23 (2012) 731–749
http://dx.doi.org/10.1016/S1047-9651(12)00061-7
1047-9651/12/$ – see front matter © 2012 Elsevier Inc. All rights reserved.

Moving?

Make sure your subscription moves with you!

To notify us of your new address, find your **Clinics Account Number** (located on your mailing label above your name), and contact customer service at:

Email: journalscustomerservice-usa@elsevier.com

800-654-2452 (subscribers in the U.S. & Canada)
314-447-8871 (subscribers outside of the U.S. & Canada)

Fax number: 314-447-8029

Elsevier Health Sciences Division
Subscription Customer Service
3251 Riverport Lane
Maryland Heights, MO 63043

*To ensure uninterrupted delivery of your subscription, please notify us at least 4 weeks in advance of move.

Printed and bound by CPI Group (UK) Ltd, Croydon, CR0 4YY

03/10/2024

01040439-0013